USAMRIID'S MEDICAL MANAGEMENT OF BIOLOGICAL CASUALTIES HANDBOOK

8TH EDITION

SEPTEMBER 2014

U.S. Army Medical Research
Institute of Infectious Diseases

Fort Detrick
Frederick, Maryland

Emergency Response Numbers

National Response Center
(for chem/bio hazards & terrorist events):..800-424-8802

National Domestic Preparedness Consortium
(for civilian use): 225-578-8187

FEMA Center for Domestic Preparedness:..866-213-9553

USAMRIID's Emergency Response Line: 888-872-7443

CDC's Emergency Operations Center
(for health professionals and government officials): 770-488-7100

U.S. Army Chemical Materiel Agency
Operations Center: ....410-436-4484 or DSN 584-4484

Handbook Reprinting Policy

The U.S. Army Medical Research Institute of Infectious Diseases, requests that users of this handbook, before distributing or reprinting parts of or this entire handbook, notify:

USAMRIID
ATTN: Division of Medicine
1425 Porter Street
Fort Detrick, MD 21702-5011

Handbook Download Site

An Adobe Acrobat Reader (pdf file) version of this handbook can be downloaded from the internet at the following url: *http://www.usamriid.army.mil*

For sale by the Superintendent of Documents, U.S. Government Publishing Office
Internet: bookstore.gpo.gov Phone: toll free (866) 512-1800; DC area (202) 512-1800
Fax: (202) 512-2104 Mail: Stop IDCC, Washington, DC 20402-0001

ISBN 978-0-16-093126-0

USAMRIID's Medical Management of Biological Casualties Handbook

Eighth Edition · September 2014

Lead Editor

Mark R. Withers, MD, MPH
COL, MC, FS, USA

Contributing Editors

LTC Derron A. Alves, VC, USA
MAJ Todd M. Bell, VC, USA
LTC Michael J. Berecz, VC, USA
LTC Taylor B. Chance, VC, USA
George W. Christopher, MD (Col, USAF, Ret.)
COL Ted J. Cieslak, MC, USA
MAJ Eric R. Fleming, MS, USA
Pamela J. Glass, PhD
Arthur J. Goff III, PhD
Mark J. Goldberg, MD
CPT John C. Gorbet MS, USA
David G. Heath, PhD
LTC Shelley P. Honnold, VC, USA
James W. Karaszkiewicz, PhD
LTC Jennifer M. Kishimori, VC, USA
Aysegul Nalca, MD, PhD
SFC Steve Phoenix, USA
Mark A. Poli, PhD, DABT
LTC Robert G. Rivard, MC, USA
Janice M. Rusnak, MD (Lt Col, USAF, Ret.)
LTC Kurt E. Schaecher, MS, USA
CAPT Darrell Singer, MC, USPHS
LTC Nancy A. Twenhafel, VC, USA
Chris A. Whitehouse, PhD

Comments & suggestions are welcome & should be addressed to

Division of Medicine
Attn: MCMR-UIM-R
U.S. Army Medical Research
Institute of Infectious Diseases (USAMRIID)
Fort Detrick, Maryland 21702-5011

Acknowledgments

Previous editions

Editors: LTC Derron A. Alves; CAPT Duane Caneva; Lt Col Bridget K. Carr; COL (Ret) Les Caudle, COL Ted J. Cieslak; CDR Ken Cole; CDR (Ret) Randall C. Culpepper; MAJ Christine A. Ege; MAJ Eric R. Fleming; Col (Ret) George W. Christopher; CAPT Robert G. Darling; COL (Ret) Zygmunt F. Dembek; COL (Ret) Edward Eitzen; Dr. Pamela J. Glass; LTC Matthew J. Hepburn; LTC Shelley P. Honnold; CPT Monique S. Jesionowski; Ms. Katheryn F. Kenyon; COL Mark G. Kortepeter; Dr. David Lange; LCDR James V. Lawler; MAJ Anthony C. Littrell; MAJ Charles L. Marchand; COL (Ret) James W. Martin; COL (Ret) Kelly McKee; CPT Vanessa R. Melanson; COL Sherman A. McCall; COL (Ret) Julie A. Pavlin; COL (Ret) Phillip R. Pittman; Dr. Mark A. Poli; LTC (Ret) Nelson W. Rebert; MAJ Roseanne A. Ressner; CPT Thomas G. Robinson; COL (Ret) John Rowe; LTC John M. Scherer; COL Scott A. Stanek; Mr. Richard J. Stevens; Dr. Bradley G. Stiles; LTC Lawrence R. Suddendorf; LTC Nicholas J. Vietri; Dr. Chris A. Whitehouse; Lt Col Jon B. Woods.

Contributors: Dr. Richard Dukes; COL (Ret) David Franz; COL (Ret) Gerald Parker; COL (Ret) Gerald Jennings; SGM Raymond Alston; COL (Ret) James Arthur; COL (Ret) W. Russell Byrne; Dr. John Ezzell; Ms. Sandy Flynn; COL (Ret) Arthur Friedlander; Dr. Robert Hawley; COL (Ret) Erik Henchal; COL (Ret) Ted Hussey; Dr. Peter Jahrling; COL (Ret) Ross LeClaire; Dr. George Ludwig; Mr. William Patrick; Dr. Mark Poli; Dr. Fred Sidell; Dr. Jonathon Smith; Mr. Richard J. Stevens; Dr. Jeff Teska; COL (Ret) Stanley Wiener; and many others. The exclusion of anyone on this page is purely accidental and in no way lessens the gratitude we feel for contributions received.

Preface to the Eighth Edition

Since the first edition *USAMRIID's Medical Management of Biological Casualties Handbook* in 1993, the awareness of, and interest in, biological weapons in the US has increased dramatically. This handbook — which has long been known informally as the "Blue Book" — was enormously successful in its seventh (2011) edition. It has been readily available online for free and is in the public domain. In addition, over 205,000 hard copies of all editions of the "Blue Book" have now been distributed to military and civilian healthcare providers around the world. This has primarily been accomplished through USAMRIID's resident and off-site Medical Management of Biological Casualties (MMBC) course.

This eighth edition has been revised and updated to better present our current understanding of the optimal medical management of diseases and syndromes caused by biological threat agents, or bio-agents. In addition to updates of the sections on individual pathogens and toxins, as well as to most of the appendices, new material on the CDC's Select Agent program, the Laboratory Response Network (LRN), the development of biosurveillance systems, and contagious casualty care has been introduced. Citations to the medical literature are now referenced by in-text superscript numbers directing the reader to the "References" appendix at the back of the book.

Our goal has been to make this reference useful for the healthcare provider on the front lines, whether on the battlefield or in a fixed clinic, where basic summary and treatment information is quickly required. We are constantly striving to make it a better product. We would like your feedback to make future editions more useful and readable. Thank you for your interest in this important subject.

The Editors

Disclaimer

The purpose of this handbook is to provide concise supplemental reading material to assist healthcare providers in the management of biological casualties. Although every effort has been made to make the information in this handbook consistent with official policy and doctrine (see FM 8-284, *Treatment of Biological Warfare Agent Casualties*, 17 JUL 2000), the information contained in this handbook is **not** official Department of the Army policy or doctrine, and should not be construed as such.

Most of the specific therapies and prophylactic regimens found in this handbook are based upon standard treatment guidelines; however, some of the regimens described here may vary from information found in those sources. This is because the clinical presentation of certain diseases caused by a weaponized biological agent (bioagent) may vary from the natural (endemic) form of the disease. For ethical reasons, human challenge clinical trials can only be performed with a limited number of these agents. Therefore, treatment and prophylaxis regimens may be derived from *in vitro* data, animal models, historical case reports of accidental occupational exposures, and other limited human data. Occasionally you will find Investigational New Drug (IND) products mentioned. They are often used at USAMRIID and the CDC to protect laboratory workers. These products are not available commercially and can only be given under a specific investigational protocol with informed consent. They are mentioned for scientific completeness and are not necessarily to be construed as recommendations for therapy. For information on their use and availability, see Appendix J ("Investigational Medical Products [INDs, etc] & Emergency Use Authorizations [EUAs]").

Executive Order 13139: Improving Health Protection of Military Personnel Participating in Particular Military Operations

On 30 September 1999, the President of the US issued Executive Order 13139, which outlines the conditions under which Investigational New Drug (IND) and off-label pharmaceuticals can be administered to US service members. This handbook discusses numerous pharmaceutical products, some of which are INDs. In certain other cases, licensed pharmaceuticals are discussed for use in a manner (or for a condition) other than that for which they were originally licensed (i.e., an "off-label" indication).

This executive order does not intend to alter the traditional physician-patient relationship or individual physician prescribing practices. Healthcare providers remain free to exercise clinical judgment and prescribe licensed pharmaceutical products as they deem appropriate for the optimal care of their patients. This policy does, however, potentially influence recommendations that might be made by US Government agencies and that might be applied to large numbers of service members outside of the individual physician-patient relationship. The following text presents a brief overview of EO 13139 for the benefit of the individual provider.

EO13139...

- Provides the Secretary of Defense guidance regarding the provision of IND products or products unapproved for their intended use as antidotes to chemical, biological, or radiological weapons;
- Stipulates that the US Government will administer products approved by the US Food and Drug Administration only for their intended use;
- Provides the circumstances and controls under which IND products may be used.
- To administer an IND product:
  - Informed consent must be obtained from individual service members
  - The President may waive informed consent (at the request of the Secretary of Defense and only the Secretary of Defense) if:
    - Informed consent is not feasible
    - Informed consent is contrary to the best interests of the service member
    - Obtaining informed consent is not in the best interests of national security.

Table of Contents

INTRODUCTION

Medical defense against the use of pathogens and toxins as battlefield weapons, or in terrorism, is a subject that remains exotic to many military and civilian healthcare providers. The US military has pursued research relevant to the medical defense against biological threat agents (bio-agents) since World War II, first in concert with an offensive weapons program, then — for the past 45 years — as a purely defensive research program. But the 2001 terrorist attacks on the US mainland, and subsequent anthrax mail attacks, galvanized national and local political leaders, including lawmakers, medical opinion makers, and the public at large, that the bio-agent threat was real and required much more planning, training, and resources for an effective response.

At the National Integrated Biodefense Campus (NIBC) at Fort Detrick, and elsewhere, USAMRIID has now been joined in a new "whole-of-government" approach, by agencies representing four federal cabinet level departments which are coordinated by the National Interagency Confederation for Biological Research (NICBR): the DoD (2 agencies), the DHHS (4), the DHS (1) and the USDA (1).[1] At the same time, there has been a widespread increase in interest among healthcare practitioners, across the academic and practice spectrum, to understand better how to manage the medical consequences of bio-agent exposure, as well as exotic natural infections, so as to minimize casualties.

Diverse measures to improve preparedness for, and response to, a bio-agent release are continuing at local, state, and federal, as well as international, levels. Training efforts have increased in both the military and civilian sectors. A week-long Medical Management of Chemical and Biological Casualties (MCBC) course, taught at both USAMRIID and USAMRICD, trains hundreds of military and civilian medical professionals every year about biological and chemical medical defense. The highly successful USAMRIID international satellite, online, and DVD courses on the Medical Management of Biological Casualties (MMBC) have reached hundreds of thousands of medical personnel over the past two decades.

By means of this handbook and the related materials and courses, practitioners may learn about effective and available medical countermeasures against many of the bacteria, viruses, and toxins of greatest concern. The importance of this education is self-evident and it is hoped that thereby practitioners will develop a solid understanding of the biological threats that our military forces, as well as civilian communities, may face.

The purpose of this handbook is to serve as a concise, pocket-sized manual that can be pulled off the shelf — or from a pocket — in a crisis to guide medical personnel in the prophylaxis, recognition, and management of biological casualties. It is designed as a quick reference and overview, and is not intended as a definitive or exhaustive textbook. A more in-depth discussion of the bio-agents covered here may be found in the US Army Surgeon General's Borden Institute *Textbook of Military Medicine: Medical Aspects of Biological Warfare* (published in 2007 and currently in revision) and in relevant infectious disease, tropical medicine, and disaster medicine textbooks.

HISTORY OF BIOLOGICAL WARFARE & THE CURRENT THREAT

The use of biological agents in warfare has been recorded throughout history.[1] During the 14th century BC, the Hittites are known to have driven diseased animals and people into enemy territory with the intent of initiating an epidemic, successfully propagating the disease we know as tularemia.[2] In the 6th century BC, the Assyrians poisoned enemy wells with rye ergot, and the Greek general Solon used the herb hellebore to poison the water source of the city of Kirra during his siege.[3] In 1346, plague broke out in the Tartar army during its siege of Kaffa (at present day Feodosia in the Crimea). The attackers hurled the corpses of plague victims over the city walls and this act is likely the reason for the entry of the "Black Death" into that city.[4] In 1422, at the siege of Karlstejn during the Hussite Wars in Bohemia, Prince Coribut hurled corpses of plague-stricken soldiers at the enemy troops, and Russian forces may have used the same tactic against the Swedes in 1710.

In 1611 at Jamestown Colony in Virginia, a toxic hallucinogenic drug derived from plants was deployed with some success against the English settlers by Chief Powhatan.[5] A century and a half later, smallpox was used as a biological weapon by the British in North America. In 1763, towards the close of the French and Indian War, Sir Jeffery Amherst recommended that a subordinate provide smallpox-laden blankets to the Native Americans remaining loyal to the French. Another subordinate, Captain Simeon Ecuyer, subsequently gave blankets and a handkerchief from a smallpox hospital to these adversaries, after which he wrote: "I hope it will have the desired effect." The subsequent outbreaks cannot with certainty be attributed to Ecuyer's actions, but the intent was entirely clear.[6] General George Washington ordered variolation (a precursor of vaccination, using material obtained from smallpox scabs) for protection of the Continental Army in 1777, in part due to devastation previously rendered on his forces by natural smallpox outbreaks and in part because of his concerns (and those of Franklin and Jefferson) for the purposeful spread of smallpox among the colonials by the British.[7]

In the 20th century, the stakes became much higher as the Germ Theory and subsequent scientific discipline of microbiology provided a new level of sophistication in the production of bio-agents for war. During World War I, operatives of Imperial Germany inoculated horses and cattle with anthrax and glanders at several ports around the world — including that of Baltimore — before the animals were shipped to France.[8] The French, for their part, began the world's first truly scientific biological weapons program targeted against human combatants, under the direction of Auguste Trillat in the early 1920s.[9] In the early 1930s, Imperial Japan began an ambitious bio-warfare program; by 1937, the notorious facility code-named "Unit 731", located 40 miles south of Harbin, in occupied Manchuria, was operational. Studies directed by Japanese general and physician Shiro Ishii continued there until it was destroyed by the allies in 1945. A post-war investigation revealed that the Japanese program researched numerous bio-agents and used POWs as research subjects. About 1,000 human autopsies were apparently carried out at Unit 731, mostly on victims exposed to aerosolized anthrax. Many more prisoners and Chinese nationals may have died in this facility, up to 3,000 in total.

The Japanese also apparently used bio-agents in the field. These instances remain history's only examples of the actual use of industrial-scale biological warfare (BW) on a battlefield or against an enemy's civilian population: the aftermath of the Battle of Khalkhin-Gol in August 1939 (where typhus, paratyphus, cholera, and dysentery were deployed as Japanese troops retreated from the Soviets), at Ning Bo in Zhejiang Province, China, in 1940, where ~1,000 civilians were sickened and perhaps 100 killed (plague fleas, typhoid and cholera in water) and in several cities of Zhejiang in 1942 (where reportedly ~1,000 Japanese troops were also inadvertently killed). The reported overflights by Japanese planes suspected of dropping plague-infected fleas may have caused the plague epidemics that ensued in China and Manchuria, with resulting untold thousands of deaths.[10] This story, still incompletely understood, has been a long time in the telling. One scholar has concluded that:

> ... the latest research ... shows that in the two bio-war campaigns alone, those in Yunnan Province in southern China and Shandong Province in the north, more than 400,000 people died of cholera. Special army forces waged germ attacks across China, at countless locations under Imperial Japan's heel of occupation, and even in unoccupied regions that were subject to fly-overs by Japanese planes. Plague literally rained down upon people's heads, sprayed from special bio-war air team planes of the military; cholera, typhoid, dysentery, anthrax, paratyphoid, glanders, and other pestilences infected their food, drinking wells, crops, and livestock .... The number of people killed by Japanese germ warfare and human experiments [was estimated] to be approximately 590,000. This is the figure that was ... mutually agreed upon at the International Symposium on the Crimes of Bacteriological Warfare ... in December 2002 in the city of Changede, Hunan Province .... The number of physicians and scientists involved in these germ attacks and in the human experiments totaled more than 20,000.[11]

By war's end, the Japanese program had also stockpiled 400 kilograms of anthrax to be used in a specially designed fragmentation bomb, although this particular weapon technology was never tested or proven operationally.

In 1942, at the direction of President Franklin D. Roosevelt, the US began its own research and development program in the use of bio-agents for offensive purposes. Similar programs had already begun in earnest two years earlier in Canada, the United Kingdom (UK), and probably several other countries. This work was started, interestingly enough, in response to a perceived German bio-warfare threat as opposed to a Japanese one. The US research program was headquartered at Camp Detrick (now Fort Detrick), and produced agents and conducted field testing at other sites until 1969, when President Nixon stopped all offensive biological and toxin weapon research and production by executive order. (The UK had discontinued its own program about 10 years earlier.) Between May 1971 and May 1972, all stockpiles of bio-agents and munitions from the now defunct US program were destroyed in the presence of monitors representing the USDA, the Department of Health, Education, and Welfare, (now the DHHS), and the states of Arkansas, Colorado, and Maryland, where bio-arsenals existed. Included among the bio-agents destroyed were *Bacillus anthracis*, botulinum toxin, *Francisella tularensis, Coxiella burnetii*, Venezuelan equine encephalitis virus, *Brucella suis* and staphylococcal enterotoxin B. The US Army began a medical defensive program against bio-agents in 1953 which continues today at USAMRIID.[12]

In 1972, the US, UK, and USSR signed the Convention on the Prohibition of the Development, Production and Stockpiling of Bacteriological and Toxin Weapons and on Their Destruction, commonly called the Biological Weapons Convention (BWC). A total of 171 countries have now added their ratification. This treaty prohibits the stockpiling of bio-agents for offensive military purposes, and also forbids research on agents for other than peaceful purposes. To strengthen efforts to combat the BW threat, signatory states agreed in November 2002 to have experts meet annually through 2006 to discuss and promote common understanding and effective action on biosecurity, national implementation measures, suspicious outbreaks of disease, disease surveillance, and codes of conduct for scientists. However, despite this historic agreement among nations, biowarfare research continued to flourish in many countries hostile to the US. Moreover, there have been several cases of suspected or actual release of biological weapons. Among the most notorious of these were the "yellow rain" (possible T-2 mycotoxin) incidents in Southeast Asia (1975-78), the use of ricin as an assassination weapon in London in 1978, and the accidental release of weaponized anthrax spores at Sverdlovsk in 1979.

Testimony from the late 1970s indicated that Laos and Kampuchea were attacked by planes and helicopters delivering colored aerosols. After being exposed, people and animals became disoriented and ill, and a small percentage of those stricken died. Some of these clouds may have been comprised of trichothecene toxins (in particular, T-2 mycotoxin). These attacks are grouped under the label "yellow rain." There has been a great deal of controversy about whether these clouds were truly biowarfare agents. Some have argued that the clouds were nothing more than feces produced by swarms of bees.

In 1978, Georgi Markov, a Bulgarian defector living in the UK, was attacked in London with a device disguised as an umbrella, which injected a tiny pellet filled with ricin toxin into the subcutaneous tissue of his leg. He died several days later. On autopsy, the tiny pellet was found and determined to contain ricin toxin. It was later revealed that the Bulgarian secret service carried out the assassination, and the technology to commit the crime was developed and supplied by the Soviet Union's secret service (KGB). (Interestingly, never-used research conducted in the US during World War I had revealed that ricin toxin-coated bullets produced shrapnel capable of causing fatal wounds.)

In April, 1979, an incident occurred in Sverdlovsk (now Yekaterinburg) in the Soviet Union which appeared to be an accidental aerosol release of *Bacillus anthracis* spores from a Soviet military microbiology facility: Compound 19. At least 77 residents living downwind from this compound developed high fever and had difficulty breathing; at least 66 cases died. The Soviet Ministry of Health blamed the deaths on the consumption of contaminated meat, and for years, controversy raged in the press over the actual cause of the outbreak. All evidence available to the US Government indicated a release of aerosolized *B. anthracis* spores. In the summer of 1992, US intelligence officials were proven correct when the new Russian President, Boris Yeltsin, acknowledged that the Sverdlovsk incident was in fact related to activities at a BW production facility. In 1994, Harvard Professor Mathew Meselson and colleagues published an in-depth analysis of the incident.[13] They documented that all of the cases occurred within a narrow zone extending 4 kilometers downwind in a southeasterly direction from Compound 19. A more recently reported incident from the Soviet Union revealed that in 1971, a field test of smallpox biological weapon near Aralsk, Kazakhstan caused an outbreak of at least 10 cases and one death. In both Sverdlovsk and Aralsk, a massive intervention by public health authorities greatly helped to lower potential disease spread and deaths.

Since the fall of the Soviet Union in 1991, something of the enormous size of Russia's former BW program, which had its origins in the 1920s, has become apparent.[14, 15] By 1960, numerous BW research facilities existed throughout the country; after 1973, they were coordinated by an agency known as Biopreparat. These programs became immense — the largest of any country in history — and at their peak were conducted at 52 clandestine research and production sites employing over 50,000 people. Annualized production capacity for weaponized smallpox, for example, was 90 to 100 tons. Yeltsin stated that he would put an end to further offensive BW research; however, the degree to which the program was scaled back is not known. Revelations from Colonel Kanatzhan Alibekov (Ken Alibek), a senior biowarfare program manager who defected from Russia in 1992, outlined a still remarkably robust BW program, which included active research into genetic engineering, binary bio-agents and chimeras, and capacity to produce industrial quantities of agents.[16] It is now known that, in the 1980s and '90s, many of these agents were genetically altered to resist heat, cold, and antibiotics. In September 1992, an agreement was signed with the US and UK promising to end BW programs and convert facilities to benevolent purposes, but compliance with the agreement — and the fate of the former Soviet bio-agents and facilities — is still mostly undocumented. (In a particularly dispiriting development, and despite overwhelming evidence to the contrary, Russian President Vladimir Putin has asserted that the USSR never pursued an offensive BW program in violation of the BWC.[17])

During United Nations (UN) inspections of former BW facilities in Iraq in 1998, it emerged that Iraqi President Saddam Hussein had had prisoners tied to stakes and bombarded with anthrax and chemical weapons for experimental purposes. These experiments began in the 1980s during the Iran-Iraq War after initial experiments on sheep and camels. Dozens of prisoners are believed to have died in agony during the program. According to an investigation by the *London Sunday Times*:

> Iranian prisoners of war are said to have been tied up and killed by bacteria from a shell detonated nearby. Others were exposed to an aerosol of anthrax sprayed into a chamber while doctors watched behind a glass screen. Two British-trained scientists have been identified as leading figures in the programme.... 10 Iranian prisoners of war were taken to a location near Iraq's border with Saudi Arabia. They were lashed to posts and left helpless as an anthrax bomb was exploded by remote control 15 yards away. All died painfully from internal haemorrhaging. In another experiment, 15 Kurdish prisoners were tied up in a field while shells containing camel pox, a mild virus, were dropped from a light aircraft. The results were slower but the test was judged a success; the prisoners fell ill within a week. Iraqi sources say some of the cruellest research has been conducted at an underground facility near Salman Pak, southwest of Baghdad. Here... experiments with biological and chemical agents were carried out first on dogs and cats, then on Iranian prisoners... secured to a bed in a purpose-built chamber, into which lethal agents, including anthrax, were sprayed from a high-velocity device mounted in the ceiling. Medical researchers viewed the results through fortified glass. Details of the experiments were known only to Saddam and an inner circle of senior government officials and Iraqi scientists educated in the West.... The facility, which is understood to have been built by German engineers in the 1980s, has been at the centre of Iraq's experiments on "human guinea pigs" for more than 10 years.[18]

In August, 1991, the UN carried out its first inspection of Iraq's biowarfare capabilities in the aftermath of the Gulf War. On August 2, 1991, representatives of the Iraqi government announced to leaders of UN Special Commission Team 7 that they had conducted research into the offensive use of *Bacillus anthracis*, botulinum toxins, *Clostridium perfringens* (presumably one of its toxins), and other bio-agents. This open admission of biological weapons research verified many of the concerns of the US intelligence community. Iraq had extensive and redundant research facilities at Salman Pak and other sites, many of which were destroyed during the war.

In 1995, further information on Iraq's offensive program was made available to UN inspectors. Iraq conducted research and development work on anthrax, botulinum toxins, *C. perfringens*, aflatoxins, wheat cover smut, and ricin. Field trials were conducted with *Bacillus subtilis* (a simulant for anthrax), botulinum toxin, and aflatoxin. Bio-agents were tested in various delivery systems, including rockets, aerial bombs, and spray tanks. In December 1990, the Iraqis filled 100 R400 bombs with botulinum toxin, 50 with anthrax, and 16 with aflatoxin. In addition, 13 Al Hussein (Scud) warheads were filled with botulinum toxin, 10 with anthrax, and 2 with aflatoxin. These weapons were deployed in January 1991 to four locations. In all, Iraq produced 19,000 liters of concentrated botulinum toxin (nearly 10,000 liters filled into munitions), 8,500 liters of concentrated anthrax (6,500 liters filled into munitions) and 2,200 liters of aflatoxin (1,580 liters filled into munitions). It appears that any subsequent BW program in Iraq was limited to research.

The 1990s also saw increasing concern over the possibility of the terrorist use of bio-agents to threaten either military or civilian populations. Extremist groups have tried to obtain microorganisms that could be used as biological weapons. The 1995 sarin nerve agent attack in the Tokyo subway system raised awareness that terrorist organizations could potentially acquire or develop weapons of mass destruction (WMD) for use against civilian populations. Subsequent investigations revealed that, on several occasions, the Aum Shinrikyo cult had attempted to release botulinum toxin (1993 and 1995) and *B. anthracis* (1995) from trucks and rooftops, efforts that were, fortunately, unsuccessful.[19]

In response, the DoD initially led a federal effort to train the first responders in 120 American cities to be prepared to act in case of a domestic terrorist incident involving WMD. This program was subsequently handed over to the Department of Justice, and then to the Department of Homeland Security (DHS). First responders, public health and medical personnel, and law enforcement agencies have dealt with the exponential increase in biological weapons hoaxes around the country over the past several years. The National Pharmaceutical Stockpile (NPS) was launched in 1999, under direction of the Centers for Disease Control and Prevention (CDC). It became the Strategic National Stockpile (SNS) in 2002 and represents the nation's repository of antibiotic, vaccines, chemical antidotes, antitoxins, and other critical medical equipment and supplies under joint control of CDC and DHS.

The events of September 11, 2001, and subsequent anthrax mail attacks brought immediacy to planning for the terrorist use of WMD in the US. Anthrax-laden letters placed in the mail caused 23 probable or confirmed cases of anthrax-related illness and five deaths, mostly among postal workers and those handling mail. On October 17, 2001, US lawmakers were directly affected by anthrax contamination leading to closure of the Hart Senate Office Building in Washington, D.C. Terrorist plots to use ricin were uncovered in England in January, 2003. Ricin was also found in a South Carolina postal facility in October, 2003[20] and the Dirksen Senate Office Building in Washington, D.C. in February, 2004. Ricin incidents continue to occur due to the ready availability of the source material from castor beans. (Most recently, in April 2013, envelopes addressed to the office of US Senator Roger Wicker and to President Barack Obama tested positive for ricin. A Mississippi man was ultimately sentenced to 25 years in prison for the crime.[21])

The National Strategy for Homeland Security (2002) and the Homeland Security Act of 2002 were developed in response to the terrorist attacks. The DHS, with over 180,000 personnel, was established to provide the unifying foundation for a national network of organizations and institutions involved in efforts to secure the nation. Over $8 billion from the DHS has been awarded since March, 2003 to help first responders and state and local governments to prevent, respond to and recover from potential acts of terrorism and other disasters. The Office for Domestic Preparedness (ODP) is the principal component of the DHS responsible for preparing the US for acts of terrorism by providing training, funds for the purchase of equipment, support for the planning and execution of exercises, technical assistance and other support to assist states and local jurisdictions to prevent, plan for, and respond to acts of terrorism.

The Public Health Security and Bioterrorism Response Act of 2002 requires drinking water facilities to conduct vulnerability assessments; all universities and laboratories that work with biological material that could pose a public-health threat have to be registered with the DHHS or the USDA; and new steps were imposed to limit access to potential bio-agents. Smallpox preparedness was implemented, including a civilian vaccination program, vaccine injury compensation program, and aid to the states. Before the March 2003 invasion of Iraq, state and local health departments and hospitals nationwide conducted smallpox vaccinations of healthcare workers and have since developed statewide bio-terrorism response plans.

According to many experts, the threat of bio-warfare has increased in recent decades, with a number of countries working on the offensive use of these agents. In 2008, according to a US Congressional Research Service report, nine countries—China, Cuba, Egypt, Iran, Israel, North Korea, Russia, Syria and Taiwan—are considered, with varying degrees of certainty, to have some BW capability.[22] (Iran and Syria have been identified as countries "aggressively seeking" biological — as well as nuclear and chemical—weapons.) The threat of the use of bio-agents against US military forces and civilians may be more acute than at any time in US history, due to the widespread availability of agents, along with knowledge of production methodologies and potential dissemination devices. There is still intense concern in the west about the possibility of proliferation or enhancement of offensive programs in countries hostile to the law-abiding democracies, due to the potential hiring of expatriate Russian scientists. There is also growing concern that the smallpox virus, lawfully stored in only two laboratories at the CDC in Atlanta and the Russian State Centre for Research on Virology and Biotechnology (Vektor), may exist in other countries around the globe. Therefore, awareness of, and preparedness for, this threat requires the ongoing education of our government officials, public health officials, healthcare providers, and law enforcement personnel and is vital to our national security.

DISTINGUISHING BETWEEN NATURAL & INTENTIONAL DISEASE OUTBREAKS

General epidemiological principles are as applicable to a biological attack — whether from bio-terrorism or biological warfare on the battlefield — as they are to natural or endemic infectious disease outbreaks. The ability to accurately determine who is at risk, and to make appropriate decisions regarding prophylaxis and other responses after a bio-agent attack, rests upon these essential tools.[1] There are, however, some important special considerations that apply to deliberate outbreaks. Because the use of a biological weapon is a criminal act, it will be very important for the evidence gathered to be usable as evidence in court. Therefore, if criminality is suspected, samples should be handled through a formal chain of custody and there must be good communication and information sharing between public health and law-enforcement authorities. In addition, because the attack may be intentional, one must be prepared for the unexpected — there is always the possibility of multiple outbreaks at different locations, as well as of the use of multiple different agents, including mixed chemical and bio-agents or multiple bio-agents.[2]

Surveillance & detection:

After a successful covert bio-agent attack, the most likely first indicator will be increased numbers of patients presenting to individual healthcare providers or emergency departments with similar clinical features, caused by the disseminated disease agent. It is axiomatic that a propagating bio-agent (bacterium or virus) has an incubation period typically lasting days, by which time the unwitting victims may have dispersed from the site of the exposure and may even have travelled significant distances. (Given a large delivered dose, however, or if the agent is a [non-propagating] toxin, this assumption cannot always be relied upon.) In the days after an unsuspected bio-attack, the possibility exists that other medical professionals, such as pharmacists or laboratorians, who may receive more than the usual numbers of prescriptions or requests for laboratory tests, respectively, may be the first to recognize that something unusual is occurring. Because animals may be sentinels of disease in humans and many of the high-threat bio-agents discussed in this book are zoonoses, it is possible that veterinarians might recognize an event in animals before it is recognized in humans.[3] Medical examiners, coroners, and non-medical professionals, such as morticians, may also be important sentinel event reporters.

To help ensure a prompt and efficient response, public officials must implement and utilize routine biosurveillance systems so that they know the background disease rates and can recognize patterns of non-specific syndromes that could represent early manifestations of a bio-agent attack. The system must be timely, sensitive, specific, and practical. To recognize any unusual changes in disease occurrence, surveillance of background disease activity should be ongoing, and any significant variation should trigger a directed examination of the facts regarding the change. In the past several years, many public health agencies have initiated syndrome-based surveillance systems in an attempt to achieve near real-time detection of unusual events. Currently, these systems collectively represent something of a hodge-podge. (See the subsequent section on "Biosurveillance".) Some collect data broadly from the US healthcare system (For example, the National Electronic Disease Surveillance System [NEDSS][4].) Others are much more narrowly focused. The exemplar of the latter approach is the sophisticated national and international surveillance systems that have been developed to detect specific circulating influenza genotypes that are not included in a current year's vaccine. (For example, the U.S. Air Force School of Aerospace Medicine [USAFSAM] performs global, laboratory-based influenza surveillance through a system of sentinel sites.) Other such systems are in varying stages of maturity. Regardless of the existence of these systems, a sudden sharp increase in illness rates, or the diagnosis of a rare or unusual case, may still be first recognized by astute individuals working as clinicians or laboratorians.

Outbreak investigation:

After detection of a potential disease outbreak, whether natural or purposeful, a thorough outbreak investigation will assist medical personnel in identifying the pathogen and lead to the institution of appropriate medical and public health interventions. The identification of the affected population, possible routes of exposure, signs and symptoms of disease, along with the rapid laboratory identification of the causative agent(s) are all essential elements of this effort. Good epidemiologic information can guide the appropriate management of those potentially exposed, as well as assist in risk communication to authorities and in formulating responses to the media.[5]

Many diseases caused by weaponized bio-agents initially present with non-specific clinical features—notably undifferentiated fevers—that may be difficult to diagnose and recognize as a biological attack. Features of the epidemic may be important in distinguishing between a natural and a terrorist or military attack. Epidemiologic clues that may suggest an intentional attack are listed in Table 1. While a helpful guide, it is important to remember that naturally occurring epidemics may have one or more of these characteristics and that a biological attack may have none. However, if many of the listed clues are recognized, one's index of suspicion for an intentionally spread outbreak should increase.[6]

Table 1. Possible Epidemiologic Clues to Intentional Bio-agent Use
• The appearence of a large outbreak of cases of a similar disease or syndrome, especially in a discrete population
• Many cases of unexplained diseases or deaths
• More severe disease than is usually expected for a specific pathogen or failure to respond to standard therapy
• Unusual routes of exposure for a pathogen, such as the inhalational route for diseases that normally occur through other exposures
• A disease case or cases that are unusual for a given geographic area or transmission season
• Disease normally transmitted by a vector that is not present in the local area
• Multiple simultaneous or serial epidemics of different diseases in the same population
• A single case of disease caused by an uncommon agent (smallpox, some viral hemorrhagic fevers, inhalational anthrax, pneumonic plague)
• A disease that is unusual for an age group
• Unusual strains or variants of organisms or antimicrobial resistance patterns different from those known to be circulating
• A similar or identical genetic type among agents isolated from distinct sources at different times or locations
• Higher attack rates among those exposed in certain areas, such as inside a building if released indoors, or lower rates in those inside a sealed building if released outside
• Outbreaks of the same disease occurring simultaneously in noncontiguous areas
• Zoonotic disease outbreaks
• A zoonotic disease occurring in humans, but not animals
• Intelligence of a potential attack, claims by a terrorist or aggressor of a release, and discovery of munitions, tampering, or other potential vehicle of spread (spray device, contaminated letter)

The first step in an outbreak investigation is to confirm that a disease outbreak has in fact occurred. Because an outbreak is defined as a higher rate of an illness than is normally seen in a given population, it is helpful to have handy background surveillance data to determine if what is being seen constitutes a deviation from the norm.[7] For example, in mid-winter, thousands of cases of influenza may not be considered an outbreak, whereas in the summer, it might be highly unusual. Moreover, even a single case of a very unusual illness, such as inhalational anthrax, might constitute an outbreak and should be viewed with high suspicion. The clinical features seen in the initial cases can be used to construct a case definition to determine the number of cases and the attack rate (i.e., the population that is ill or meets the case definition divided by the population at risk). The case definition allows investigators who are separated geographically to use the same criteria when evaluating the outbreak. The use of objective criteria in the case definition is critical to determining an accurate case number, as additional cases may be found and some cases may be excluded. This is especially true as the potential exists for panic and for subjective or routine complaints to be confused with actual disease.

Outbreak description & analysis:

Once the attack rate has been determined, an outbreak can be described in terms of time, place, and person. These data will provide crucial information in determining the potential source of the outbreak. The epidemic curve is calculated based upon cases over time. In a point-source outbreak, which is the most likely type in a biological attack or bio-terrorism situation, individuals are exposed to the disease agent in a fairly short time and in a restricted geographic venue. The early phase of the epidemic curve may be compressed compared to a natural disease outbreak. In addition, the incubation period could be shorter than for a natural outbreak if individuals are exposed to higher inocula of the bio-agent than would occur in the natural setting. The peak may occur in days or even hours, especially if a toxin (as opposed to a propagating bio-agent) is used. Later phases of the curve may also help determine if the disease is able to spread from person to person. Determining whether the disease is contagious will be extremely important for crafting effective disease control measures, such as deciding whether isolation, or even quarantine, is justified. If the agent(s) is released at multiple times or sites, additional cases and multiple sequential peaks in the epidemic curve may also occur, something that happened with the mailed anthrax letters in 2001.

Once the disease agent is recognized, appropriate prophylaxis, treatment, and other measures to decrease disease spread, can be instituted. These may need to be modified as additional data on the agent (strain, anti-infective susceptibilities, etc.) come to light. The ultimate test of whether control measures are effective will be simply careful observation to see if they reduce ongoing illness or spread of disease.

Finally, it is important to understand that although the recognition of and preparation for a biological attack will be similar to that for any infectious disease outbreak, the surveillance, response, and other demands on resources will likely be of an unparalleled intensity. Public anxiety will be greater after an intentionally caused event; therefore, a sound risk-communication plan that involves public health authorities will be vital to an effective response and to allay the fears of the public. A strong public-health infrastructure—with an effective epidemiological investigation capability, practical training programs, and preparedness plans—is essential to the prevention and control of disease outbreaks, whether they are naturally-occurring or purposeful.

BIOSURVEILLANCE

Syndromic Surveillance

The need to rapidly detect an intentionally caused disease outbreak has prompted a search for faster and more reliable methods for disease surveillance. "Syndromic surveillance" typically refers to the automated analysis of routinely collected health data that are available even before specific diagnoses are made. The rapid expansion of such surveillance systems in recent years can be attributed to 1) increasingly available and timely electronic data entered into accessible databases, 2) advances in informatics and statistics for data extraction, normalization, and detection of aberrations in temporal or spatial data, and 3) growing concerns about the threat of epidemics, influenza pandemics, bio-terrorism and biowarfare. In many situations, syndromic surveillance systems may not detect outbreaks faster than traditional epidemiological surveillance methods. However, these systems may be able to provide information that can assist with the outbreak investigation, situational awareness, tracing the spread of outbreaks and the effectiveness of countermeasures.

Data that arise from an interaction with the health care system, but do not include confirmed or definitive diagnoses, can include early, non-specific diagnoses, such as "gastroenteritis," or procedures from initial encounters, such as "stool culture." They can be recorded as text in an electronic record, or through codes such as the International Classification of Diseases (ICD) or Current Procedural Terminology (CPT). A chief complaint such as "cough" can be entered in an Emergency Department electronic medical record, or "rash, unknown etiology" entered in a billing database. These data can also include initial impressions from emergency medical personnel on ambulance runs or calls to nurse advice lines or doctor's offices for information. Pre-encounter information obtained about the health of a population before presentation to a health care provider includes over-the-counter pharmacy sales for items such as cough syrup or anti-diarrheal medication. Behavioral changes can be detected in school or work absenteeism rates or internet queries. In general, the closer the data source is to a medical encounter (chief complaints, provider initial impressions, laboratory test orders), the more reliable the information.

To be analyzed for anomalies and compared to expected illness rates, indicator health events must be grouped into syndromes. Most data types, including pharmacy sales and prescriptions, laboratory tests, ambulance runs, chief complaints and diagnostic codes can be grouped into syndromes. Common syndrome groups include respiratory, gastrointestinal, rash, neurological, and febrile illnesses. A syndrome grouping schema based on ICD-9 codes, with an emphasis on bio-terrorism detection, is available.[1]

The most commonly promoted use of syndromic surveillance in a bio-terrorism or biological warfare context is for early detection of an attack. Timely awareness of an increase in disease incidence can assist in mobilizing resources and potentially decrease associated morbidity and mortality. There are many examples of retrospective studies showing that syndromic surveillance can provide early warning of large community-wide disease outbreaks when compared to traditional disease reporting. Furthermore, it is assumed that such an alert could effect earlier etiologic diagnoses, and early institution of preventive measures such as vaccination and antibiotic prophylaxis, as well as prioritization of these measures to affected communities in time to reduce morbidity and mortality.

The characteristics of an outbreak that make it most likely to be detected by syndromic surveillance are 1) narrow distribution of the incubation period, 2) longer prodrome, 3) absence of a pathognomonic clinical sign that would speed diagnosis, and 4) diagnosis that is dependent on the use of specialized tests that are unlikely to be ordered. Not all biowarfare or terrorism-caused outbreaks will have these characteristics. In addition, early detection may or may not assist with determining whether the outbreak is the result of an intentional biological attack. Any disease outbreak must be investigated by appropriate public health officials, and law enforcement will only be involved if evidence arises that points to illegal activity. Early detection alone does not ensure recognition of a biological attack, but data in a syndromic system may help find clues that suggest an intentional event.

Besides early detection, syndromic surveillance systems can assist with the evaluation of the effectiveness of countermeasures, and provide support to epidemiological investigations by finding potential cases that have recently presented and have the same syndromic presentation as those already identified. It can also be used for situational awareness — providing reassurance during periods of high concern such as large public events or when bio-agents have been used on a small scale, such as the anthrax-laced letters mailed from New Jersey in 2001 or the ricin-laced letters mailed from Tennessee in 2013. With the use of environmental sensors for bio-terrorism detection in large metropolitan areas, potential alerts can be shared with public health officials who can then carefully monitor syndromic data in the same geographic area.

National Strategy for Biosurveillance

Protecting the health and safety of the American people through a well-integrated national biosurveillance (BSV) enterprise has become a top national security priority. This requires a focus on core functions if progress is to be made. It also necessitates an embrace of an "all-of-Nation" approach, and indeed a global health security intent, since the effects of any deliberate CBRN (chemical, biological, radiological, or nuclear) attack or accident, or emerging infectious disease, can easily transcend national borders. There exists an imperative that the Federal government expand its efforts to detect rapidly a potential incident of national significance affecting human, animal, or plant health, whether resulting from a bio-terror attack or other CBRN threat, an emerging infectious disease, pandemic, or a food-borne illness. Rapid detection is critical to save lives and improve incident outcomes, and the United States serves as a key participant and leader in an international network of BSV centers operating across the globe.[2-5]

A National Strategy for Biosurveillance (NSB)[6], initiated by the Obama Administration in the summer of 2012, seeks to leverage existing capabilities across the Nation, yet emphasizes a discrete focus on specified core functions. It articulates that essential information can be derived from a specific set of questions to speed the detection of a deliberate or accidental CBRN incident or naturally occurring disease outbreak. This Strategy further articulates that when the collection and sharing of this essential information is prioritized, decision making can be expedited at all levels of government and beyond. While other activities are integral to everyday local BSV efforts that can and should continue, the NSB calls for a national focus on fewer issues so that more can be achieved collectively. This approach also seeks to inspire new thinking and revised methodologies to "forecast" that which we cannot yet prove, so that timely decisions can be made to save lives and reduce impacts during an emergency incident. It is a national plan of action to protect the health, well being, and safety of the American people as part of the greater global community.

The NSB, defines "biosurveillance" as "the process of gathering, integrating, interpreting, and communicating essential information related to all-hazard threats or disease activities affecting human, animal, or plant health to achieve early detection and warning; contribute to overall situational awareness of the health aspects of an incident; and enable better decision-making at all levels". The NSB specifies the US Government's approach to strengthening our national BSV enterprise. It describes a core set of functions critical to success as:

1. Scan and discern the environment;
2. Identify and integrate essential information;
3. Inform and alert decision-makers; and
4. Forecast and advise potential impacts.

The approach builds on existing BSV concepts and capabilities to enable more rapid detection, knowledge, and characterization of human, animal, and plant disease activities to enhance situational awareness. The NSB is consistent with the *National Strategy for Countering Biological Threats*[7], which emphasizes information sharing among Federal departments and agencies to identify biological threats.

In the context of the 2012 launch of the NSB, the Office of Management and Budget (OMB) asked the DoD to review its BSV programs, prioritize missions and desired outcomes, evaluate how DoD programs contribute to these, and assess the appropriateness and stability of the Department's funding system for biosurveillance. In support of this strategy, the DoD is endevouring to strengthen its BSV capabilities to enhance all-hazards incident management by providing essential information for timely decision-making at all levels, whether an incident is deliberate, accidental, or naturally occurring.

The Deputy Secretary of Defense (DEPSECDEF) published interim DoD guidance for implementing the NSB[8] in the summer of 2013. The DoD defines "biosurveillence" the same way as does the NSB. The interim DoD guidance states that Combatant Commands (CCMDs) will continue updating directed plans and corresponding capability gaps for improved analysis of data and reporting generated by ongoing BSV-related activities. CCMDs will also identify requirements and gaps for improved integration of data and reporting generated by ongoing BSV-related activities. For the Military Services, it states that Secretaries of the Military Departments, in coordination with their Surgeons General (SGs), will make their BSV-related data, reporting and analyses available for integration at the tactical, operational, and strategic levels. DoD BSV activities include the areas of Comprehensive Health Surveillance (CHS); Force Health Protection (FHP), food protection and zoonotic disease surveillance; CBRN detection and monitoring; intelligence; law enforcement; and installation environmental and wildlife monitoring.

During 19–21 February 2014, USSTRATCOM J85, in partnership with USPACOM, led a table top exercise (TTX) gathering over 135 DoD BSV "key stakeholders" and decision-makers in an informal setting to generate discussion of BSV "lines of communication" (LOCs) and "information exchanges" (IEs) using hypothetical scenarios. Participants represented organizations from across the DoD BSV stakeholder community. In addition, there were representatives from the DHS, DHHS (CDC, etc), members of the US intelligence community, national laboratories and academia. During the TTX, players applied their specific knowledge in response to a series of scenario questions presented by a facilitator. Exercise information collected on the BSV information flow within the DoD BSV stakeholder community was used to create the baseline operational assessment (BOA) report, which will become a key document moving forward.

Development, implementation, and refinement of the NBS are all ongoing. The Federal government seeks to galvanize jurisdictions across the nation to further extend and integrate a distributed national BSV enterprise. The NSB embraces the need to engage in surveillance for weapons of mass destruction (WMD) threats and a much broader range of human, animal, and plant health challenges, including emerging infectious diseases, pandemics, agricultural threats, and food-borne illnesses.

TEN STEPS IN THE MANAGEMENT OF POTENTIAL BIOLOGICAL CASUALTIES

Military medical personnel will require a firm understanding of certain key elements of biological defense to manage effectively the consequences of a biological attack amid the confusion that prevails on the modern battlefield. Civilian providers who might be called upon to respond to a terrorist attack potentially employing biological agents require a similar understanding. Familiarity with the symptomatology, pathogenesis, transmissibility, and available diagnostic and treatment options for each of the potential bio-agents thus becomes imperative. Acquiring such an understanding is relatively straightforward once the identity of the agent is known; many references[1], including this handbook, exist to assist medical personnel in standard-of-care, pathogen-specific therapy. A larger problem presents itself, however, when the identity of a causative agent is unknown. In some cases, an attack may be threatened, but it may remain unclear whether such an attack has actually occurred. Similarly, it may be unclear whether casualties that do present are suffering from the intentional release of a bio-agent or a chemical agent, or whether they are due to a naturally occurring infectious disease outbreak (such as an exotic emerging infectious disease) or an accidental toxic industrial exposure. We recommend here a ten-step process to guide medical personnel in the evaluation and management of outbreaks of unknown origin and etiology. We feel that such an algorithmic approach — which incorporates elements of the Advanced Trauma Life Support (ATLS) course sponsored by the American College of Surgeons[2] — is desirable when dealing with the unknown, especially under austere conditions or amid the expected chaos of the modern battlefield. The development of this algorithmic approach has been detailed elsewhere[3-6] and a greatly expanded version of this construct is available in one of the Borden Institute's *Textbook of Military Medicine* (*TMM*) volumes.[7]

I. Maintain an index of suspicion. In the case of chemical or conventional warfare and terrorism, the sinister nature of an attack may be immediately obvious. Victims would likely succumb in close temporal and geographic proximity to a dispersal or explosive device, "clustered" in time and space. Complicating the discovery of the existence of a biological attack, however, is the fact that bio-agents possess inherent incubation periods. These incubation periods, typically days to even weeks in length, permit the wide dispersal of victims (both spatially and temporally) after exposure and infection. Moreover, they make it likely that the "first responder" to a biological attack would not be a traditional first responder (fireman, policeman, paramedic), but rather fixed facility medics, or primary care providers (physicians, PAs, nurses), emergency department personnel, and public health officials. In such circumstances, the maintenance of a pre-existing "index of suspicion" is essential if a timely diagnosis is to be made and prompt therapy instituted.[8] This is especially the case at lower echelons of care, remote from diagnostic and consultative resources.

Moreover, for many of the diseases typically regarded as potential bio-weapons, very early intervention is mandatory if a good patient outcome is to be achieved. Anthrax, botulism, plague, and smallpox are readily prevented if patients are provided proper anti-infectives, antisera, and/or vaccination promptly after exposure. Conversely, all of these diseases may prove fatal if prophylaxis or therapy is delayed until full-blown symptoms develop. Unfortunately, symptoms in the early, or prodromal, phase of these illnesses are non-specific, making diagnosis difficult. Furthermore, many bio-agent caused diseases, such as brucellosis, Q-fever, and Venezuelan equine encephalitis (VEE), tend to present simply as undifferentiated fevers. In such cases, epidemiologic clues might prove quite helpful in placing the available information in the proper context. (See the section on "Distinguishing Between Natural & Intentional Disease Outbreaks", above).

II. Protect yourself. Before medical personnel approach a potential biological (or chemical or radiological) casualty, they must first take steps to protect themselves. These steps may involve a combination of physical, chemical, and immunologic forms of protection. On the battlefield, "physical protection" typically consists of a protective mask ("gas mask"). Designed primarily with chemical vapor hazards in mind, the M-40/42, M-45, and M-50 series masks certainly provide adequate protection against all aerosolized BW threats. In fact, a HEPA-filter (or even a simple surgical) mask will often afford adequate protection against all bio-agents, although not against chemical threats. "Chemical protection" refers, in general, to the pre-exposure and/or post-exposure administration of antibiotics; such strategies are discussed on a bio-agent-specific basis in the relevant sections of this book. "Immunologic protection" principally involves active vaccination and as yet applies mainly to protection against just two bio-agents: anthrax and smallpox. Again, specific vaccination strategies are discussed throughout this book. Obviously, not all of these protective strategies would be applicable in every situation.

III. Assess the patient. This initial assessment is somewhat analogous to the primary survey and 'ABCDE' algorithm of ATLS management. As such, airway adequacy should be assessed and breathing and circulation problems addressed before attention is given to specific management. This initial assessment is conducted before decontamination is accomplished and should thus be brief, but the need for decon and for the administration of antidotes for rapid-acting chemical agents (nerve agents and cyanide) should be determined at this time.[9]

IV. Decontaminate as appropriate. Decon plays a very important role in the approach to chemical casualty management. The incubation period of biological agents, however, makes it unlikely that victims of a biological attack will present for medical care until days after exposure. (The biological toxins are an exception to this.) At such a late point — given that the victim has likely bathed and changed clothing several times, effectively accomplishing "self-decontamination" — the need for further intervention in this regard is likely minimal or non-existent. In those exceptional cases where decon is warranted, simple soap and water bathing or showering will usually suffice. Certainly, standard military decon solutions (such as hypochlorite solution), typically employed in cases of chemical agent contamination, will be effective against all biological agents. In fact, even 0.1% bleach reliably kills anthrax spores, the hardiest of bio-agents. However, the use of caustic substances, especially on human skin, is rarely warranted after a biological exposure. More information on decon for bio-agents (and on the management of scenarios involving announced threats, empty letters, suspicious packages, and delivery devices) is included in the section on "Decontamination" in this book as well as in Reference 1. It should also be kept in mind that a biological attack constitutes a criminal act and that hasty or ill-considered decon risks destroying valuable forensic evidence.

V. Establish a diagnosis. With decon (where warranted) accomplished, a more thorough attempt to establish a diagnosis can be carried out. This attempt, somewhat analogous to the secondary survey used in the ATLS approach, should involve a combination of clinical, epidemiological, and laboratory examinations. Medical history data of potential interest to the clinician should also be gathered and the ATLS "A.M.P.L.E." mnemonic provides a helpful approach to this. Information about illnesses among other unit members or co-workers, the presence of unusual munitions or dispersal devices, food and water procurement sources, vector exposure, vaccination history, travel history, occupational duties, and MOPP (or other PPE) status may all be relevant. Physical exam at this point should concentrate on the pulmonary and neuromuscular systems, as well as unusual skin or bleeding manifetations.

Resources available to a clinician naturally vary at each echelon of care. At higher echelons, a full range of lab capabilities might enable prompt definitive diagnoses. At lower echelons, every attempt should be made to obtain diagnostic specimens from representative patients and these should be forwarded through lab channels. Nasal swabs (important for culture and PCR, even if the clinician is unsure *which* organisms are present), blood cultures, serum, sputum cultures, blood and urine for toxin analysis, throat swabs, and environmental samples should all be considered according to the context. In no case, however, should the performance (or unavailability) of lab studies delay expeditious empiric diagnosis and therapy.

Table 1. Diagnostic Matrix: Chemical & Biological Casualties

	Rapid-Onset	Delayed-Onset
Respiratory Casualties	Nerve Agents Cyanide Mustard Lewisite Phosgene SEB Inhalation	Inhalational Anthrax Pneumonic Plague Pneumonic Tularemia Q Fever SEB Inhalation Ricin Inhalation Mustard Lewisite Phosgene
	Rapid-Onset	**Delayed-Onset**
Neurological Casualties	Nerve Agents Cyanide	Botulism (Peripheral symptoms) VEE (CNS symptoms)

While awaiting lab confirmation, a physician should attempt to make a clinical (presumptive) diagnosis. Access to infectious disease, preventive medicine, and other specialists, can assist in this process if one is working at a higher echelon of care. At lower echelons, the clinician should, at the very least, be conversant with the concept of syndromic diagnosis. Chemical and bio-agent diseases can be generally divided into those that present "immediately" with little or no incubation period (principally the chemical agents) and those with a considerable delay in presentation (principally the biological agents). Moreover, bio-agent-induced diseases are likely to present as one of a limited number of clinical syndromes. For example, plague, tularemia, and staphylococcal enterotoxin (SEB) disease all may present as pneumonia. Botulism and VEE may present with peripheral and central neuromuscular findings, respectively. This situation lends itself to the construction of a simple contingency table (diagnostic matrix) as shown in Table 1. Even basic syndromic diagnosis, however, is complicated by the fact that the "incapacitating" bio-agents (VEE, Q-fever, brucellosis) present simply as undifferentiated febrile illnesses, and persist that way, whereas the "lethal" bio-agents (anthrax, plague, tularemia, smallpox) present as undifferentiated febrile prodromes initially, but then progress, sometimes quite dramatically.

VI. Render prompt treatment. Unfortunately, it is precisely in the prodromal phase of many diseases that therapy is most likely to be effective. For this reason, empiric therapy of "pneumonia" or undifferentiated febrile illness on the battlefield, or in a potential bio-terrorism scenario, might be indicated under certain circumstances. Table 2 was constructed by eliminating from consideration those diseases for which definitive therapy is not warranted, not available, or not essential. Empiric treatment of respiratory casualties — patients with undifferentiated fevers who might have prodromal anthrax, plague, or tularemia would be managed similarly — might then be entertained. Doxycycline, for example, is effective against most strains of *Bacillus anthracis, Yersinia pestis,* and *Francisella tularensis,* as well as against *Coxiella burnetii,* and the *Brucellae.* Other tetracyclines and fluoroquinolones might also be considered. Similarly, rapid-onset respiratory casualties might be treated empirically using a cyanide antidote kit, while rapid-onset neurological casualties might warrant prompt empiric therapy with a nerve agent antidote kit (NAAK). Keep in mind that such empiric therapy is in no way a substitute for a careful and thorough diagnostic evaluation, when the environment is permissive of such.

Table 2. CW & BW Diseases Potentially Requiring Prompt Empiric Therapy

Respiratory Casualties	Rapid-Onset	Delayed-Onset
	Cyanide	Inhalational Anthrax Pneumonic Plague Pneumonic Tularemia
Neurological Casualties	Rapid-Onset	Delayed-Onset
	Nerve Agents	Botulism

VII. Practice good infection control. Standard Precautions (see Appendix H) provide adequate protection against most infectious diseases, including those potentially employed in a biological attack.[10] Anthrax, tularemia, brucellosis, glanders, melioidosis, Q-fever, the alphaviral encephalitides, and the toxin-mediated diseases are not generally contagious, and victims can be safely managed using standard precautions. This procedure should be familiar to all medical providers. Under certain circumstances, however, one of three forms of Transmission-based Precautions (again, see Appendix H) would be warranted. Smallpox patients should, wherever possible, be managed using Airborne Precautions (including, ideally, a HEPA filter mask). Pneumonic plague warrants the use of Droplet Precautions (which include, among other measures, the wearing of a simple surgical mask), and certain viral hemorrhagic fevers mandate the use of Contact Precautions.

VIII. Alert the proper authorities. In any military context, the command should immediately be notified of casualties potentially exposed to chemical or biological agents. The relevant clinical laboratory should also be notified. This will enable lab personnel to take proper precautions when handling specimens and will also permit the optimal use of available diagnostic assays and cultures. Chemical Corps and preventive medicine personnel should be contacted to assist in the delineation of contaminated areas and the search for additional victims.

In a civilian context, such notification would typically be made through local and/or regional health department channels. In the U.S., the larger cities often have their own health departments. In most other areas, the county health department represents the lowest echelon public health jurisdiction. In some rural areas, practitioners would access the state health department directly. Once alerted, local and regional health authorities can become well-versed in procedures for requesting additional support from their superiors. Every medical practitioner should have points of contact at such agencies readily available and should be familiar with mechanisms for engaging with them *before* a crisis arises in their community.

IX. Assist in the epidemiologic investigation and manage the psychological consequences. All health care providers must have a basic understanding of epidemiological principles.[11] Even under austere conditions, a rudimentary outbreak investigation may assist in diagnosis and in the discovery of additional bio-agent victims.[12] Clinicians should, at the very least, query patients about illness onset and symptoms, potential exposures, ill unit members or co-workers, food/water sources, unusual munitions or spray devices, and vector exposures. Early discovery of additional cases through an expedient outbreak investigation might, in turn, inform the need for post-exposure prophylaxis (PEP), thereby preventing additional morbidity and mortality. Public health officials would normally conduct more formal and thorough epidemiologic investigations and should be contacted as soon as one suspects the possibility of a biological attack. In a military setting, preventive medicine officers, field sanitation personnel, epidemiology technicians, environmental science officers, and veterinary officers are all available to assist the clinician in initiating an epidemiologic investigation.

In addition to implementing specific medical countermeasures and initiating the outbreak investigation, the clinician must be prepared to address the psychological effects of a known, suspected, or feared exposure. Such exposure (or threat of exposure) will likely provoke anxiety, even panic, in a community, and may result in overwhelming numbers of patients seeking urgent medical evaluation. Many of these may have unexplained symptoms and many may demand antidotes, antibiotics, or other therapies. Moreover, symptoms due to anxiety and autonomic arousal, as well as the side effects of PEP may suggest prodromal disease due to bio-agent exposure, and may pose challenges in differential diagnosis. This "behavioral contagion" is best prempted by robust, proactive, risk communication from public health and other governmental authorities.[13] This should include a realistic assessment of the risk of exposure, information about the resulting disease, steps to be taken, and points of contact for suspected exposure. It must be timely, accurate, consistent, and well coordinated.

Effective risk communication is predicated upon the pre-existence of detailed risk communication plans (many are available from the CDC) as well as various tactical approaches. Similarly, plans must be made to rapidly deploy resources for the initial evaluation and administration of PEP. (Ideally, this will be decentralized to unit level on the battlefield or to residential areas in a civilian context.) Finally, plans must be made to proactively develop patient and contact tracing and vaccine screening tools, to access stockpiled vaccines and medications, and to identify and prepare local facilities and health care teams for the management of mass casualties.

X. Maintain Proficiency and Spread the Word. Fortunately, the threats of biological warfare and bio-terrorism have to date remained theoretical ones for almost all medical personnel. Inability to continually practice casualty management, however, can lead to a rapid loss of knowledge and skills. Medics and corpsmen must maintain proficiency in dealing with this low-probability — but high-consequence — problem. This can be done, in part, by availing oneself of several resources.[14-16] The USAMRIID web site[17] provides a wealth of information, including the full text of this handbook, as well as links to many other useful sites. Numerous satellite television broadcasts sponsored by USAMRIID, as well as other video course resources, provide in-depth discussion and training in medical biodefense. CD, DVD, and other training aids are also available, and the previously mentioned field manuals[1] and relevant *TMM* volume[6, 18] summarize bio-agent disease management guidelines. Finally, medical personnel, once cognizant of the threat and enlightened as to how to deal with it, must ensure that their less informed colleagues receive training as well. It is only through this ongoing education that personnel will be prepared for the threat posed by biological weapons. By familiarizing yourself with the contents of this handbook, you will have taken a significant step towards such readiness.

BACTERIAL AGENTS

Bacteria are unicellular microbes that vary in shape and size from spherical cells (cocci) with a diameter of 0.5-1.0 µm (micrometer), to long rod-shaped organisms (bacilli) which may be from 1 to 5 µm. Chains of some bacilli may exceed 50 µm in length. The shape of the bacterial cell is determined by the rigid cell wall. The interior of the cell contains the nuclear material (DNA), cytoplasm, and cell membrane; all are necessary for the life of the bacterium. Many bacteria also have glycoproteins on their outer surfaces which aid in attachment to cell-surface receptors on other organisms. Under special circumstances, some types of bacteria (such as *Bacillus anthracis*) can sporulate (transform into spores). The spore form of the bacterial cell is much more resistant to cold, heat, drying, chemicals, UV light, and other radiation than is the vegetative bacterium itself. Spores are a dormant form of the bacterium and, like the seeds of plants, they can wait and germinate when conditions are more favorable. Aerosolized spores that are 1-5 µm in size may be inhaled deeply into the terminal bronchioles and alveoli of the lungs of humans and animals.

The term rickettsia generally applies to very small, gram-negative coccobacilli of the genera *Rickettsia* and *Coxiella*. Rickettsiae are distinct from classical bacteria in their inability to grow (with rare exceptions) in the absence of a living eukaryotic host cell (typically an endothelial cell). Like the classical bacteria, however, rickettsiae are susceptible to treatment with antibiotics.

Bacteria generally cause disease in human beings and animals by one of two mechanisms: (1) invasion (infection) of host tissues, with propagation there, and (2) production of poisons (toxins) that destroy or disrupt host tissues. Many pathogenic bacteria demonstrate both approaches. The diseases they produce often respond to specific therapy with antibiotics or antitoxins.

A number of bacteria have been weaponized by major state bio-weapons programs in the past. Imperial Japan weaponized and deployed the agents of plague, cholera, typhoid, dysentery, anthrax, paratyphoid, and glanders before and during World War II. During the Cold War, the former US and UK bio-warfare programs weaponized the brucella, anthrax, tularemia, and Q-fever agents. In addition to these four bacterial agents, the Soviet Union is known to have added plague and glanders to its stockpiles.

One should distinguish between the name of the disease-causing organism and the name of the disease it causes (in parentheses below). This manual covers several of the bacteria or rickettsiae considered to be potential threat bio-agents: *Bacillus anthracis* (anthrax), *Brucella* spp. (brucellosis), *Burkholderia mallei* (glanders), *Burholderia pseudomallei* (melioidosis), *Yersinia pestis* (plague), *Francisella tularensis* (tularemia), and *Coxiella burnetii* (Q-fever). Three of the bacterial toxins are also discussed in a separate section on toxins below.

Anthrax

Summary

Signs and symptoms of inhalational anthrax (IA): Incubation period is generally 1 to 6 d, although longer periods have been noted. Fever, malaise, fatigue, dry cough, and mild chest discomfort progress to severe respiratory distress with dyspnea, diaphoresis, stridor, cyanosis, and shock. Death typically occurs in 24 to 36 h after onset of severe symptoms.

Diagnosis: Physical findings are non-specific. A widened mediastinum and pleural effusions may be seen on CXR or CT scan in later stages of illness. The organism is detectable by Gram stain of blood, blood culture, serum levels of anthrax-specific Protective Antigen (PA) and/or Lethal Factor (LF), serology, PCR, and immunohistochemistry.

Treatment: Although effectiveness may be limited after symptoms are present, high-dose IV ciprofloxacin or doxycycline combined with one or two additional antibiotics are indicated. An FDA-approved monoclonal antibody (Raxibacumab) and an anthrax immune globulin (AIGIV; used only under an IND or EUA) are also available and should be used with antibiotics. Intensive supportive therapy will be necessary.

Prophylaxis: An FDA-licensed vaccine (*BioThrax*) is available. Schedule is 0.5 ml IM at 0 and 4 wks, then 6, 12, and 18 mos (primary series), followed by annual boosters for pre-event prophylaxis. For known or imminent exposure (post-exposure prophylaxis; not FDA-approved), `schedule is 0, 2 and 4 wks SQ in combination with PO ciprofloxacin or doxycycline for 60 d. The vaccine schedule is then resumed at 6 mos. Raxibacumab is FDA-approved for PEP only if other therapies are not available or appropriate.

Isolation and decontamination: Standard precautions for healthcare workers. Avoid invasive procedures or autopsy; but if unavoidable, personal protective equipment (PPE) is mandatory; all instruments and the proximate environment should be thoroughly disinfected with a sporicidal agent (e.g., hypochlorite).

Overview

Bacillus anthracis, the causative agent of anthrax, is a Gram-positive, sporulating rod. The spores are the usual infective form. Naturally occurring anthrax is primarily a zoonotic disease of herbivores, with cattle, sheep, goats, and horses serving as the usual domesticated animal hosts, but other animals may be infected. Humans generally contract the disease when handling contaminated hair, wool, hides, flesh, blood, and excreta of infected animals and from manufactured products such as bone meal. Infection is introduced through scratches or abrasions of the skin, wounds, inhaling spores, eating insufficiently cooked infected meat, or by fly bites. The primary concern for intentional infection by this organism is through inhalation after aerosol dissemination of spores. All human populations are susceptible. The spores are very stable and may remain viable for many years in soil and water. They resist sunlight for varying periods.

History & Significance

Anthrax can be produced in either a wet (slurry) or dry (powder) form, stabilized for weaponization, and delivered as an aerosol cloud either from a line source (e.g., boat or aircraft moving upwind of a target), or as a point source (from a spray device). Historically, coverage of large ground areas was also planned by national programs using multiple spray bomblets disseminated from missile warheads at a predetermined height above the ground[1,2] Such anthrax bombs, however, were never deployed on a battlefield. Anthrax was weaponized by the US from the 1940s to the '60s when the US offensive BW program was terminated. Other countries, including the Soviet Union and Iraq, have also weaponized it. In 2001, anthrax spores were delivered in the US mail, resulting in 22 cases of confirmed or suspected anthrax disease, of which 5 died. [3,4] Anthrax bacteria are easy to cultivate and spore production is readily induced. Moreover, the spores are highly resistant to sunlight, heat, and disinfectants — properties which create concerns for environmental persistence after an attack.

Clinical Features

Anthrax presents as three distinct clinical syndromes in humans: cutaneous, gastrointestinal, and inhalational disease.[5]

Cutaneous anthrax. The cutaneous form—also referred to as "malignant pustule"—is the most common naturally occurring form of anthrax. It occurs most frequently on the hands and forearms of persons working with infected livestock or livestock products, but during epizootics it has been transmitted to humans by the bites of flies, and more recently occurred in as many as 11 people exposed to anthrax spores in the US mail After a 1 to 12 d (usually 5 to 7 d) incubation period, a painless or pruritic papule forms at the site of exposure, enlarging into a round ulcer by the next day.[6] Vesicles or bullae containing clear or serosanguinous fluid and bacilli may form on the edge of the ulcer, which can be surrounded by various degrees of non-pitting edema. The ulcer subsequently dries and forms a coal-black scab (eschar), which falls off over the ensuing 1 to 2 wks. Regional lymphadenopathy with associated systemic symptoms can occur. If untreated, this local infection may disseminate into a fatal systemic infection in 10 to 20% of cases. Treated, the case fatality rate (CFR) is < 1%.

Gastrointestinal (GI) anthrax is rare in humans, and is contracted by eating insufficiently cooked meat from infected animals. Infection is thought to occur as a result of the ingestion of viable vegetative organisms rather than spores. Both forms of

GI anthrax, oropharyngeal and intestinal, have incubation periods of 1 to 6 d. Disease in ***oropharyngeal*** anthrax is heralded by the onset of fever and severe pharyngitis, followed by oral ulcers which progress from whitish patches to tan or gray pseudomembranes. These lesions vary in location but often form unilaterally over a palatine tonsil. Other signs and symptoms include dysphagia, regional nonpurulent lymphadenopathy, and severe neck swelling (often unilateral). Edema can lead to airway compromise, and disease can progress to sepsis, with CFR of 10 to 50%. ***Intestinal*** anthrax begins with fever, nausea, vomiting, and focal abdominal pain. These symptoms can progress to hematemesis, hematochezia or melena, massive serosanguinous or hemorrhagic ascites, and sepsis. Overall CFR is > 50%. Some evidence exists for a mild, self-limited gastroenteritis syndrome associated with intestinal anthrax, but this is poorly described.

Inhalational anthrax (IA). Endemic inhalational anthrax ("woolsorter's disease") is also an extremely rare infection contracted by inhaling *B. anthracis* spores. It has historically occurred in an occupational setting, mainly among workers who handle infected hides, wool, and furs. Because of the rarity of human IA, a single case of this disease should be presumed to be as a result of intentional exposure to anthrax until proved otherwise. After an incubation period of 1 to 6 d*, a non-specific febrile syndrome begins. Fever, malaise, headache, fatigue, and drenching sweats are often present, sometimes in association with nausea, vomiting, confusion, a nonproductive cough, and mild chest discomfort. Physical findings are typically non-specific in the early phase of the disease. Patients are often tachycardic, but may have normal lung physical exams. Chest radiographs or CT scan may show subtle changes including slightly widened mediastinum, (hemorrhagic mediastinitis) or pleural effusions. These initial symptoms generally last 2 to 5 d and can be followed by a short period of apparent improvement (hours to 2 to 3 d), culminating in the abrupt development of severe respiratory distress with dyspnea, diaphoresis, stridor, and cyanosis. Septicemia, shock, and death usually follow within 24 to 36 h after the onset of respiratory distress unless dramatic life-saving efforts are initiated. Historically, IA has been complicated by hemorrhagic meningitis in up to 50% of cases and GI hemorrhage in 80%. In the anthrax letter attacks in 2001, victims developed IA following exposure to envelope contents. The CFR among victims was only 45%, despite previously reported CFRs for IA of > 85%. The improved outcome was likely a reflection of rapid and aggressive treatment regimens and advancements in intensive care medicine.

* During the accidental Sverdlovsk outbreak in the Soviet Union in 1979, persons are reported to have become ill up to 6 wks after an aerosol release. Studies performed in nonhuman primates demonstrate that anthrax spores remain in the lung for up to 100 d.

Diagnosis

All forms of anthrax are diagnosed using a combination of clinical and laboratory findings.

Cutaneous anthrax. The key to diagnosis centers upon the presence of the characteristic painless skin lesion which progresses to a vesicle, ulcer, then eschar, with surrounding edema. While arachnid bites, trauma, burns or cutaneous tularemia may look similar, these are typically painful lesions. Known exposure history or risk factors may also be present. To perform Gram stain and bacterial culture of the lesion, samples should be collected by using two dry Dacron or rayon swabs, ideally with the fluid of an unopened vesicle. If no vesicle is present, apply moistened swabs (sterile saline) under the edge of an eschar or in the base of an ulcer. One swab is sent for Gram stain and culture, the other for PCR testing. Gram stain often demonstrates large Gram-positive bacilli if the patient has not yet received antibiotics. If the Gram stain and culture are negative, collect a 4-mm punch biopsy (or two if both eschar and vesicle are present) of the leading margin of the lesion for general histology and immunohistochemical staining. Blood culture should be performed in all patients suspected of having anthrax.

Gastrointestinal anthrax. History of exposure to, or ingestion of, the meat of sick animals should be elicited. Clinical suspicion should be elevated for multiple cases of similar disease. ***Oropharyngeal*** disease can mimic diphtheria. Vaccination and travel history should be queried. Gram stain and culture of the oral lesion may be positive for *B. anthracis* if collected before initiation of antibiotics. ***Intestinal*** anthrax may mimic acute gastroenteritis, acute abdomen with peritonitis (focal with rebound tenderness), or dysentery. Abdominal radiographs are non-specific, sometimes showing diffuse air-fluid levels, bowel thickening, and peritoneal fluid. Surgical findings may include hemorrhagic mesenteric adenitis, serosanguinous to hemorrhagic ascites, bowel ulceration (usually ileum and cecum), edema, and necrosis. Stool culture may identify bacilli with intestinal anthrax. Peritoneal fluid and ascities fluid should be evaluated by culture, Gram stain, immunohistochemistry, and PCR. Blood should be collected for culture, serology (paired frozen sera 3–4 wks apart, –70°C) and PCR (lavender tube, refrigerated) in patients with either form of GI disease.

Inhalational anthrax. Early IA is a non-specific syndrome which may be difficult to distinguish clinically from other illnesses. Notably absent in IA are upper respiratory symptoms (rhinorrhea, coryza, congestion) usually present in patients with influenza. Pneumonia generally does not occur; therefore, lung exam may be unrevealing and organisms are not typically seen in the sputum. Patients suspected of having IA should have a complete blood count (CBC), blood culture, and serum electrolytes. White blood cell count is typically elevated only slightly at presentation (mean 9,800/µL in the 2001 cases) with a neutrophil predominance. Hemoconcentration may be evidenced by elevated serum sodium and hematocrit. Mildly elevated serum aspartate aminotransferase (AST) and alanine aminotransferase (ALT) may be present as well as hypoalbuminemia. *B. anthracis* will be detectable even in the early phase of disease by routine blood culture and may even be seen with Gram stain of blood later in the course of the illness; however, even one or two doses of antibiotics will render blood (and other sites) sterile. In patients with neurologic symptoms, cerebrospinal fluid (CSF) may show evidence of hemorrhagic meningitis with numerous Gram-positive bacilli. Pleural effusions may be large and bloody and may also contain numerous Gram-positive bacilli. Blood, CSF, and pleural effusions may be evaluated by Gram stain, immunohistochemistry, and PCR. Acute and convalescent serum may be collected for serology. All patients suspected of having IA should have a CXR to screen for widened mediastinum, enlarged mediastinal lymph nodes, and pleural effusions. In suspected cases CXR and chest CT scan should be performed. In the attacks of 2001, CXR and/or chest CT were abnormal in all cases.

Medical Management

Inhalational anthrax. Early initiation of appropriate antibiotics is paramount for patient survival of IA. Initial therapy for patients with a strain of unknown antibiotic susceptibilities should include ciprofloxacin (400 mg IV q 12 h for adults, and 10–15 mg/kg IV q12 h (up to 1 g/d) for children) OR doxycycline (200 mg IV load, followed by 100 mg IV q12 h for adults and children ≥ 8 yrs and > 45 kg, and 2.2 mg/kg q12 h for children < 8 yrs (up to 200 mg/d))* PLUS one or two additional antibiotics effective against anthrax. Some additional antibiotics to which naturally occurring strains are susceptible include imipenem, meropenem, daptomycin, quinupristin-dalfopristin, linezolid, vancomycin, rifampin, macrolides (e.g., erythromycin, azithromycin, and clarithromycin), clindamycin, chloramphenocol, and aminoglycosides (e.g., gentamicin). While the optimal combination antibiotic therapy for IA is not known, many infectious disease (ID) physicians have suggested a combination of a quinolone, clindamycin, and rifampin for susceptible strains. Penicillin (or other beta-lactam antibiotics) should NEVER be used as monotherapy for severe anthrax disease as the *B. anthracis* genome encodes for both constitutive and inducible beta-lactamases and resistance may occur *in vivo* despite apparent *in vitro* susceptibility. Antibiotic choices must be adjusted for strain susceptibility patterns, and consultation with an ID physician is imperative.

If meningitis is suspected, at least one antibiotic with good CSF penetration (e.g., rifampin or chloramphenicol) should be used, as quinolones and tetracyclines do not enter the CSF well. Generally, ciprofloxacin or doxycycline use is avoided during pregnancy and in children due to safety concerns; however, a consensus group and the American Academy of Pediatrics have suggested that they should still be used as first

* Other quinolone antibiotics (levofloxacin, trovofloxacin) or tetracyclines (minocycline, tetracycline) would likely be effective as well, although they have not been specifically approved by the FDA for this purpose.

line therapy in life-threatening anthrax disease until strain susceptibilities are known. In fact, ciprofloxacin has been approved by the FDA for prophylaxis and treatment of anthrax in children. Recommended treatment duration is ≥ 60 d, and should be changed to oral therapy as clinical condition improves.

Raxibacumab, a monoclonal antibody, is approved by the FDA for the treatment of IA in combination with recommended antibiotic regimens (see above).[7,8,9] It is given as a single dose of 40 mg/kg IV over 2 h and 15 min (diluted in 0.9% Sodium Chloride Injection, USP, normal saline) to a final volume of 250 mL. Diphenhydramine, 25 to 50 mg should be given within 1 h prior to *Raxibacumab* to reduce the risk of infusion reactions. Dosing for children is weight based: Greater than 50 kg, 40 mg/kg; between 15 kg and 50 kg, 60 mg/kg; and 15 kg or less, 80 mg/kg. Consult the package insert for final infusion volume for children.

In the event of a mass-casualty situation IV antibiotics may not be available. In this case oral ciprofloxacin OR doxycycline may have to suffice as initial therapy. The doses for ciprofloxacin are 500 mg PO bid for adults, and 10–15 mg/kg PO bid (up to 1 g/d) for children. The doses for doxycycline are 200 mg PO initially then 100 mg PO bid thereafter for adults (or children > 8 yrs and > 45 kg), and 2.2 mg/kg PO bid (up to 200 mg/d) for children < 8 yrs.

Supportive therapy for shock, fluid volume deficit, and adequacy of airway may be needed. In the IA cases from the 2001 attacks, aggressive drainage of pleural effusions seemed to improve clinical outcome. Corticosteroids may be considered as adjunct therapy in patients with severe edema or meningitis, based upon experience in treating other bacterial diseases. Human anthrax immune globulin can be obtained as a therapy for IA under an IND from the CDC (see Appendix J).

Cutaneous anthrax. Uncomplicated cutaneous anthrax should be treated initially with either ciprofloxacin (500 mg PO bid for adults or 10–15 mg/kg/d divided bid [up to 1 g/d] for children) or doxycycline (100 mg PO bid for adults, 5 mg/kg/d divided bid for children less than 8 yrs (up to 200 mg/d)). If the strain proves penicillin susceptible, then the treatment may be switched to amoxicillin (500 mg PO tid for adults or 80 mg/kg PO divided tid [up to 1.5 g/d] for children). While the *B. anthracis* genome encodes for beta-lactamases, the organism may still respond to penicillins (such as amoxicillin) if slowly growing as in localized cutaneous disease. In the event the exposure route is unknown, or suspected to be intentional, antibiotics should be continued for ≥ 60 d. If the exposure is known to have been due to contact with infected livestock or their products, then 7 to 10 d of antibiotics may suffice. For patients with significant edema, non-steroidal anti-inflammatory drugs (NSAIDS) or corticosteroids may be of benefit. Debridement of lesions is not indicated. If systemic illness develops, then IV antibiotics should be administered as for IA, as discussed above.

Gastrointestinal anthrax. Documentation of clinical experience in treating oropharyngeal and intestinal anthrax is limited. Supportive care to include fluid for shock and airway management should be anticipated. Both forms of GI disease should receive the IV antibiotic regimen described for IA above. For oropharyngeal anthrax, airway compromise is a significant risk, and consideration should be given for the early administration of corticosteroids to reduce the development of airway edema. If, despite medical therapy, airway compromise develops, early intubation should be considered. Incision and drainage of affected lymph nodes is not generally indicated. No specific guidance exists for drainage of ascites in patients with intestinal anthrax. However, large fluid collections could at a minimum compromise respiration and consideration should be given to therapeutic—and potentially diagnostic—paracentesis.

Infection control. Standard precautions are recommended for patient care in all forms of anthrax disease. There are no data to suggest direct person-to-person spread from any form of anthrax. However, for patients with systemic anthrax disease—especially before antibiotics are initiated—invasive procedures, autopsy, or embalming of remains could potentially lead to the generation of infectious droplets; thus, such procedures should be avoided when possible. If unavoidable, all instruments and materials used should be autoclaved or incinerated, and the immediate environment where the procedure took place should be thoroughly disinfected with a sporicidal agent. Chlorine, in the form of sodium or calcium hypochlorite (bleach), can also be used, but with the caution that the activity of hypochlorites is greatly reduced in the presence of organic material. The US Environmental Protection Agency has endorsed the use of bleach to destroy anthrax.

Any clinical laboratory should be warned before the delivery of suspected anthrax specimens, as growth of *B. anthracis* in culture necessitates biosafety level–2 (BSL–2) precautions.

Experience of anthrax in livestock indicates that incineration of carcasses and sterilization of contaminated ground is the environmental control method of choice. Formerly, a recommendation was deep burial (> 6 feet deep) in pits copiously lined with sodium hydroxide (lye); however, this practice may still leave a significant proportion of viable spores. This has led a consensus group to recommend "serious consideration" of cremation of human anthrax victim remains.

Prophylaxis

Vaccine: A licensed vaccine—*BioThrax®* or Anthrax Vaccine Adsorbed (AVA) Emergent Biosolutions, Rockville, MD—is derived from sterile culture fluid supernatant taken from an attenuated (non-encapsulated) strain of anthrax. Therefore, it does not contain living or dead organisms. The schedule consists of five 0.5–ml IM total doses: one each at 0 and 4 wks; then 6, 12, and 18 mos, followed by yearly boosters. Current DoD policy for missed doses (for those individuals required to remain immune) is to administer the missed dose ASAP and reset the timeline for the series based upon the most recent dose.[10] In 2005, the FDA officially determined (after a second exhaustive review) that AVA is properly licensed for the prevention of anthrax, regardless of the route of exposure. It is licensed only for pre-exposure prophylaxis of anthrax in adults (ages >18 and < 65). It is available for pre-exposure use in children and post-exposure prophylaxis (PEP—administered SQ) in adults and children only under an IND protocol or an Emergency Use Authorization (EUA) through the CDC or DoD. As with all vaccines, the degree of protection depends upon the magnitude of the challenge dose of pathogen received; vaccine-induced protection could presumably be overwhelmed by extremely high spore challenge. Thus, even fully vaccinated personnel should receive antibiotic PEP if exposed to aerosolized anthrax, IAW the guidelines below.[11,12,13,14]

Contraindications for use of AVA include hypersensitivity reaction to a previous dose of vaccine and age < 18 or > 65 yrs. Reasons for temporary deferment of the vaccine include pregnancy, active infection with fever, or a course of immune-suppressing drugs such as steroids. Reactogenicity is mild to moderate. Up to 30% of recipients may experience mild discomfort at the inoculation site for up to 72 h (e.g., tenderness, erythema, edema, pruritus), fewer experience moderate reactions, while < 1% may experience more severe local reactions, potentially limiting use of the arm for 1 to 2 d. Modest systemic reactions (e.g., myalgia, malaise, low-grade fever) are uncommon, and severe systemic reactions such as anaphylaxis, which precludes subsequent vaccination, are rare. The vaccine should be stored between 2 and 6°C (refrigerator temperature, not frozen).

Current DoD policy requires AVA administration to active-duty personnel (without specific contraindications) as well as some emergency-essential DoD civilians and contractors, who deploy for > 15 consecutive d or > 15 cumulative d over 12 mos, to designated "higher-threat" areas. The vaccination series should be initiated, when feasible, > 45 d before deployment. (Details of the DoD [and service-specific] guidance can be found elsewhere.[15]) AVA is recommended for persons who handle high concentrations of spores and potentially infected animals and those who work in spore-contaminated areas.

AVA is maintained in the US Strategic National Stockpile (SNS) for PEP use in the event of a large biological attack, under either an IND protocol or an EUA.

Antibiotics: No antibiotic is approved for pre-exposure prophylaxis of anthrax. Thus, official DoD policy is not to initiate prophylactic antibiotics until AFTER an attack is suspected to have occurred. After a suspected exposure to aerosolized anthrax of unknown antibiotic susceptibility, prophylaxis with ciprofloxacin (500 mg PO bid for adults, and 10–15 mg/kg PO bid [up to 1 g/d] for children) OR doxycycline (100 mg PO bid for adults or children >8 yrs and >45 kg, and 2.2 mg/kg PO bid [up to 200 mg/d] for children < 8yrs) should be initiated immediately. Should an attack be confirmed as anthrax, antibiotics should be continued for variable lengths of time dependent upon the patient's vaccination status. If antibiotic susceptibilities allow, patients who cannot tolerate tetracyclines or quinolones can be switched to amoxicillin (500 mg PO tid for adults and 80 mg/kg divided tid [up to 1.5 g/d] in children).

AVA is a critical part of PEP for inhaled anthrax; without vaccination, victims inhaling anthrax spores are unlikely to develop the immunity necessary to prevent disease caused by spores that germinate after antibiotics are discontinued. The Advisory Committee on Immunization Practices (ACIP) recommends a post-exposure regimen of 60 d of appropriate antimicrobial prophylaxis combined with three doses of AVA (0, 2, and 4 wks) for previously unvaccinated persons aged >18 yrs. The licensed vaccination schedule can be resumed at 6 mos. The first dose should be administered within 10 d. Persons for whom vaccination has been delayed should extend antimicrobial use to 14 d after the third dose (even if this practice might result in use of antimicrobials for > 60 d).[16] Patients who were either partially* or fully vaccinated† before the attack should continue with the licensed vaccination schedule and take antibiotics for at least 60 d. Upon discontinuation of antibiotics, a patient should be closely observed. If clinical signs of anthrax occur, empiric therapy for anthrax is indicated, pending definitive diagnosis. Optimally, patients should have medical care available upon discontinuation of antibiotics from a fixed medical care facility with intensive care capabilities and infectious disease consultants.

Antitoxins: *Raxibacumab*, a monoclonal antibody, is approved by the FDA for prophylaxis of IA in adults and children when alternative treatments are not available or are contraindicated.[7,9] (See "Medical Management" section above for dosing.)

* Partially vaccinated = received < five IM priming doses or have not received all annual boosters

† Fully vaccinated = completed the five dose IM series and are up to date on all annual boosters

Brucellosis

Summary

Signs and symptoms are usually non-specific: fever, headache, myalgias, arthralgias, back pain, profuse sweats, chills, weight loss, and malaise. Onset may be acute or insidious. Fever may be intermittent or continuous and recrudescence is common even after antibiotic treatment. Subclinical infections are common. Osteoarticular complications, notably sacroiliitis, occur with some degree of frequency and are responsible for much of the disability associated with Brucella infection. Other manifestations include depression and mental status changes, epididymoorchitis, and localized suppurative infection. Morbidity may be pronounced; fatalities are uncommon.

Diagnosis requires a high index of suspicion, as most infections present as non-specific febrile illnesses or are asymptomatic. Lab diagnosis can be made by serum agglutination tests, ELISA, immunofluorescence, and by standard culture. Blood cultures often require extended incubation to become positive, even up to 30 d. Bone marrow cultures may produce a higher yield. Other body fluids may be tested depending on the sites affected (e.g., synovial, pleural, CSF).

Treatment with doxycycline and rifampin (or other antibiotics) for 6 wks is usually sufficient. More prolonged regimens may be required for patients with complications such as hepatitis, splenitis, meningoencephalitis, endocarditis, or osteomyelitis.

Prophylaxis: No human vaccine is available. Chemoprophylaxis should be considered for high-risk exposures in the following situations: (1) inadvertent wound or mucous membrane exposure to infected livestock tissues and body fluids and to livestock vaccines; (2) exposure to lab aerosols or to secondary aerosols generated from contaminated soil in calving/lambing areas; and (3) confirmed bio-warfare/bio-terrorism exposure.

Isolation and decontamination: Brucella is spread readily via bodily fluids and certain aerosols, but not by respiratory droplets; standard precautions are thus adequate for the protection of healthcare workers. If an attack with a Brucella sp. is suspected, special care should be taken to avoid the generation of secondary aerosols. Contact surfaces that are free of organic matter can be decontaminated with a 0.5% hypochlorite solution; higher concentrations (> 5%), or other disinfectants, should be used where organic matter cannot be effectively reduced or controlled.

Overview

Brucellosis is a zoonotic disease caused by infection with one of several species of the genus *Brucella*, a group of facultative intracellular gram-negative cocco-baccillary organisms. Four of the six described species are known to infect humans (Table 1).

Table 1. Characteristics of brucellosis in animals & humans

Brucella spp.	1° Reservoir	2° Hosts	Geographic Distribution	Human Exposure Activity	Pathogenicity To Humans
B. abortus	Cattle, Bison, Deer	Goat, Sheep, Dog, Human	Worldwide	Raw dairy foods, animal husbandry, laboratory	Moderate
B. melitensis	Goat, Sheep	Dog, Human	Latin America, Asia, Mediterranean	Raw dairy foods, animal husbandry, laboratory	Highest
B. suis	Pig (feral, and domestic)	Dog, Human, Cattle	SE Asia, Scattered & Midwest US, S America	Pork slaughter, processing, feral pig hunting, laboratory	High
B. canis	Dog, Coyote		Scattered	Dog breeding & whelping	Moderate

Brucellosis can be thought of as a venereal disease of livestock and, as such, primarily affects the reproductive system of these animals producing septic abortion, retained fetal membranes, orchitis, and infection of the male accessory sex glands. Transmission occurs primarily via the ingestion of organisms contained in fetal membranes, aborted fetuses, and uterine discharges, and occasionally from dams to nursing young. Brucellae may also enter the body through mucous membranes, conjunctivae, and wounds.

Zoonotic transmission to humans has occurred via contact with infected tissues, blood, urine, semen, and gynecologic secretions.[1] Veterinarians, slaughterhouse workers, ranchers, animal husbandry workers, and hunters have consequently been infected in occupational and recreational settings. Transmission to humans also occurs via the ingestion of raw milk and other dairy products from infected animals. Though less common, airborne infections have also occurred in livestock husbandry settings (inhalation of contaminated particles from soil and bedding in birthing areas) and in lab settings. Finally, accidental percutaneous exposure to modified-live livestock vaccines (e.g., veterinarians) has also occurred.

Infections among abattoir and lab workers suggest that the inhalation of as few as 10 organisms is sufficient to cause disease in humans. Subclinical infections are relatively common. Brucellosis has a low case fatality rate (5% of untreated cases), with rare deaths caused by complications such as endocarditis or meningitis. When disease is naturally occurring, the incubation period may be several days to several months. However, large aerosol doses—as would be expected in a bio-warfare scenario—would shorten the incubation period, lead to higher clinical attack rates, and result in more prolonged, incapacitating, and disabling disease than in the natural form.

History & Significance

Jeffrey Allen Marston first described the disease manifestations associated with *Brucella melitensis* infection among British soldiers on Malta during the Crimean War (1853-56; Florence Nightingale may have been the most famous victim of the so-called "Malta fever" or "Crimean fever" during that conflict). Goats were identified as the source of this outbreak and restrictions on the consumption of unpasteurized dairy goat products soon decreased the incidence among military personnel. *Brucella abortus* was first isolated by David Bruce—hence the genus designation—in 1897. The extraordinary infectivity[2], as well as stability in aerosol form and resistance to dessication, led bioweaponeers in the UK to focus on the brucellae during World War II and, in 1954, *B. suis* became the first agent weaponized by the US at its Pine Bluff Arsenal located in Arkansas. Moreover, Ken Alibek, a Soviet defector and former official with the Russian bioweapons program, began his career by perfecting the culture of the brucellae. It has been alleged that the South African Defense Forces, in the apartheid era, experimented with weaponized *B. melitenisis*. Conversely, their long and variable incubation periods, coupled with the large percentage of asymptomatic infections, mitigate against the use of the brucellae as weapons.

Human brucellosis is now rare in the US with about 100 cases reported annually, mostly from CA, FL, TX, and VA. The majority of these are associated with the ingestion of unpasteurized dairy products made outside of the US and privately imported (thus escaping FDA and USDA regulatory food-safety measures). Rare infections may still occur in meat processing or livestock handling settings in areas with herds or flocks that are not certified "brucellosis-free" by regional animal health authorities. Human brucellosis is endemic in some Mediterranean basin nations, as well as India, Mexico, South and Central America and many of the republics of the former Soviet Union.[3] Disease incidence and prevalence vary regionally, with some reporting annual incidences of over 80 cases per 100,000 population. Persistent foci of enzootic disease among sheep and goats plague the Middle East today and serologic evidence of *Brucella* spp. exposure among humans on the Arabian peninsula was near 20% with more than 2% having active disease in one recent WHO study. A few regions in Kuwait have reported annual incidences as high as 128 cases per 100,000 population. These findings highlight a risk to military personnel in the region.[4]

Clinical Features

Brucellosis is a systemic disease with protean manifestations that can involve virtually any organ system[5, 6]; disease type and severity vary with the infecting *Brucella* species. *B. melitensis* is the most pathogenic for humans, in whom infection is associated with an acute course and disabling complications. *B. suis* infection is associated with localized abscess formation and a chronic course. *B. abortus* and *B. canis* infections are associated with frequent relapses and insidious onset.

Untreated, *Brucellae* localize in the reticuloendothelial system, primarily the liver, spleen, and bone marrow, where granuloma formation ensues. Large granulomas serve as a source for persistent bacteremia. The incubation period of brucellosis is typically 3 or 4 wks, but can range from as few as 5 d to many mos. Illness onset can be abrupt, or come insidiously over wks or mos. Non-specific symptoms such as fever (90-95%), malaise (80-95%), sweats (40-90%), and myalgias/arthralgias (40-70%), are typical. Fever is typically intermittent, and can assume an undulant (wave-like) pattern in patients with chronic, untreated infection. Fatigue, chills, and backache are not unusual. Neuropsychiatric symptoms including depression, headache, and irritability, are common.[7] GI symptoms (abdominal pain, anorexia, constipation, diarrhea, vomiting) are reported in nearly 70% of adult cases. Cough, dyspnea, chest pain, and testicular pain occur less frequently. Common physical findings include hepatomegaly (10-70%) and/or splenomegaly (10-30%), arthritis (up to 40%), weight loss, and adenopathy (10-20%).

Osteoarticular complications of brucellosis, seen in 20-60% of cases, include bursitis, tenosynovitis, arthritis, osteomyelitis, sacroiliitis, discitis, and paravertebral abscess. Sacroiliitis typically presents acutely with fever and focal lower back pain and occurs in up to 30% of cases, predominantly in young men. Arthritis of large, weight-bearing joints of the lower extremities may occur in 20%. Arthritis is usually monoarticular, but can be polyarticular up to 30%. Spondylitis or vertebral osteomyelitis may affect from up to 30% of all cases of brucellosis. Patients with spondylitis tend to be older and have a more chronic, destructive disease course than those with sacroiliitis or peripheral arthritis; the lumbar vertebrae are most commonly affected.

GI disease can manifest as ileitis, colitis, or granulomatous or mononuclear infiltrative hepatitis. As a rule, hepatitis only progresses to cirrhosis if pre-existing liver disease (e.g., hepatitis C or alcoholic liver disease) is present. Pulmonary disease occurs in 1 to 5% of cases and may take the form of solitary nodules, lung abscesses, miliary lesions, bronchopneumonia, enlarged hilar lymph nodes, or pleural effusions. Rare patients have succumbed to ARDS associated with pulmonary brucellosis.[8] While inhalational exposure to *Brucella* has been described in lab and abattoir workers, this route of infection has not proven to lead with regularity to any specifically pneumonic form of disease.

Epididymoorchitis has been described in 2 to 20% of male brucellosis patients and typically presents acutely with scrotal pain and swelling, as well as unremitting fever. Orchitis is unilateral in the majority of cases. Neurologic disease can take the form of meningitis, encephalitis, peripheral neuropathy, brain or epidural abscesses, radiculo-neuropathies or meningovascular syndromes. However, direct CNS invasion occurs in < 5% of brucellosis cases. Behavioral disturbances and psychoses appear to occur unrelated to the degree of fever and may be only occasionally associated with the afore-mentioned neural syndromes during acute phases. Endocarditis occurs in < 2% of cases, but accounts for the majority of brucellosis-related deaths. Acute brucellosis during the first 2 trimesters of pregnancy has been reported to lead to spontaneous abortion in up to 40% of cases if untreated.

Diagnosis

A high index of suspicion is necessary in order to make a diagnosis of brucellosis. A history of contact with susceptible animals, or of consumption of unpasteurized dairy products (including goat), and travel to endemic areas, should prompt consideration of brucellosis. Patients presenting with fever, night sweats, undue fatigue, GI symptoms, anorexia, weight loss, headache, arthralgias, and hepatosplenomegaly should also lead to the consideration of this diagnosis. Additionally, patients with some of the aforementioned complications, such as sacroiliitis or epididymoorchitis merit consideration for brucellosis testing. Brucellosis is a well-established diagnosis in patients with fever of unknown origin, and a thorough review of risk factors seeking a potential exposure to *Brucella* species should be conducted in such patients.

The leukocyte count in brucellosis is usually normal but may be low; anemia, neutropenia, and thrombocytopenia occur in some cases. AST and ALT may be mildly elevated; the ESR is normal or only mildly elevated in the majority of cases. Under the microscope, *Brucella* species are small, non-motile, non-encapsulated, non-spore forming, slow-growing, coccobacilli gram-negative intracellular aerobes. Modern automated blood culture systems will grow brucellae within 7 d in 95% of cases, although misidentification is common. Blood and bone marrow cultures taken during the acute febrile phase of illness yield the organism in most cases. CSF, synovial fluid, and urine cultures may prove useful in patients with appropriate clinical signs. Bone marrow and liver biopsies (to detect granulomatous disease) may be useful in select circumstances. Clinical labs should always be alerted if a diagnosis of brucellosis is suspected. This permits the use of selective isolation media and the implementation of BSL-3 containment.

Several laboratory studies may be employed in the definitive diagnosis of brucellosis: culture, serologic testing, immunoflourescence (IF) and molecular diagnostics. Each modality has limitations. Blood cultures are typically negative in patients taking antibiotics. (In many countries, antibiotics can easily be obtained without a prescription, and are frequently obtained by patients before presentation to healthcare facilities, hampering diagnosis in many enzootic areas.) Widely-used agglutination tests often give false-positive results in these areas, owing to remote exposure to brucellae; such tests can also be unreliable in patients with relapsed infection. A presumptive diagnosis of brucellosis can be made using a serum agglutination test (SAT) for IgM and IgG, and a tube agglutination method for anti-O polysaccharide antibody is available; titers of > 1:160 by each indicate active disease. An ELISA is also available, and CSF as well as joint fluid may be used for antibody testing with some test kits. IF staining of biopsy-obtained tissue can be used to demonstrate organisms in select cases. Molecular diagnostics, usually involving PCR, can have false-negative results, possibly due to inhibitors of PCR in the patient's blood.

Because all modalities have shortcomings, multiple categories of tests may be enlisted to establish the diagnosis. Definitive lab criteria include: 1) isolation of *Brucella* sp. from a clinical specimen; 2) > a fourfold rise in *Brucella* sp. agglutination titer between acute and convalescent sera obtained > 2 wks apart and performed at the same lab; 3) demonstration by IF of *Brucella* sp. in a clinical specimen. A probable case is one that is clinically compatible and epidemiologically linked to a confirmed case or that has supportive serology (i.e., *Brucella* agglutination titer of > 1:160 in one or more serum specimens obtained after onset of symptoms). A confirmed case is a clinically compatible case that is lab-confirmed.

Imaging studies may help to localize seats of infection. Persistent fever after therapy or the prolonged presence of significant musculoskeletal complaints should prompt CT or MR imaging. ^{99m}Technetium and ^{67}gallium scans may reveal sacroiliitis or other axial skeletal infections. CXR in brucellosis patients may be unremarkable even in the presence of respiratory symptoms. ECG may reveal evidence of endocarditis. Vegetative lesions are most common on the aortic valve (sinus of Valsalva), followed by the mitral valve. Testicular ultrasound may be helpful in distinguishing *Brucella* epididymoorchitis from testicular abscess or tumor.

Clinically, identification to the genus level is adequate to initiate therapy for brucellosis. Species identification is epidemiologically necessary and helps to inform prognosis; however, it requires more specialized analyses.

Medical Management

Historically, the most effective proven treatment for acute brucellosis in adults has been the combination of doxycycline 100 mg PO bid for 4 to 6 wks plus streptomycin 1 g IM daily for the first 2 to 3 wks.[9] As streptomycin is no longer widely available, gentamicin probably represents a suitable alternative. For uncomplicated acute brucellosis, however, combinations of oral antibiotics are usually sufficient and have cure rates approaching those of the doxycycline-aminoglycoside combinations. The most widely recommended combination for adults and children > 8 yrs old is doxycycline (100 mg PO bid for adults, 2.2 mg/kg PO bid [up to 200 mg/d] for children) + rifampin (600-900 mg/d PO qd for adults,15-20 mg/kg [up to 600-900 mg/d] for children) for 4 to 6 wks; a fluoroquinolone (e.g., ofloxacin or ciprofloxacin) + rifampin or TMP-SMX + rifampin may be appropriate alternatives. Relapse rates of 5 to 10% for most combination oral regimens and higher for monotherapy (up to 30% with TMP-SMX alone) complicate therapy. During pregnancy and for children < 8 yrs old, the combination of TMP-SMX and rifampin has been advocated.

Acute, complicated brucellosis (e.g., skeletal disease, endocarditis) often requires long-term triple-drug therapy for effective cure. A combination of oral rifampin and doxycycline (or TMP-SMX in children < 8 yrs old), plus IM streptomycin (or gentamicin) for the first 2 to 3 wks has been used most frequently. For skeletal disease, 6 to 8 wks of antibiotics may be necessary for cure; persisting musculoskeletal complaints may be present in patients with chronic infection and sacroiliitis. Patients with meningoencephalitis or endocarditis should receive > 90 d of therapy and may require > 6 mos. Endocarditis typically responds poorly to antibiotics alone and generally requires surgical excision of the affected valve. Necrotizing orchitis and other suppurative complications of brucellosis may also require surgical management.

Patient education is a critical component of medical management and must include emphasis on the importance of antibiotic compliance. Periodic follow-up is also critical, and referral to medical specialists may be indicated. As is the case with all bacterial bio-agents, antibiotic resistance can be engineered into the organism, and thus determination of antibiotic susceptibilities in an intentional attack with *Brucella* would be paramount.

Infection control: Standard precautions are adequate in managing brucellosis patients, as the disease is not generally transmissible from person-to-person. Masks, gloves, and eye protection are indicated when performing respiratory procedures and when handling body fluids. BSL-3 containment practices should be used when handling suspected *Brucella* sp. cultures in the laboratory because of potential aerosol exposure.[10]

Prophylaxis

No licensed human brucellosis vaccine is available.[11] Livestock vaccines are available; these live vaccines are potentially hazardous to humans and are thus tightly controlled by regional animal health authorities.

Optimal chemoprophylaxis following known or suspected exposure to brucellae remains a matter of dispute. The CDC interim recommendations for high-risk exposures to are: doxycycline 100 mg PO bid plus rifampin 600 mg PO qd.

Most developed countries have largely eradicated brucellosis from domestic cattle, sheep, and goat herds via multifaceted control programs, including periodic testing and slaughter of positive and contact animals and periodic batch testing of raw milk. Travelers to developing countries should be aware of prevalent foodborne and endemic brucellosis risks. The risk of foodborne brucellosis is reduced by avoiding unpasteurized dairy products, particularly in areas where brucellosis is known to still occur in livestock.

Brucellosis is a reportable human and livestock disease in the US and in many other countries.

Glanders & Melioidosis

Summary

Symptoms and signs: Incubation periods after inhalation are usually < 14 d, but may range from days to weeks for glanders and days to decades for melioidosis. Onset of symptoms may be abrupt or gradual. Respiratory tract disease can produce fever (usually > 102°F), rigors, sweats, myalgias, headache, productive or nonproductive cough, pleuritic chest pain, and cervical lymphadenopathy. Pneumonia can progress rapidly and lead to metastatic infection, causing hepatosplenomegaly and generalized papular/pustular eruptions. Both diseases are usually fatal without treatment.

Diagnosis: *Burkholderia mallei* and *B. pseudomallei* (agents of glanders and melioidosis, respectively) are gram-negative bacilli; methylene blue or Wright's stain of exudates may disclose a "safety-pin" bipolar appearance. CXR may show infiltrates with consolidation and cavitation, multiple small lung abscess, or miliary lesions. Abdominal and pelvic ultrasound, CT or MRI may reveal splenic, hepatic, or prostatic abscesses. Standard cultures and PCR can identify both agents.

Treatment: Initial therapy can consist of IV ceftazidime, meropenem, or imipenem, followed by prolonged oral antibiotic therapy. Surgical drainage is indicated for large abscesses. Life-long follow-up is advised after treatment for melioidosis due to a 10% risk of relapse.

Prophylaxis: No vaccines are currently available. There are no human data or FDA-approved regimens for post-exposure prophylaxis, although TMP-SMX shows promise in animal studies and is recommended after accidental laboratory exposures, and should be considered ASAP after a biological attack with either agent. (See also Appendix I.)

Isolation and decontamination: Standard precautions are recommended for health cre workers, with contact precautions added for patients with skin lesions. Person-to-person airborne or droplet transmission is unlikely. Cultures must be handled under BSL-3 conditions. Environmental decon using a 0.5% to 1.0% hypochlorite solution is effective.

Overview

The etiologic agents of these two diseases are the gram-negative bacilli *Burkholderia mallei* (glanders) and *Burkholderia pseudomallei* (melioidosis).

The natural reservoir of *B. mallei* is limited to horses, mules, and donkeys. Transmission to humans is infrequent, possibly due to low bacterial loads in lesion discharge and because strains virulent for equids are often less virulent for humans. Cases have occurred among horse and donkey caretakers, abattoir workers, veterinarians, and microbiologists. In the past, humans seldom became infected, despite frequent and often close contact with infected animals. This may be due to exposure to low concentrations of organisms from infected sites in ill animals and because strains virulent for equids are often less virulent for humans. The low transmission rates of *B. mallei* to humans from infected horses is exemplified by the fact that in China, during World War II, 30% of tested horses were positive for glanders, but human cases were rare. Acute presentations are more common in mules and donkeys, with death typically occurring within 3 to 4 wks. Chronic disease is more common in horses and humans, and can cause multiple skin nodules that ulcerate and drain, induration and nodular lesions of superficial lymphatic vessels of the extremities, regional lymphadenopathy, and abscesses of internal organs. The cutaneous and lymphatic disease in horses is known as "farcy."[1]

B. pseudomallei is widely distributed in water and soil in tropical and subtropical regions. It spreads to humans by inoculation of abraded or lacerated skin, ingestion of contaminated food or water, or by inhalation. Melioidosis is endemic in Southeast Asia and northern Australia, where it is most prevalent during the rainy season among people who have direct contact with wet soils. Most exposed persons do not develop disease; asymptomatic seroconversion is common in endemic regions. Most (50-80%) patients have predisposing conditions including diabetes mellitus, alcoholism, cirrhosis, renal disease, thallassemia, cystic fibrosis, or impaired immunity. Clinical presentations vary from mild disease to overwhelming sepsis with up to a 90% case fatality rate (CFR) and death 24 to 48 h after onset.[2, 3] Aerosols from cultures are highly infectious to lab workers. BSL-3 containment practices are required when working with cultures of these organisms. Clinical chemistries, hematology, and other laboratory tests may be done under BSL-2 conditions. Person-to-person spread is rare.

Because of their virulence, potential transmission by environmental aerosols, lack of available vaccines, and difficult treatment regimens, *B. mallei* and *B. pseudomallei* have been considered potential bio-agents.

History & Significance

B. mallei (glanders) was one of the first bacterial agents to be weaponized in a modern bio-warfare program. During World War I, German agents in Baltimore and other seaports allegedly inoculated horses, mules and donkeys intended for export to Allied forces in Europe. The intent was to disrupt military logistics, as these animals were essential to transportation before the large-scale availability of motorized vehicles. The results of these alleged biological attacks are unknown. The Japanese allegedly infected horses, civilians, and prisoners of war with *B. mallei* at the Pinfang Institute during World War II. The US also studied this agent as a possible biowarfare weapon in 1943 and '44, but did not weaponize it. The Soviet Union is believed to have identified *B. mallei* as a potential bio-agent after World War II. Glanders has been eliminated from

North America, Europe, and Australia, but sporadic cases still occur among equids in Asia, Africa, the Middle East, and South America. Human cases are rare. A laboratory-acquired case occurred at USAMRIID in 2000.[1,4,5]

B. pseudomallei (melioidosis) is a leading cause of community-acquired pneumonia and sepsis in northern Australia, and has accounted for 20% of community-acquired sepsis in northern Thailand. Pulmonary melioidosis occurred among US forces during the Vietnam conflict, thought to have been due to inhalation of aerosols of contaminated soil and water generated by helicopter prop blast in irrigated rice fields. Due to activation of latent infection, French and later US soldiers returning from Vietnam would infrequently develop disease (the "Vietnamese time-bomb") years after exposure. *B. pseudomallei* was also studied by the US as a potential bio-agent, but never weaponized. It has been reported that the Soviet Union studied and weaponized *B. pseudomallei.*[6]

Clinical Features

Incubation periods vary by portal of entry, inoculum, virulence, and host factors. Animal models of high dose inhalational exposure to either *B. mallei or B. pseudomallei* are usually followed by incubation of 1 to 4 d. In the few well-documented human cases of glanders due to respiratory exposure, incubation varied from 10 to 14 d. Incubation following mucus membrane or skin exposure is usually in the range of 1 to 21 d, but can be several mos. The incubation of naturally acquired melioidosis is more difficult to determine, because exposure in endemic regions may be continuous. Documented incubations of clinically overt melioidosis are typically 1 to 21 d, although periods of several mos can occur. Uncommonly, patients may present with either disease years after exposure due to activation of latent infection, in the case of melioidosis usually after the onset of diabetes or other risk factors.[1-3]

The manifestations of both glanders and melioidosis are protean; disease can be acute or chronic, localized or systemic, or progress from one form to another. Inhalation of aerosols produced by bio-weapons containing high inocula of *B. mallei* or *B. pseudomallei* could presumably produce any of these syndromes, although acute respiratory or systemic syndromes would be most likely.

Acute glanders and melioidosis after intentional high-inoculum aerosol exposure can be expected to have similar clinical presentations; differentiation will depend upon laboratory studies. Pneumonia would likely develop. Patients would likely present within a few days of exposure with the acute onset of fever, chills, malaise, myalgias, and shortness of breath, with or without cough and pleuritic chest pain. Sputum is often purulent, and hemoptysis may occur. CXR findings vary and may disclose unilateral or bilateral, multifocal, nodular, or lobar consolidation, often progressing to abscess formation and cavitation.

Septicemia may occur at any time, regardless of the portal of entry, and cause fever, rigors, night sweats, myalgia, anorexia, and headache. Bacteremia may cause diffuse seeding of the skin, leading to a regional or generalized papular and/or pustular rash. Disseminated infection may produce abscesses of internal organs (especially liver, spleen, and lungs) and skeletal muscles. These abscesses may result in hepatosplenomegaly and abdominal tenderness. Osteomyelitis, brain abscess, and meningitis have been reported. Disseminated infection carries a high risk of septic shock, end-organ failures, and death.

Rarely, these diseases present as a focal abscess without an antecedent illness or obvious site of primary inoculation; most commonly in melioidosis this is as a primary purulent parotitis in children (more common in Thailand) or as a primary prostatic abscess (more common in northern Australia).

Clinical presentations may suggest other bio-agents in the differential diagnosis. A rapidly progressive pneumonia accompanied by sepsis, with respiratory secretions demonstrating gram-negative bacteria with "safety pin" appearance on Wright's stain suggests pneumonic plague, while a diffuse papular or pustular rash may suggest smallpox.

Natural disease due to both organisms is described in the literature.[1-3] Differences between the clinical presentations of glanders and melioidosis may result from mucocutaneous or low inoculum exposures, and are described below.

Glanders. Cutaneous exposure typically leads to local inflammatory nodules with subsequent lymphangitis (sometimes with a sporotrichoid nodular presentation) and regional lymphadenitis. Nodules typically ulcerate and drain. Conjunctivitis can result in photophobia, lacrimation, and purulent discharge. Acute or subacute constitutional symptoms may develop, and can include fever (low-grade or recurring), rigors, sweats, headache, fatigue and myalgias.

Inhalational exposure may produce either upper or lower respiratory tract disease. Rhinitis or pharyngitis may feature constitutional symptoms, headache, purulent exudates, and cervical lymphadenopathy. Chronic infection and erosion of the nasal septum and turbinates can lead to severe disfigurement.

Chronic disease occurs in half of all natural cases and is eventually fatal without treatment. Chronic infections may feature spontaneous clinical remission followed by relapse. CFRs dropped to 20% for localized disease, and to 40% overall, after sulfadiazine therapy became available. Experience during the modern antibiotic era is, however, very limited.

Melioidosis. Mucocutaneous exposure may lead to local nodules/abscesses and regional lymphadenitis. Cutaneous disease may result from local inoculation or from bacteremic seeding of the skin.

Inhalational exposure, either through near drowning or via infectious aerosols, may result in respiratory diseases that can range from a mild bronchitis to a chronic subacute pneumonia, or a severe acute necrotizing pneumonia and septic shock.

Sputum is often purulent, and hemoptysis may be present. Radiographic findings commonly feature lobar or segmental consolidation with a predilection for the upper lobes, or multiple, widespread 0.5 to 1.0 cm nodules, or cavitation. Chronic pulmonary disease can follow acute pneumonia, or reactivate years after exposure, with clinical and radiographic findings mimicking those of tuberculosis. Cutaneous and internal (especially hepatic, splenic, and prostatic) abscesses can occur up to wks or mos after exposure or acute disease.

Septicemic melioidosis presents with fever, rigors, night sweats, myalgia, anorexia, and headache. Additional features can include papular or pustular skin lesions, diarrhea, and hepatosplenomegaly. Dissemination is likely to produce cutaneous and internal (especially liver and spleen) abscesses even wks to mos later. Prostatic abscess occurs in 2 to 15% of cases. Poor prognostic indicators include positive blood cultures within 24 h of incubation and neutropenia. Without proper treatment, most septicemic patients will die within 2 or 3 d. With treatment, CFRs are approximately 40% in Thailand and 14% in Australia.[3] Relapse occurs in approximately 10% of survivors.[3,7,8]

Diagnosis

Microbiology. Gram stain of lesion exudates reveals small irregularly staining, gram-negative bacilli. Methylene blue or Wright's stain may reveal bipolar "safety pin" staining. The organisms can be cultured from abscesses/wounds, secretions, sputum (in pneumonia), and sometimes blood and urine with standard media. Primary isolation requires 48 to 72 h in agar at 37.5° C; automated blood culture methods are typically more rapid. Selective media (e.g., Ashdown's medium for *B. pseudomallei*) may be necessary for isolation from non-sterile sites (sputum, pharynx swabs).

Blood cultures for *B. mallei* are rarely positive. In contrast, blood cultures for *B. pseudomallei* are often positive and urine culture may be positive, especially if prostatitis or renal abscesses are present. The laboratory should be alerted if these diagnoses are being considered, because of the occupational health hazards posed by these organisms, and because some automated culture systems may misidentify *B. pseudomallei* as *Pseudomonas* spp.[2] Cultures must be performed under BSL-3 precautions due to the high aerosol risk to lab workers.

PCR is rapid and specific, but may be less sensitive than cultures, especially for evaluating blood samples. Rapid immunoassays for *B. pseudomallei* capsular antigens are available in some reference laboratories.

Serologic tests are of limited utility, particularly in endemic areas where backround seroprevalence is high.[2,3,10] Indirect hemaglutination assays are the most frequently used serologic tests in endemic regions, but are poorly standardized and difficult to perform.[8,9] Currently available tests do not distinguish between the two etiologic agents, and are considered inadequate as a sole method of laboratory confirmation.[2,9,10]

For *B. mallei,* agglutination tests are not positive for 7 to 10 d (or up to 3 wks), and a high background titer in normal sera (1:320 to 1:640) makes interpretation difficult. Complement fixation (CF) tests are more specific, but less sensitive, and may require 40 d for conversion. CF tests are considered positive if the titer is > 1:20. For *B. pseudomallei,* a fourfold increase in titer supports the diagnosis. A single IgM titer > 1:160 with a compatible clinical picture suggests active infection; IgG is less useful in endemic regions due to high seroprevalence.

Other laboratory studies. Clinical chemistries, hematology, and similar clinical laboratory tests not involving cultures may be done under BSL- 2 conditions. Findings may include leukocytosis, anemia, coagulopathy, and abnormal hepatic and renal function tests. In septicemic glanders, mild leukocytosis with a shift to the left or leukopenia with a relative lymphocytosis may occur. In systemic melioidosis, significant leukocytosis with left shift is common, and leucopenia (neutropenia) is a poor prognostic indicator; anemia, coagulopathy, and evidence of hepatic or renal dysfunction may be present.

Radiographic studies. CXRs may demonstrate lobar or segmental consolidation, diffuse nodular opacities, cavitary lesions, pleural effusions and empyemas. Hilar adenopathy is infrequent.[11] Abdominal and pelvic imaging (CT or MRI imaging, or abdominal and pelvic/transrectal ultrasounds) should be considered for all patients with suspected glanders or melioidosis to exclude hepatic, splenic or prostatic abscesses.

Pathology. Melioidosis can cause granulomatous lesions suggesting tuberculosis. This can make diagnosis difficult, especially in areas where both melioidosis and tuberculosis are endemic, such as Thailand.[12]

Medical Management

Supportive Care. Ventilatory support may be necessary for severe pneumonia. Septicemic patients often require aggressive care including fluid resuscitation, vasopressors, and management of coagulopathy. Large abscesses and empyemas should be drained; prostatic and parotid abscesses in patients with melioidosis are unlikely to resolve without surgical intervention. Surgical therapy is not necessary for multiple small hepatic or splenic abscesses, which respond to prolonged antibiotic therapy.

Antimicrobials. Antibiotic regimens for melioidosis are based on clinical trials and medical experience in Thailand and Australia. Although experience with human glanders is limited due to its low incidence during the antibiotic era, the same treatment regimens are recommended for both diseases as these organisms have similar antibiotic susceptibility patterns. (Unlike *B. pseudomallei*, however, natural *B. mallei* strains generally remain susceptible to aminoglycosides and macrolides *in vitro.*) Revision of empiric therapy is guided by antibiotic susceptibilities of bacterial isolates.

Initial therapy. All cases of both diseases, regardless of clinical severity, should be treated with IV therapy for > 10 to 14 d and until the patient shows clinical improvement, followed by oral eradication therapy for > another 3 mos.[2,3] Antibiotic regimens include either ceftazidime (50 mg/kg [up to 2 g]) IV every 6 to 8 h or meropenem (25 mg/kg [up to 1 g]) IV every 8 h. Imipenem (25 mg/kg [up to 1 g]) IV every 6 h is an acceptable alternative, but carries a higher risk of CNS toxicity and is more difficult to dose in renal failure. Meropenem is advised for patients with CNS involvement. A switch to meropenem is indicated if the patient has positive blood cultures after 7 d of therapy, or clinically deteriorates (e.g., develops organ failure or a new focus of infection) at any time during ceftazidime therapy. If ceftazidime or a carbapenem are not available, ampicillin/sulbactam or other intravenous beta-lactam/beta-lactamase inhibitor combinations may be viable, albeit less-proven alternatives. IV therapy may be extended (4 to 8 wks) for critical illness, severe pulmonary disease, deep-seated abscesses, bone, joint, or CNS involvement.[2,3,8,13] Fever can persist for prolonged periods during appropriate therapy, and does not necessarily indicate treatment failure. Median time to fever resolution is 9 d, but can be significantly longer in patients with large, undrained abscesses.

Maintenance therapy. Upon completion of IV therapy, oral maintenance therapy with TMP/SMX (2 X 160-800 mg [960 mg tablets if > 60 kg]) every 12 h should be continued for 3 to 6 mos.[2,3,13] Maintenance therapy of severe disease should continue for > 20 wks to reduce the risk of relapse. Toxicity screening during TMP/SMX maintenance therapy or post-exposure prophylaxis should include complete blood counts, renal function tests and serum electrolytes (weekly during the first 2 to 3 wks, then biweekly). Folate supplementation (5 mg/d) should be considered for those at risk for folate deficiency.[13] *Augmentin* is advised for resistant isolates or if the patient is intolerant of TMP/SMX, and is used during pregnancy and for children < 8 yrs old.[3] Life-long follow-up is indicated for melioidosis patients to identify relapse.

Isolation precautions. Person-to-person spread is rare. Standard precautions (i.e., the use of disposable surgical masks; face shields, gloves and gowns, when appropriate, to prevent splashing of mucous membranes and skin) are sufficient to prevent transmission to those caring for patients. Droplet, airborne, or airborne-plus-contact precautions should be used, respectively, if pneumonic plague, pulmonary tuberculosis, or smallpox are serious considerations in the differential diagnosis.[4,16] Environmental decontamination using a 0.5% to 1.0% hypochlorite solution is effective.

Prophylaxis

Vaccine: There are currently no vaccines available for human use.

Antibiotics: There are no human data or FDA-approved PEP regimens. TMP-SMX has been effective in limited animal studies[14], and should be strongly considered following a bio-warfare attack. Recommendations for PEP following lab accidents advise TMP/SMX (2 X 160-800 mg (960 mg tablets if > 60 kg]) every 12 h, with *Augmentin* 20.5 mg/kg every 8 h as an alternative, especially during pregnancy or for children < 8 yrs old.[8,13] Toxicity screening and folate supplementation should be considered as discussed for maintainence therapy. Doxycycline 2.5 mg/kg (up to 100 mg) every 12 h may be considered[8,13], although it has resulted in high relapse rates in animal studies.[13,15] Fluoroquinolones are not recommended, due to poor performance in animal studies of PEP, and high relapse rates during clinical trials for therapy.[8,13] Optimal duration of PEP is unknown, but 3 wks is recommended by expert consensus.[8,13]

Plague

Summary

Signs and symptoms: *Bubonic plague* is characterized by swollen painful lymph nodes ("buboes") — often in the inguinal area — high fever, and malaise. It may progress spontaneously to the *septicemic* form (septic shock, thrombosis, disseminated intravascular coagulation) or the *pneumonic* form (secondary pneumonic plague) with cough, dyspnea, and hemoptysis.

Primary pneumonic plague (the expected form following a bio-agent attack) begins with a sudden onset of symptoms after an incubation period of 1 to 6 d. These include high fever, chills, headache, malaise, followed by cough (often producing blood), progressing rapidly to dyspnea, stridor, cyanosis, and death. GI symptoms are often present. Death results from respiratory failure, circulatory collapse, and a bleeding diathesis. Plague meningitis is also possible.

Diagnosis: Suspect plague if large numbers of previously healthy individuals suddenly develop severe pneumonia, especially if hemoptysis is prominent and Gram-negative coccobacilli are present in sputum. Presumptive diagnosis can be made by Wright, Giemsa, Wayson, or methylene blue stain of blood, sputum, CSF, or lymph node aspirates. Immuno-diagnosis may be helpful, but definitive diagnosis requires culture of *Yersinia pestis* from one of those sites.

Treatment: Early administration of antibiotics is critical, as pneumonic plague is invariably fatal if this is delayed for > 1 d after onset of symptoms. The treatment of choice is parenteral streptomycin or gentamicin, with doxycycline, ciprofloxacin, and levofloxacin representing acceptable alternatives. Duration of therapy is between 10 and 14 d. For plague meningitis, chloramphenicol is added to the regimen.

Prophylaxis: For asymptomatic persons exposed to a plague aerosol or to a suspected pneumonic plague case, doxycycline 100 mg PO bid is given for 7 d, or for the duration of the period of exposure plus 7 d. Alternative antibiotics include ciprofloxacin, tetracycline, or chloramphenicol. No vaccine is currently available for plague prophylaxis. (The previously available licensed, killed vaccine was effective against natural bubonic plague, but not against aerosol exposure.) No prophylaxis is required for asymptomatic contacts of individuals with bubonic or septicemic plague without pneumonia.

Isolation and decontamination: Standard precautions are used by medical personnel for bubonic or septicemic plague and respiratory droplet precautions are required for a suspected or known pneumonic plague case. *Y. pestis* can survive in the environment for varying periods, but is susceptible to heat, disinfectants, and exposure to sunlight. Soap and water are effective for decontamination if needed.

Overview

Yersinia pestis is a rod-shaped, non-motile, non-sporulating, Gram-negative bacterium of the family *Enterobacteraceae.* It causes plague, a zoonotic disease of rodents (rats, mice, ground squirrels, etc). Humans typically develop disease through contact with infected rodents or, more commonly, their fleas.[1] The biting fleas transmit bacteria to humans, who then typically develop the bubonic form of plague. The bubonic form may progress to the septicemic and/or pneumonic forms. Larger outbreaks of human plague often follow epizootics in which large numbers of host rodents die off, leaving their fleas in search of other sources of a blood meal.[2] Pneumonic plague would be the predominant form of disease expected after purposeful aerosol dissemination. All human populations are susceptible. Recovery from the disease is followed by immunity, but the duration of this in humans is currently unknown. (Antibody to F1 can be found in humans more than 10 yrs following infection.[3]) The organism remains viable in unchlorinated water, moist soil, and grains for several weeks. At near freezing temperatures, it will remain alive for mos to yrs, but it is killed by 15 min of exposure to 55° C. It also remains viable for some time (hours to days) in dry sputum, flea feces, and buried bodies, but is killed within several hours of exposure to sunlight.

History & Significance

Historically, *Y. pestis* has been the cause of several human pandemics and countless deaths.[4] Plague is now endemic worldwide, yet is responsible for only sporadic human disease (200-4,500 human cases including 30–200 deaths reported to the WHO annually). Before and during World War II, the Japanese Imperial Army released plague-infected fleas from aircraft over Chinese cities producing outbreaks and deaths.[6] This method was cumbersome and unpredictable. Later, the Soviet Union had several institutes and thousands of scientists dedicated to their ultimately successful project to create and produce an effective *Y. pestis* munition.[5] The US worked with plague as a potential bio-agent in the 1950s and '60s, but never successfully weaponized it before the its offensive biowarfare program was terminated. Both the US and USSR developed reliable and effective delivery methods for aerosolizing the organism. The terrorist potential of plague was highlighted in 1995 when Larry Wayne Harris was arrested in Ohio for the illicit procurement of a *Y. pestis* culture through the mail. The contagious nature of pneumonic plague, whether through zoonotic or person-to-person transmission, makes it particularly concerning as a biological weapon.[7]

Clinical Features

Human plague can present in one of three predominant forms: bubonic, septicemic, and pneumonic. The vast majority of the 1 to 40 human cases reported annually in the US are from the desert southwest, where plague is endemic in rural rodent populations.[8] Most naturally occurring human cases in the US are bubonic (80–85%);

primary septicemic cases are less common (15%); and primary pneumonic cases are quite rare (1–2%).[9]

Bubonic plague may occur after an infected flea vector bites a human host. The disease begins after a typical incubation period of 2 to 8 d, with acute and fulminant onset of nonspecific symptoms, including high fever (up to 40° C), severe malaise, headache, myalgias, and — in 25 to 50% — nausea and vomiting.[2] Up to half of patients will have abdominal pain. Simultaneous with, or shortly following, the onset of these nonspecific symptoms, the characteristic bubo develops – a swollen, extremely painful, infected lymph node.[2] Buboes may be from 1 to 10 cm in diameter with erythema of the overlying skin and variable degrees of surrounding edema. They rarely become fluctuant or suppurate, and lymphangitis is uncommon. They are most commonly seen affecting the femoral or inguinal lymph nodes since the legs are the most commonly flea-bitten part of the adult human body. But any lymph nodes can be involved, including intra-abdominal nodes (presumably through hematogenous extension) which can present as a febrile patient with an acute abdomen. The liver and spleen are often tender and palpable. One quarter of patients will have some type of skin lesion: a pustule, vesicle, eschar or papule (containing leukocytes and bacteria) in the lymphatic drainage of the bubo, and presumably representing the site of the inoculating flea bite. Bacteremia is common, as greater than 80% of blood cultures are positive for the organism in patients with bubonic plague. However, only about a quarter of bubonic plague patients progress to clinical septicemia, typically within 2 to 6 d of symptom onset in untreated patients. The case fatality rate (CFR) of untreated bubonic plague is approximately 60%, but this is reduced to < 5% with prompt, effective therapy.

Septicemic plague. In cases that progress to secondary septicemia, as in primary septicemia, the symptoms and signs are similar to other Gram-negative septicemias: high fever, chills, malaise, hypotension, tachycardia, tachypnea, nausea, vomiting, and diarrhea. All age groups can be affected, but the elderly seem to be at increased risk. Plague septicemia can produce thrombi in the acral vessels (presumably assisted by a low-temperature-activated coagulase protein produced by the organism), possibly leading to necrosis and gangrene, and disseminated intravascular coagulation (DIC); thus, black necrotic appendages may be accompanied by more proximal, purpuric lesions due to endotoxemia in advanced disease. Organisms can spread via the bloodstream to the lungs and, less commonly, to the CNS and elsewhere. Untreated septicemic plague is virtually 100% fatal, while treated disease carries a CFR of 30 to 50%.

Pneumonic plague is an infection of the lungs due to either inhalation of the organisms (primary pneumonic plague), or spread to the lungs from bacteremia (secondary pneumonic plague). Secondary pneumonic plague has been a complication in 12% of bubonic cases in the US over the past 50 yrs. (28% of human plague cases resulting from exposure to plague-infected domestic cats in the US in recent decades presented as primary pneumonic plague; 25% of these human cases were in veterinarians or their assistants.) Person-to-person spread of pneumonic plague has not occurred in the US since 1925. After an incubation period varying from 1 to 6 d for primary pneumonic plague (usually 2-4 d, and presumably dose-dependent), onset is acute and often fulminant. The first signs of illness include high fever, chills, headache, malaise, and myalgias, followed within 24 h by tachypnea and cough, progressing to hemoptysis.[2] Although bloody sputum is characteristic, it can sometimes be watery or, less commonly, purulent. Nausea, vomiting, diarrhea, and abdominal pain, may all be present. Rarely, a cervical bubo might result from an inhalational exposure. CXR findings are variable, but most commonly reveal bilateral infiltrates, which may be patchy or consolidated. The pneumonia progresses rapidly, resulting in dyspnea, stridor, and cyanosis. The disease terminates with respiratory failure and circulatory collapse. The CFR for treated pneumonic plague patients in the US is approximately 50%; if untreated, however, it is nearly 100%. (In the US in the past 50 yrs, 4 of the 7 pneumonic plague patients [57%] died.) Recent data from the ongoing Madagascar epidemic, which began in 1989, corroborate that figure; the CFR associated with respiratory involvement was 57%, while that for uncomplicated bubonic plague was 15%.

Pneumonic plague is the only form of the disease which readily spreads from person to person. From the sparse historical data available on past cases, the average secondary infection rate is 1.3 cases per primary case (range: 0 to 6). Transmission has been greatest under crowded, cold, and humid conditions.[10] The majority of secondary cases have been in caregivers at home (80%) or medical professionals (14%) after close proximity (< 2 meters) with the primary cases.

Plague meningitis is a rare complication (up to 6% of patients with septicemia, more commonly in children), most often occurring in bubonic or septicemic plague patients a week or more into illness. Typically these patients have been receiving sub-therapeutic doses of antibiotics or bacteriostatic antibiotics which do not cross the blood brain barrier well (e.g., tetracyclines). Signs and symptoms are consistent with subacute bacterial meningitis, and CSF demonstrates a leukocytosis with neutrophil predominance and perhaps Gram-negative coccobacilli.

Other syndromes. Plague can also present as a primary pharyngitis and tonsillitis, usually with swollen and inflammed anterior cervical lymph nodes.[11] This rare form of plague is acquired from inhalation or ingestion of plague coccobacilli.[12] The clinician should be aware of asymptomatic pharyngeal colonization by *Y. pestis* in people with close contact to pneumonic or bubonic cases of plague.[13]

Nonspecific laboratory findings in all forms of human plague include a leukocytosis, with a total WBC up to 20,000 cells per ml or more with increased band forms, and > 80% polymorphonuclear cells. Platelet counts can be normal or low. Increased fibrin split products and elevated partial thromboplastin time, indicating a low-grade DIC, can also be seen. The blood urea nitrogen, creatinine, transaminases, and bilirubin may also be elevated, consistent with multiorgan failure.

Diagnosis

Clinical diagnosis. Diagnosis of plague is based primarily on clinical suspicion. A patient with a painful lymph node accompanied by fever, severe malaise and possible rodent exposure in an endemic area should raise suspicion of bubonic plague. The sudden appearance of large numbers of previously healthy patients with severe, rapidly progressive pneumonia with hemoptysis strongly suggests pneumonic plague as a result of an intentional aerosolization.

Laboratory diagnosis. A presumptive diagnosis can be made microscopically by identification of the coccobacillus in Wright, Giemsa, Wayson's or methylene blue stains, or more specific immunofluorescence antibody-stained smears from lymph node needle aspirate, sputum, blood, or CSF samples. Although a Gram stain should be used for classification purposes, it should not be used to seek the "safety pin" appearance characteristic of *Y. pestis.* This characteristic morphology is sometimes not apparent on Gram stain[14] and to an inexperienced microscopist, other members of the *Enterobacteriaceae* may seem to have it, especially in the early log phase of growth.[15] Bubo aspirates can be obtained by inserting a 20 gauge needle on a 10 ml syringe containing 1 ml of sterile saline; saline is injected and withdrawn until blood tinged. Definitive diagnosis relies on culturing the organism from clinical specimens. The organism grows slowly at normal incubation temperatures (optimally, 25 to 28° C), and may be misidentified by automated systems (often as *Y. pseudotuberculosis)* because of delayed biochemical reactions. It may be cultured on blood agar, MacConkey agar, or infusion broth. It will also grow in automated culture systems. Any patient with suspected plague should have blood cultures performed (at 28° and 35°C); as bacteremia can be intermittent, multiple cultures should be obtained, preferably before receipt of antibiotics (clinical severity permitting). Confirmatory diagnosis via culture commonly takes 48 to 72 h (cultures should be held for 5 to 7 d); thus specific antibiotic therapy for plague must not be withheld pending culture results. Confirmatory culture-based diagnosis is made by specific bacteriophage lysis of the organism, along with PCR to identify *Y. pestis*-specific genes, available at many reference laboratories, especially those participating in the CDC-sponsored Laboratory Response Network (several major civilian and military medical centers). The clinician should be aware of a recent history of the misidentification of *Y. pestis* as *Pseudomonas luteola, Acinetobacter lwoffi,* and *Y. pseudotuberculosis* by automated bacterial identification systems.

Most naturally occurring strains of *Y. pestis* produce an F1-antigen *in vivo,* which can be detected in serum samples by specific immunoassay. A single anti-F1 titer of >1:10 by agglutination testing is suggestive of plague, while a single titer of >1:128 in a patient who has not previously been exposed to plague, or has not previously received a plague vaccine, is more specific; a fourfold rise in acute vs. convalescent antibody titers in patient serum is probably the most specific serologic method to confirm diagnosis, albeit only retrospectively. Most patients will seroconvert within 1 to 2 wks of disease onset, but a minority require 3 or more wks.

Most clinical assays can be performed in BSL-2 laboratories, but procedures producing aerosols, or yielding significant quantities of organisms, require BSL-3 containment.

Medical Management

Antibiotics. Prompt initiation of appropriate antibiotics is paramount for reducing mortality; this is especially true in primary pneumonic plague, for which CFRs approach 100% if adequate therapy is not initiated within 24 h of onset of symptoms. Initial empiric therapy for systemic disease caused by *Y. pestis* includes at least one of the following antibiotics:[16]

Preferred

- Streptomycin (FDA approved)*, 1 g IM bid (15 mg/kg IM bid for children (up to 2 g/d)), or
- Gentamicin 5 mg/kg IM or IV qd, or 2 mg/kg loading dose followed by 1.7 mg/kg IM or IV q 8 h (2.5 mg/kg IV q 8 h for children), adjusted for renal clearance, or

Alternatives

- Doxycycline (FDA approved), 100 mg IV q12 h or 200 mg IV qd for adults or children ≥ 45 kg (2.2 mg/kg IV q 12 h for children < 45 kg), or
- Ciprofloxacin 400 mg IV every 12 h for adults (for children use 15 mg/kg IV q 12 h [up to 1 g/d]), or
- Chloramphenicol, 25 mg/kg IV, then 15 mg/kg IV q 6 h (adjusted for serum levels, & not for children < 2 yrs old)
- Levofloxacin (recently FDA approved), adult & pediatric patients > 50kg; 500mg administered by slow IV infusion over 60 min q 24 h for 10 to 14 d. Pediatric patients < 50kg & > 6 mos of age: 8 mg/kg (not to exceed 250 mg per dose) by slow IV infusion every 12 h for 10 to 14 d.

IV antibiotics can be switched to PO administration as the improvement in the patient's clinical course dictates, to complete 10 to 14 total d of therapy. For treatment of plague meningitis, add IV chloramphenicol. Patients with uncomplicated bubonic plague often demonstrate resolution of fever and other systemic symptoms in 3 to 5 d,

* Streptomycin has historically been the drug of choice for plague and is the only aminoglycoside antibiotic approved by the FDA for its treatment; however, because it may not be readily available immediately after a large-scale biowarfare attack, gentamicin and other alternative drugs should be considered first.[17]

while more complicated cases—including septicemic and pneumonic plague—often result in extended hospital courses.

It is imperative that antibiotics be adjusted to the demonstrated susceptibility patterns of the infecting organism; naturally occurring strains have been reported which are resistant to streptomycin, tetracyclines, and chloramphenocol, and it is anticipated that weaponized plague could be intentionally rendered antibiotic resistant. Despite typically good *in vitro* susceptibilities to penicillins and cephalosporins, these drugs are generally felt to be ineffective for plague; in fact, animal studies suggest that beta-lactam antibiotics may accelerate mortality in bacteremic mice. Macrolide antibiotics are ineffective for plague.

Supportive therapy includes IV crystalloids and hemodynamic monitoring. Although low-grade DIC may occur, clinically significant hemorrhage is uncommon, as is the need to treat with heparin. Endotoxic shock is common, but pressor agents are rarely needed. Finally, buboes rarely require any form of local care, but instead recede with systemic antibiotic therapy. In fact, incision and drainage poses an infection risk to others in contact with the patient due to possible aerosolization of the bubo contents. Needle aspiration is recommended for diagnostic purposes and may provide symptomatic relief.

Infection control. Use standard precautions for bubonic and septicemic plague patients. Suspected pneumonic plague requires strict isolation with respiratory droplet precautions for > 48 h after initiation of antibiotic therapy, or until sputum cultures are negative in confirmed cases. Historically, epidemics of pneumonic plague have subsided rapidly with implementation of such relatively simple infection control measures. Pneumonic plague patients being transported should wear a surgical mask when feasible. If competent vectors (fleas) and reservoirs (rodents) are present, measures must be taken to prevent local disease cycles.[17] These might include: use of flea insecticides, rodent control measures (after or during flea control), and flea barriers for patient-care areas.[18]

Prophylaxis

Chemoprophylaxis.

Pre-exposure: No antibiotic is licensed by the FDA for use before exposure to plague. However, chemoprophylaxis with doxycycline (or ciprofloxacin) may protect against plague based upon *in vitro* susceptibilities.

Post-exposure: Face-to-face contacts (< 2 meters) of patients with pneumonic plague, or persons possibly exposed to a plague aerosol (i.e., in a bio-agent attack), should be given antibiotic prophylaxis for 7 d or the duration of risk of exposure plus 7 d. If fever or cough occurs in these individuals, a full treatment course is warranted.

- Preferred empiric prophylaxis
- Doxycycline 100 mg PO bid for adults & children > 45 kg (for children <45 kg use 2.2 mg / kg PO bid), or

Alternatives

- Ciprofloxacin 500 mg PO bid for adults (20 mg/kg PO bid [up to 1 g/d] for children)
- Chloramphenicol 25 mg/kg PO qid

Other tetracyclines and fluoroquinolones could potentially be substituted for doxycycline and ciprofloxacin, respectively. TMP/SMX may represent a second-line alternative, should susceptibilities allow. Chemoprophylaxis is generally not recommended after contact with bubonic or septicemic plague patients; however, individuals making such contacts, especially if sharing the same environment in which the patient received a natural exposure, should be observed for symptoms for a week. If symptoms occur, start treatment antibiotics while awaiting results of diagnostic studies.

Immunoprophylaxis.
Vaccines: No vaccine is currently available for prophylaxis of plague. A licensed, killed whole-cell vaccine was formerly manufactured by Greer and available in the US between 1946 and 1998. It offered protection against bubonic plague, but was not effective against aerosolized *Y. pestis.*

The plague bacterium secretes several virulence factors—such as Fraction 1 (F1) and V (virulence) proteins—which as subunit proteins are immunogenic and possess protective properties. As combined recombinant (fusion) proteins, these have been the focus of vaccine development and have shown promise in preclinical studies and in Phase 1 and Phase 2 clinical trials. Recently, an F1-V antigen (fusion protein) vaccine developed at USAMRIID[19] provided 100% protection in monkeys against a high-dose aerosol challenge.[20]

Passive: There is no passive immunoprophylaxis (i.e., immune globulin) available for pre- or post-exposure management of plague.

Q-Fever

Summary

Signs and symptoms: Q-fever may initially present with either acute or chronic manifestations; long-term sequelae may be considered a third form. Route and magnitude of exposure largely determine the dominant clinical feature (e.g., pneumonia follows an aerosol exposure). Up to 60% of human infections are clinically inapparent. A non-specific flu-like illness predominates in the remaining 40% with a minority developing immunosuppression, pneumonia or hepatitis. Incubation period is estimated at 1 to 5 wks (10 to 17 d is most typical) and the duration of symptoms ranges from a few days to a few mos. Chronic disease may manifest many mos or yrs after the primary infection; the most frequent and serious presentation being endocarditis, which is usually fatal if not treated.

Diagnosis: The combination of frequent subclinical disease, sporadic local occurrence and non-specific signs and symptoms makes Q-fever diagnosis problematic. Careful history may reveal risk factors (e.g., working around livestock, travelling in endemic areas) during natural infection. The gold standard for acute disease is a fourfold increase in phase II IgG antibody titer by indirect immunofluorescence assay (IFA) of paired acute and convalescent specimens; however, a negative acute titer does not rule out acute Q fever (seroconversion may be delayed). Other relevant lab approaches include PCR, *C. burnetii* blood or tissue culture (requires a BSL-3 facility), and immunohistochemistry.

Treatment: Acute patients should receive antibiotic treatment, optimally begun within the first 3 d of illness. If acute Q fever is suspected, this should not be withheld pending results of lab tests, nor treatment discontinued on account of initially negative serology. Doxycycline (100 mg q12 h) for > 14 d is the treatment of choice. For acute patients with pre-existing disease, such as valvulopathy, 12 to 18 mos of doxy with hydroxychloroquine (200 mg q8 h) may be necessary. Chronic Q fever should be treated only after lab diagnostic confirmation and may require individualized treatment plans based on disease severity, underlying immune and valvular status, and response to prior treatment. Generally, the same two drugs are administered for 18 mos.

Prophylaxis: A licensed vaccine (*Q-Vax*) is available in Australia and Europe. A formalin-inactivated whole cell IND vaccine is available in the US for at-risk personnel on an investigational basis only. (Pre-vaccination screening is essential as those who were previously exposed to Q-fever, or to a Q-fever vaccine, may develop severe local or systemic disease following vaccination.) Post-exposure prophylaxis in suspected *C. burnetii* exposures has recently been called into question (see main text).

Isolation and decontamination: Standard precautions are recommended for HCWs dealing with suspected or confirmed cases. For autopsies, precautions should be taken to prevent aerosolization of body fluids. Culturing of the organism requires a BSL-3 facility. Q-fever is primarily considered to be a zoonotic disease, with human-to-human, or tick-to-human transmission very rare. Patients are not required to wear masks. The spore form of the organism is very hardy and can survive for yrs in the environment. It can probably survive direct UV light, dilute bleach and typical disinfectants. Autoclaving and boiling for 10 min will kill the organism. Decontamination may be attempted with a 1:100 *Lysol* solution, 1% sodium hypochlorite solution, 5% hydrogen peroxide, or 70% ethanol. The M291 skin decontamination kit will not neutralize the organism.

Overview

Q-fever is a zoonotic disease caused by the obligate intracellular, gram-negative bacterium *Coxiella burnetii.*[1-4] A nationally notifiable disease in the US, Q-fever is found world-wide (exception: New Zealand). Its natural reservoirs include sheep, cattle, goats, rabbits, cats, dogs, rodents, birds and ticks. The organism localizes in the gravid uterus and mammary glands of infected animals and is shed in very high numbers at parturition, whether at or before term. Infection in livestock occasionally results in abortion, stillbirth, and dystocia, but is most often asymptomatic. Direct animal contact is not required for transmission to humans. Human infection is typically via aerosolization of infectious particles, especially in premises contaminated with fetal membranes, birth fluids, aborted fetuses, and excreta from infected animals in locations where infected animals and their by-products are processed, as well as at necropsy sites. Transmission to humans may also occur by ingesting contaminated raw milk and cheese, through blood product transfusions and bone marrow transplantations, vertically (mother to offspring), and by ticks. Person-to-person transmission through sexual contact is rare but considered possible. Tick bites are believed to be important in maintaining disease in livestock and wild animal reservoirs, but not in human disease. *C. burnetii* may be found in high numbers in tick feces with consequent environmental contamination.

Humans acquire Q-fever primarily by inhaling the aerosolized organism.[1,2] The infectious dose is extremely low; a single bacterium may lead to infection in 50% of people (ID_{50} = 1 organism). Concentrations of the organism in a single gram of placental tissue may be as high as 10^9. Infected livestock, even if asymptomatic, shed large numbers of organisms in placental tissues and body fluids including milk, urine, and feces. The spore-like form of *C. burnetii* can persist in the environment for mos making it highly suitable for aerosol delivery (weaponization). Direct exposure to aerosols, or to sites contaminated by them, is a significant risk factor. Farmers, abattoir workers, and hunters are at greatest risk. *C. burnetii* is also a significant hazard for the lab personnel who work with it.

History & Significance

Q-fever was first described in 1935 in Brisbane, Australia, by Edward Holbrook Derrick after an outbreak of febrile illness among abattoir workers. It was called "Query fever" because the causative agent was initially unknown. No diagnosis could be made based on the varied patient histories, physical exam findings and investigations. In 1937, Australian researchers Frank Macfarlane Burnet and Mavis Freeman identified a fastidious, intracellular bacterium in guinea pigs that had been injected with body fluids from Derrick's patients. Almost at the same time, in the US, a rickettsia-like bacterium was isolated from ticks by Herald Cox. These agents were later determined to be identical. Burnet was first to isolate and describe the organism in 1937, and Cox described vector transmission from ticks in 1938. Owing to the transmission properties described above, the US, UK, and USSR researched, weaponized and stockpiled *C. burnetii* during the Cold War.

C. burnetii is currently classified by the CDC as a Category B pathogen (see Appendix B). Even with low mortality and moderate morbidity rates, the number of individuals seeking treatment (required or not) could be immense. During 2007-2010, the largest Q-fever natural outbreak ever reported involved ~ 4,000 human cases in the Netherlands.[5,6] Dairy goat farms, located near densely populated areas, were the presumed source of human exposures via the windborne route. In the most affected areas, up to 15% of the population was involved with a hospitalization rate of 20% of known cases. This outbreak is expected to result in more cases of chronic Q fever among cases and risk groups in the coming years. Additionally, a substantial number of acute Q-fever cases have been reported in both US and UK military personnel during deployments in support of Operation Iraqi Freedom and Operation Enduring Freedom.[2,7-9,11] Tick bites, sleeping in barns, and environmental exposure due to helicopter-generated (prop blast) aerosols have been linked to these cases.

Clinical Features

As Derrick discovered when attempting to diagnose the original patients, it is really not possible to describe a "normal" clinical presentation of the disease. A health care provider will likely be forced to make a presumptive diagnosis that includes Q-fever as a "rule out". With varying incubation periods (generally 2 or 3 wks) highly dependent on the size of the inoculum, and a vague flu-like illness being the most common presentation in acute cases, a clinical diagnosis without additional diagnostic testing is exceptionally difficult. For naturally occurring outbreaks, in which numbers of human cases are typically low (the recent Dutch epidemic notwithstanding), the majority of cases may go undiagnosed. Approximately 75% of outbreak victims have been male, with a preponderance in those over 15 yrs of age. With the intentional release of large numbers of bacteria, there may be more uniformity in the clinical presentations, as there is expected to be some correlation between the severity and physical manifestation of disease to this route and magnitude of exposure.

Acute Q-fever: Historically, up to 60% of acute infections show no clinical sign of disease. This may not hold true in an intentional release, as the exposure levels are potentially much higher. In natural outbreaks, 40% develop a non-specific flu-like illness, which can include severe headache, joint and/or muscle pain, and fever.[1, 3] Fever is variable, lasting mos in untreated patients, but otherwise reaching a peak of 102-105° F° after 3 d, then returning abruptly to normal after 5 to 14 d in treated individuals. The severe headache may radiate to the jaw mimicking migraine or toothache. Pneumonia (with or without pleural effusion) is an important clinical manifestation in acute cases and may be accompanied by a cough (often productive).[1] Hepatitis (ALP, ALT, and AST reaching 2-3X ULN) is also a common clinical finding. Weight loss may occur due to non-specific gastrointestinal illness (e.g., diarrhea, vomiting). Up to 20% of adults (and 50% of children) will develop a skin rash.[1] Overall, however, infected children are less likely to have symptoms and have a milder illness. Around 2% of acute cases will develop myocarditis (± pericarditis and pericardial effusion), which is their leading cause of death. Less frequent acute manifestations include aseptic meningitis and encephalitis, orchitis, lymphadenopathy, bone marrow necrosis, and cholecystitis. Abortion is virtually inevitable if infection occurs during the first trimester of pregnancy.[1, 12]

Chronic Q-fever is uncommon (< 10% of acute cases), but is potentially a much more serious condition than the acute form. It manifests from a few mos to 20 yrs or so following an acute infection. Individuals with pre-existing heart disease (especially mitral and/or aortic insufficiency, mitral or aortic prosthesis, and arterial aneurysms) are pre-disposed to developing endocarditis, the most serious complication of chronic Q fever which, if left untreated, is usually fatal.[1, 2, 12-14] In addition to valvulopathies, pregnancy and immunosuppression are known risk factors for chronic disease. Other reported chronic manifestations include chronic hepatitis, chronic vascular infections, osteomyelitis, osteoarthritis, and chronic pulmonary infections. Although rare, osteomyelitis is one of the most frequent sequelae in children.[15] Chronic Q-fever may also result in abortion, premature birth, or low birth weight, if the disease recrudesces during pregnancy.

Diagnosis

The Q-fever differential diagnosis is extensive due to its vague clinical symptomatology. A characteristic pattern of cases associated with a geographic area or compressed time period should raise suspicion. For military personnel, other bio-agents that have overlapping symptoms should be also considered (e.g., anthrax and plague and tularemia pneumonias). Definitive diagnosis requires laboratory testing. Any potential amplification of *C. burnetii* must be performed in a BSL-3 facility due to its highly infective nature.

Serology: Indirect immunofluorescence assay (IFA) is the current reference method for diagnosis of Q-fever.[1,2] Serum antibody detection, in addition to allowing for disease identification, may be useful in determining if the disease is acute or chronic. Serologic testing should be obtained at time of clinical presentation and 4 to 6 wks later (convalescent samples); patients with negative convalescent samples should not be diagnosed with Q fever.[2] Seroconversion, or a fourfold rise in titer (which requires a baseline and repeat testing in 2 to 4 wks), indicates an acute infection.[1,2]

Two antigenic phases of *C. burnetii* infections exist: phase I (virulent) and phase II (avirulent).[1,2] Acute Q-fever cases usually exhibit a much higher antibody level to phase II antigen (first detected during the second week of illness). Specific IgM against phase II antigen may be detectable as early as the second week after onset of illness, with a concomitant increase in phase II IgG, and remain elevated for up to 3 mos. Combined detection of IgM, IgA, and IgG improves assay specificity and provides accuracy in diagnosis. Antibodies to phase I antigens of *C. burnetii* generally take longer to appear and indicate continued exposure to bacteria. High levels of antibody to phase I in later isolates in conjunction with constant or falling levels of antibody to phase II suggest chronic Q-fever (Table 1). Antibodies to phase I and II antigens may persist for mos or yrs after initial infection. Elevated IgG of > 1:200 and IgM > 1:25 to phase II also supports an acute infection.[1] In chronic disease states, a 1:800 to 1024 IgG or > 1:59 IgA against phase I antigen suggest a chronic infection exists. In some chronic cases, phase II IgG titers equal or exceed phase I IgG titers; however, this is generally an exception. An ELISA is available at USAMRIID in which a single serum specimen can be used to reliably diagnose acute Q-fever as early as 10 to 14 d into illness.

Table 1. Antibodies generally present during acute and chronic Q-fever infection

	IgA Phase		IgM Phase		IgG Phase	
Infection Stage	I	II	I	II	I	II
Acute			X	X		X
Chronic	X				X	

PCR detection (conventional, Light-Cycler Nested, or real time) allows for rapid, sensitive and specific detection of *C. burnetii* origin DNA in samples ranging from serum to whole blood (in anticoagulant tubes) to tissue biopsies (to include excised heart valves).[1,2] As there are usually bacteria present in the serum in acute infection, PCR allows for detection well before serum antibodies against Q-fever emerge. Therefore, *C. burnetti* DNA may be detected by real time PCR (RT-PCR) prior to positive serology. In chronic Q fever cases, PCR can be performed on CSF, pleural fluid, bone marrow, bone marrow biopsies, and liver biopsies.

Culture should be performed in dedicated bio-containment laboratories. Isolating the bacterium from tissue samples is highly specific, but the process lacks sensitivity.[1, 2] Standard plate or liquid media will not support the growth of *C. burnetii*, as the bacterium is an obligate intracellular organism and requires mammalian cells to replicate. Bacterial isolation and amplification may be carried out using HEL cells and Shell Vial centrifugation. Blood cultures on standard media are invariably negative, as *C. burnetii* will only grow in living cells or organisms. In patients with chronic Q-fever endocarditis, routine blood cultures are negative.

Blood chemistry/CBC: CBC is usually unremarkable; leukocytosis being an exception (14 to 21×10^9/L) in about 25% of cases. Thrombocytopenia may also be seen in up to a third of patients in the acute phase, with thrombocytosis developing during the recovery phase. ESR typically is mildly elevated. Abnormal liver enzymes are the most common abnormal blood chemistry finding, showing a 2- or 3-fold elevation in ALP and the transaminases in up to 85% of patients.[1, 16] Bilirubin is usually normal. Hepatitis patients, and those with chronic Q-fever, frequently have circulating autoantibodies, including anti-smooth muscle, anti-cardiolipin, anti-phospholipid, anti-clotting factor (liver biopsy may risk hemorrhage), and antinuclear antibodies. Endocarditis usually causes a significantly elevated ESR, often with anemia, thrombocytopenia, and polyclonal hypergammaglobulinemia. Mild lymphocytic pleocytosis is common in the CSF of patients with meningoencephalitis.

Imaging studies: CXR is non-specific and may be normal in up to 10% of those with acute Q-fever. Pleural effusions are rare. Pericardial effusion may suggest pericarditis and/or myocarditis. A transesophageal echocardiogram (TEE) and/or transthoracic echocardiogram (TTE) help identify non-asymptomatic heart disease that could pre-dispose individuals to develop chronic Q-fever especially if valvular defects are suspected.[2] Though TEEs are more sensitive, TTEs should be considered in patients with acute Q fever, especially those with significant murmurs on physical exam or with a history of valvulopathy. TEE, more sensitive in finding small subendothelial valvular lesions, should be performed in patients with negative or inconclusive TTE findings but still suspected of endocarditis. Negative TTE or TEE should not rule out a diagnosis of chronic Q fever endocarditis.[1, 2] Sonography may reveal granulomatous lesions, particularly of the liver, even in asymptomatic patients.

Other studies: Sputum examination is unremarkable even in patients with productive cough. Liver or bone biopsies in patients with hepatitis or osteomyelitis, respectively, may reveal non-specific granulomas. Generally, *C. burnetti* antigen will not be detected by immunohistochemistry but should still be considered with microscopic examination. However, in chronic cases, immunohistochemistry performed on heart valve specimens may detect *C. burnetti* antigen in patients with culture negative endocarditis.[1]

Medical Management

An infectious disease (ID) specialist should be consulted in any patient, especially one with a history of acute Q fever. Standard precautions are recommended for HCWs dealing with suspected or confirmed cases.

Acute Q-fever

Adults: The treatment of choice is doxycycline 100 mg PO twice q12 h for > 14 d.[1,2,14] Moxifloxacin 400 mg q d for 14 d could be used as an alternative. These are most effective if begun within 3 d of the onset of symptoms. Relapse is not uncommon and may be associated with an antibiotic regimen discontinued within 2 wks. Treatment is not beneficial after the symptoms of acute infection have resolved and, therefore, should not be administered then. In cases with known valvulopathy or such discovered on exam, 12 mos of prophylactic therapy with hydroxychloroquine (HCQ) and doxy should be considered following consultation with an ID specialist.[2] TMP-SMX is used for acute symptomatic Q fever in pregnant women and children (an ID specialist should be consulted for dosage and length or treatment during pregnancy). Follow-up serological testing is recommended in all patients treated for acute Q fever. Pregnant women diagnosed with acute Q fever should be treated with TMP-SMX throughout the duration of the pregnancy.

Children aged < 8 yrs with uncomplicated acute Q-fever may be treated with TMP-SMX or a shorter duration (5 d) of doxy.[1]

Chronic Q-fever

Due to variation in the acute and chronic clinical course, disease severity, immune and valvular status, and an individual's response to treatment, successful treatment of chronic Q-fever is difficult and should be done in conjunction with an ID specialist. Doxy 100 mg PO q 12 h, with HCQ 200 mg PO tid, for > 18 mos is recommended for adults, especially those with endocarditis.[1,2] A similar approach is recommended with osteoarticular infections with surgical debridement. Routine eye examinations should be performed to monitor for HCQ- and doxy-associated ocular toxicity (e.g., photosensitivity and hypersensitivity to sunlight) or visual field changes.[2,17] Alternatively, combination therapy of doxy with a fluoroquinolone has been evaluated; but may not be as effective (i.e. more relapses) when compared to the doxy/HCQ combo. Due to the *in utero* effects of TMP-SMX and doxy, acute Q-fever infection during pregnancy requires special attention. These women should have specific serum antibody titers determined post-partum; then those with evidence of chronic Q-fever are often treated with > 12 mos of doxy and HCQ.[1,2] For all forms of chronic Q-fever, specific serum antibody titers are followed; but the optimum length of serologic follow-up remains to be determined. The current recommendation in cases of proven Q-fever endocarditis is serologic testing for 5 yrs (or longer) based on the individual's response to therapy.[2,15,16] A four-fold decrease in the phase I IgG and IgA titers and the disappearance of phase II IgM at 1 yr have been suggested as evidence of cure.

Long term sequelae

A chronic fatigue syndrome has been reported as a possible long-term complication of acute Q-fever infection.[1] It may include fatigue, muscle and joint pain, night sweats and behavioral changes (mood and sleep patterns) and may strike up to 20% of those with a history of acute infection. Specific organ involvement is not apparent, nor has the pathogenesis been elucidated. Diagnosis is based on characteristic clinical signs > 1 yr after acute Q fever infection with adequate treatment, elevated antibody titers, and absence of clinical and lab evidence of chronic Q fever (with organ involvement).[1] Treatment is largely symptomatic and may require a combination of physical and pharmacological interventions.

Prophylaxis

Immunoprophylaxis: A licensed Q-fever vaccine (*Q-Vax*) for humans is available in Australia and Eastern Europe[1, 20]. It is not commercially available in the US where most workers in high-risk occupations are not vaccinated. Administration in already immune or pre-sensitized individuals may cause severe local induration, sterile abscess formation, and necrosis at the inoculation site. Determination of prior exposure is accomplished by an intradermal skin test using 0.02 mg of vaccine. Vaccination with a single dose of this killed suspension of *C. burnetii* provides complete protection against naturally occurring Q-fever, and > 95% protection against aerosol exposure. Protection lasts for > 5 yrs. A formalin-inactivated whole cell IND vaccine for humans is available in the US for at-risk personnel on an investigational basis only; it is managed at USAMRIID. (There are no approved veterinary Q-fever vaccines in the US, although two are commercially available in Europe.)

Chemoprophylaxis, begun 8 to 12 d post-exposure, has been considered effective—either doxycycline 100 mg PO q 12 h, or tetracycline 500 mg PO q6 h, for 5 to 7 d. For pregnant women, although there are no official guidelines, TMP-SMX (160 mg/800 mg PO bid) may be considered for the duration of the pregnancy. Based on a 1956 challenge trial, however, it is believed that commencing prophylaxis within 7 d of exposure is not effective and may prolong the onset of clinical disease.[21] (Such prophylaxis prevented symptomatic illness—but not infection—in this study.) Whether chemoprophylaxis after an episode of Q-fever decreases the incidence of endocarditis in high-risk patients is not known.

In 2013, based on the weakness of the available data, the CDC's Q-fever Working Group failed to endorse the use of chemoprophylaxis for lab workers after a known or potential exposure. The use of PEP after a bio-terrorism release of *C. burnetii*—provided that the timing of exposure were known—has received some support from authorities.[22] However, even this was questioned by the CDC WG and the benefit of any kind of PEP against *C. burnetii* was repudiated.[1]

Isolation, Decon & Control

Standard precautions alone are recommended for HCWs dealing with suspected or confirmed cases. Patients are not required to wear masks. For autopsies, or when handling surgical or tissue biopsies, precautions should be taken to prevent aerosolization of body fluids. Q-fever is primarily considered to be a zoonotic disease, with human-to-human, or tick-to-human transmission very rare. The spore form of the organism is very hardy and can survive for yrs in the environment. It can probably survive direct UV light, dilute bleach and typical disinfectants. Autoclaving and boiling for 10 min will kill the organism in samples no longer needed. Culturing of the organism requires a BSL-3 facility.

Decontamination may be attempted with a 1:100 *Lysol* solution, 1% sodium hypochlorite solution, 5% hydrogen peroxide, or 70% ethanol. The M291 skin decontamination kit will not neutralize the organism.

Human Q fever infection is a notifiable disease in the U.S. Surveillance and reporting of Q fever are essential components of public health education and disease prevention efforts. As with many zoonotic outbreaks, investigations must be coordinated with animal health authorities to determine whether the source is naturally occurring or the result of an intentional release.[1] Animal health authorities can also help to control outbreaks that may be propagated by intentionally or unintentionally infected livestock sources, and ensure that dairy products are pasteurized and from approved sources.

Tularemia

Summary

Signs and symptoms: Historically, tularemia has been characterized as either an "ulceroglandular" or a "typhoidal" syndrome. Typhoidal tularemia presents with fever, chills, headache, malaise, and often a non-productive cough and chest discomfort, but without an obvious portal of entry. Ulceroglandular tularemia presents similar systemic symptoms, but includes an obvious portal of entry, usually a local ulcer with regional lymphadenopathy. Other clinical forms are known to exist.

Diagnosis: The large differential diagnosis involving both typhoidal and pneumonic syndromes make the initial approach difficult. CXR may reveal a pneumonic process, hilar lymphadenopathy, or pleural effusion. Routine culture (blood, sputum, ulcers and pharyngeal sites) is definitive, but requires precautions. Presumptive tests include direct fluorescence antibody (DFA) and PCR. The diagnosis can be established retrospectively by serology.

Treatment: Early treatment with parenteral antibiotics (streptomycin or gentamicin) is very effective for naturally acquired disease.

Prophylaxis: Following exposure to a susceptible strain, a 2 wk course of doxycycline or ciprofloxacin can be administered orally as post-exposure prophylaxis. For at-risk workers, a live-attenuated vaccine is available, but only through an IND protocol.

Isolation and decontamination: Standard precautions are recommended for healthcare workers. Organisms are relatively easy to render harmless by heat and standard disinfectants.

Overview

Francisella tularensis, the causative agent of tularemia, is a small, aerobic non-motile, gram-negative coccobacillus. Tularemia—also known as "rabbit fever" and "deer fly fever"—is a zoonotic disease that humans can acquire by several routes; it can present with different clinical syndromes, all of which usually include systemic symptoms (described below). Tularemia can present as ulceroglandular disease ("glandular" refers to regional lymphadenopathy) following skin or mucous membranes contact with tissues or body fluids of infected animals (e.g., rabbits), or from bites of infected arthropods (e.g., ticks, deerflies, or—only in Eurasia—mosquitoes). Less commonly, it can present as typhoidal disease in which a clinically obvious portal of entry is absent. As part of typhoidal disease, pneumonia may occur after apparent inhalation of contaminated aerosols. Typhoidal disease may also occur after apparent ingestion of contaminated foods or water.[1, 2, 3, 5]

F. tularensis is found throughout the temperate northern hemisphere and it typically causes only sporadic human disease (~ 125 cases/yr in the US).[6] It exists in at least two variants, or biovars: Biovar A, the more virulent form which is the predominant cause of human disease in North America; and Biovar B, a less virulent form which predominates in northern Europe and Asia.[3] Organisms can remain viable for long periods in water, mud, and animal carcasses even if frozen.[5] They are easily killed by heat and disinfectants.[7]

History & Significance

F. tularensis was identified as a distinct organism in 1911 during an investigation of a plague-like disease in ground squirrels in Tulare County, California. A US Public Health Service physician, Edward Francis, established the cause of the "deer fly fever" as *Bacterium tularense* and subsequently devoted his life to researching the organism and disease[8]; hence the organism was later renamed *Francisella tularensis*. During the German siege of Stalingrad in WWII, there were perhaps hundreds of thousands of human cases, many of which were pneumonic, leading to speculation that the epidemic may have resulted from the Soviet Union's intentional use of tularemia as a biological weapon. However, in the area before the siege, an ongoing epizootic in rodents was in progress and thousands of human cases were documented. These facts and the harsh local conditions predisposing to disease spread suggest a likely natural cause for this epidemic.[9]

F. tularensis was successfully weaponized by both the US and the USSR during the early Cold War (late 1940s and '50s).[3] Indeed, it was a particularly virulent American strain that the Soviets weaponized after it was given to them by US scientists in 1949, before relations significantly worsened. Ironically, the tularemia vaccine later developed in the US (known as LVS) was built upon a strain obtained from the Soviets in the 1950s.[4]

Clinical Features

After an incubation period of 3 to 6 d (range 1-21 d; a shorter incubation period is likely associated with a higher infectious dose), onset is usually acute. Tularemia may appear in any of several forms, which can generally be grouped as either typhoidal or ulceroglandular.[1] In humans, as few as 10 organisms will cause disease if injected intradermally, 10 to 50 organisms cause illness via inhalation, whereas ~ 10^8 organisms are required with oral ingestion.[5]

Typhoidal tularemia (~25% of naturally acquired cases) occurs mainly after inhalation of infectious aerosols but can occur after any route of exposure (i.e., intradermal or GI exposure). The disease manifests as a nonspecific syndrome consisting of abrupt onset of fever (38-40°C), chills, headache, cough, myalgias, and malaise; but unlike most other forms of tularemia, it presents without an obvious portal of entry or peripheral lymphadenopathy. Occasionally patients will present with nausea, vomiting, diarrhea, or abdominal pain. Case fatality rates (CFRs) may be 30–60% in untreated naturally acquired cases, but 1–3% with optimal treatment. Survivors of untreated tularemia may have symptoms which persist for wks to mos with progressive debilitation. Fatality is higher if pneumonia is also present; the pneumonic form of disease would most likely occur after an aerosol bio-warfare attack. Severe typhoidal disease may be complicated by meningitis, pericarditis, endocarditis, or septicemia; renal and hepatic damage may also occur.[3, 5]

Ulceroglandular tularemia (~75% of naturally acquired cases) is most often acquired through inoculation of the skin or mucous membranes with blood or tissue fluids of infected animals, or by a bite of an infected insect. It is usually characterized by systemic symptoms as described above for typhoidal disease, along with the concurrent appearance of a painful papule at the site of inoculation. The papule progresses rapidly to pustule, then a painful ulcer, and is accompanied by development of painful regional lymphadenopathy. Enlarged nodes can become fluctuant and spontaneously drain even when the patient has been taking antibiotics, and if untreated, can persist for mos or even yrs.[1]

In a small minority of cases the site of primary inoculation is the eye (***oculoglandular disease***); this occurs after inoculation of the conjunctivae by contaminated hands, by splattering of infected tissue fluids, or via infectious aerosols. Patients have unilateral painful purulent conjunctivitis with preauricular or cervical lymphadenopathy. Chemosis, periorbital edema, and small nodular granulomatous lesions or ulcerations of the conjunctiva are noted in some patients.[3, 5]

Pharyngitis can occur in up to 25% of patients with tularemia (i.e., ***oropharyngeal disease***), and may follow ingestion of contaminated food or water. It usually presents as an acute exudative pharyngitis or tonsillitis, sometimes with ulceration, and associated painful cervical lymphadenopathy.[1] It may occur as a syndrome of penicillin-unresponsive pharyngitis and be mistaken for infectious mononucleosis or other viral pharyngitis.[5]

Pulmonary involvement is seen on CXR in ~ 45% of naturally occurring cases of tularemia.[1,10] Clinically, it may vary from asymptomatic or mild or to severe or fulminant. Manifestations may include non-productive cough, pleuritic chest pain, and dyspnea; purulent sputum or hemoptysis are uncommon. 30% of patients with CXR findings, however, may be asymptomatic. Pulmonary involvement is most common in typhoidal tularemia (83% of cases), in part indicating direct inhalation of organisms, but it is seen in 31% of ulceroglandular disease, likely indicating hematogenous seeding of the lungs.[1] Untreated, tularemic pneumonia may have CFRs approaching 60%.

Diagnosis

Clinical approach. A clue to the diagnosis of tularemia after a bio-warfare attack with *F. tularensis* might be a large number of temporally clustered patients presenting with similar nonspecific febrile systemic illnesses progressing rapidly to life-threatening pleuropneumonitis.[3] Some patients may exhibit a temperature/pulse mismatch (Faget sign; seen in up to 40% in naturally acquired disease). The fever and other systemic features classically respond dramatically (within 24 to 48 h) to administration of an appropriate antibiotic. (Patients may remain febrile for weeks, however, if treated with [for example] a penicillin or cephalosporin alone.)

A CXR is mandatory in patients for whom systemic tularemia is suspected, even in the absence of pulmonary symptoms or findings. CXR patterns may include: pulmonary infiltrates (unilobar or multilobar/diffuse), pleural effusion, hilar adenopathy, or, less commonly, an oval density or cavitation.[5, 10]

In an isolated case, the differential diagnosis of tularemic pneumonia is large and includes both typhoidal syndromes (e.g., typhoid fever, rickettsia, or malaria) and pneumonic processes (e.g., pneumonic plague, influenza, Q-fever, SEB intoxication, and various causes of community acquired pneumonia [*Mycoplasma pneumoniae, Chlamydophila pneumoniae*, psittacosis, legionellosis, and others]). Inhalational anthrax and pulmonary TB should also be considered, along with other viral and fungal lung infections.[3,5] Even after an aerosol bio-warfare attack, a subset of patients would also be expected to present with ulceroglandular disease.

Laboratory diagnosis. Initial clinical lab findings are generally nonspecific. Peripheral WBC counts usually range from 5,000 to 22,000 cells per microliter. Differential cell counts may be normal however lymphocytosis may be seen. Hematocrit, hemoglobin, and platelet levels are usually normal. Mild elevations in lactose dehydrogenase, serum transaminases, and alkaline phosphatase are common. Rhabdomyolysis may be associated with elevations in serum creatine kinase and urinary myoglobin levels.[1]

Tularemia can be definitively diagnosed by recovering the organism in culture from blood, ulcers, conjunctival exudates, pharyngeal exudates, sputum, gastric washings, and CSF. Recovery may even be possible after the institution of appropriate antibiotic therapy. However, unless tularemia is suspected, delays in diagnosis are probable as the organism grows poorly on standard media. It produces small, smooth, opaque colonies after 48 to 72 h on media containing cysteine or other sulfhydryl compounds (e.g., glucose cysteine blood agar, thioglycollate broth). Physicians, however, should notify the lab that tularemia is suspected so that special precautions can be taken. Since culturing the organism can present a hazard to laboratory personnel, definit-ive isolation should be attempted only in a Level B laboratory with BSL-3 containment.[3, 11] Thus state health authorities, or if unavailable the CDC (at 800-CDC-INFO; 800-232-4636), should be contacted to receive specimens.

A presumptive diagnosis of tularemia can be made by examining specimens using special techniques such PCR or direct immunofluorescence immunoassay (DFA).[3]

Diagnosis of tularemia can also be confirmed serologically (bacterial agglutination or ELISA) by showing a 4-fold rise in antibody titer between specimens collected at presentation and again > 2 wks later. Because of the time delay, serology is usually not useful to immediately confirm the diagnosis.[3] Antibodies to *F. tularensis* appear within the first week of infection but levels adequate to allow confidence in the specificity of the serologic diagnosis (titer > 1:160) do not appear until > 2 wks after infection. Because cross-reactions can occur with *Brucella* spp., *Proteus* OX19, and *Yersinia* organisms and because antibodies may persist for years after infection, diagnosis should be made only if a 4-fold or greater increase in the tularemia tube agglutination or microagglutination titer is seen during the course of the illness. Titers are usually negative the first week of infection, positive the second week in 50-70% of cases and reach a maximum in 4-8 wks.

Medical Management

Treatment. Initial empiric therapy for systemic disease caused by *F. tularensis* includes at least one of the following antibiotics.[3]

Preferred:

- Streptomycin[*,†], 1 g IM bid (15 mg/kg IM bid for children), or
- Gentamicin[†] 5 mg/kg IM or IV qd (2.5 mg/kg IM or IV q8 h for children), or

Alternatives:

- Doxycycline[‡], 100 mg IV q12 h for adults or children ≥ 45 kg (2.2 mg/kg IV q12 h for children < 45 kg), or
- Ciprofloxacin[†] 400 mg IV q12 h for adults (for children use 15-20 mg/g IV q12 h [up to 1 g/d]), or
- Chloramphenicol[‡], 15-25 mg/kg IV q6 h

IV antibiotics can be switched to the oral route following improvement in the patient's course. Length of therapy depends upon the antibiotic used. Streptomycin, gentamicin, and ciprofloxacin should be continued for > 10 d. Doxycycline has been associated with relapse and should be continued for 14 to 21 d (or longer). Chloramphenicol (at a higher dose, along with streptomycin) is usually reserved to

---

* Streptomycin his historically been the drug of choice for tularemia and is the only aminoglycoside antibiotic approved by the FDA for treatment of tularemia; however, because it may not be readily available immediately after a large-scale bio-warfare attack, gentamicin and other alternative drugs should be considered first.

† Streptomycin, gentamicin, and ciprofloxacin are bacteriocidal.

‡ Doxycycline and chloramphenicol are bacteriostatic.

treat meningitis.[5] Since the intentional use of tularemia as a bio-weapon could employ a strain of organism that is resistant to our preferred antibiotics, testing the strain for antibiotic susceptibilities is paramount. A clinical clue to resistance would be failure of the patient to improve dramatically after 24 to 48 h of appropriate antibiotics.[3]

Infection control. As there are apparently no documented cases of human-to-human transmission of tularemia, neither isolation nor quarantine is necessary. Standard precautions are appropriate for care of patients including those with pneumonia or draining lesions.[11] Heat and disinfectants easily inactivate the organism.[7]

Prophylaxis

Vaccine. A live-attenuated tularemia vaccine (Live Vaccine Strain, or LVS) has been offered to at-risk workers since the 1960s under an IND protocol with informed consent. Administered by scarification, it has been given to > 5,000 persons without significant adverse reactions. It prevents typhoidal, and ameliorates ulceroglandular, forms of lab-acquired tularemia. It has been associated with a marked decrease in the incidence of such infections compared to historical controls.[13] Currently, no licensed tularemia vaccine is available in the US or EU.

Immunoprophylaxis. There is no passive immunoprophylaxis (i.e., specific parenteral immune globulin) available for pre- or post-exposure management of tularemia.

Pre-exposure chemoprophylaxis. No antibiotics are licensed by the FDA for use before exposure to tularemia. Based on *in vitro* susceptibilities, however, cipro or doxy may offer protection.

Post-exposure chemoprophylaxis. Initial empiric PEP against *F. tularensis* includes one of the following antibiotics.[3]

Preferred:

- Doxycycline 100 mg PO bid for adults and children ≥ 45 kg (for children < 45 kg use 2.2 mg/kg PO bid), or
- Ciprofloxacin 500 mg PO bid for adults (15-20 mg/kg PO bid (up to 1 g/d) for children)

PEP should ideally begin within 24 h of exposure and continue for > 14 d. These oral antibiotic dosages may also be appropriate for treatment in mass casualty settings in which the optimal drugs, IV antibiotics, are not available in quantity.

Chemoprophylaxis is generally not recommended after potential natural (tick bite, rabbit, or other animal) exposures.

VIRAL AGENTS

Viruses are considered the smallest and simplest infectious agents, excepting possibly prions, and consist only of genetic material, either RNA or DNA, surrounded by a protein coat. In some cases, the virion (viral particle) is also surrounded by an outer lipid bilayer. Viruses are much smaller than bacteria, varying in size from 0.02 μm to 0.2 μm (1 μm = 1/1000 mm). They are intracellular parasites and lack a system for their own metabolism. Therefore, they require host cell synthetic machinery for replication and survival, which means that, unlike bacteria, viruses cannot be cultivated in synthetic nutritive solutions.

The origins of viruses in evolutionary history are unclear: some may have evolved from plasmids—fragments of DNA that move between cells—while others may have developed from bacteria. Viruses spread in several ways: they are often transmitted from plant to plant by insects that feed on sap; among animals they can be transmitted by blood-sucking insects. (Such disease-bearing organisms are known as *vectors.*) Influenza and smallpox viruses are spread when coughing or sneezing aerosolizes them into suspended "droplet nuclei" impervious to gravity, which are then inhaled deeply into lungs. Norovirus and rotavirus, common causes of viral gastroenteritis, are transmitted by the fecal–oral route and are passed from person to person by contact, entering the body in food or water. Others are transmitted through sexual contact and by exposure to infected blood.

The types of host cells that viruses infect include animal, plant, and even bacteria. Because a very specific interaction occurs between the virus and the host cell, every virus requires its own special type of host cell for replication. Virus replication usually brings about changes in the host cell that eventually lead to cell death. Viral infections in animals and humans typically provoke an immune response that eliminates the infecting virus. (Immune responses can also be deliberately produced by vaccines, which confer an artificially acquired immunity to a specific viral infection.) However, some viruses, including those that cause AIDS and viral hepatitis, evade these immune responses and result in chronic infections. Antibiotics, developed to kill or impede bacteria, have no effect on viruses, but several effective antivirals have been developed and received widespread use.

A number of viruses have been weaponized by major state bio-weapons programs of the past. During the Cold War, the former US and UK bio-warfare programs weaponized Venezuelian equine encephalitis (VEE) virus. In addition to VEE, the Soviet Union is known to have maintained smallpox and Marburg virus stockpiles. This handbook covers three types of viruses which could potentially be employed as bio-agents: smallpox, alphaviruses (e.g., VEE), and the hemorrhagic fever viruses (e.g., Ebola, Marburg).

Smallpox (*Variola*)

Summary

Signs and symptoms begin with malaise, fever, rigors, vomiting, headache, and backache. Two to 3 d later, skin lesions appear, quickly progress (more or less simultaneously) from macules to papules, and eventually to pustular vesicles. They are "centrifugal" (more abundant on the extremities and face than the trunk).

Diagnosis, initially, must be clinical. Neither electron nor light microscopy is capable of discriminating *Variola* (smallpox) from vaccinia, monkeypox, or cowpox. Vaccinia and cowpox disease in humans are typically localized and self-limiting except in the immune compromised or those with some other underlying conditions (i.e. eczema). Variola and monkeypox viruses typically cause widespread systemic disease. Clinical management of suspected monkeypox is the same as for smallpox. PCR is accurate in discriminating *Variola* from other orthopoxviruses.

Treatment: At present, there is no FDA-approved chemotherapy for any orthopoxvirus. Currently, three IND products — cidofovir, CMX001, and ST-246 — have demonstrated efficacy in *Orthopox* virus animal models including *Variola* and have been used to treat disseminated vaccinia infection under an emergency IND (EIND). Thus, treatment remains mainly supportive.

Prophylaxis: Immediate vaccination or revaccination should be instituted for all personnel exposed to smallpox virus. This is most effective during the first 4 d after exposure.

Isolation and decontamination: Patients should be considered infectious from the onset of a rash until all scabs have separated and should be isolated under both contact and airborne precautions. Strict quarantine of asymptomatic contacts for 17 d after exposure may be advisable but could prove difficult to enforce. A reasonable alternative would be to require contacts to check their temperatures daily. Any fever above 38°C (101°F) during the 17 d after exposure to a confirmed smallpox case would suggest secondary infection. The febrile contact should then be isolated immediately, ideally at home, until the diagnosis is either confirmed or ruled out. Isolation should continue until all scabs have separated.

Overview

Smallpox was caused by an *Orthopoxvirus* called *Variola.* Two strains existed, *Variola major*—with a fatality rate of 10 to 30%—and the milder *Variola minor,* which killed < 1% of its victims.[1] Following aerosol exposure, droplet nuclei containing virus were inhaled into the lower respiratory tract, travelled to regional lymph nodes, and there replicated causing primary viremia and systemic disease. Despite global eradication of smallpox and continued availability of a vaccine, the potential weaponization of

Variola may continue to pose a military or terrorist threat. Of special concern are the aerosol infectivity of the virus, the relative ease of large-scale virus production, and an increasingly *Orthopoxvirus*-naive populace. Although the fully developed cutaneous eruption of smallpox is unique, earlier stages of the rash could be mistaken for chicken pox (varicella). Secondary spread would constitute a nosocomial hazard from the time of onset of a patient's exanthem until the scabs have separated.[2] Quarantine is recommended for secondary contacts for 17 d post-exposure. Vaccination and vaccinia immune globulin each possess some efficacy in post-exposure prophylaxis.[3] Three antivirals (cidofovir, ST-246 and CMX001), currently IND products, may also be of benefit, but are not currently licensed and would have to be used under an EIND.[4]

History & Significance

Smallpox, an ancient disease, was responsible for an estimated 300–500 million deaths worldwide during the 20th century. Earlier, smallpox-laden objects are believed to have been used by the British Army as a crude bio-weapon against Native Americans and, later, the rebelling American colonials feared its use by the British during the American Revolution.[5] The United States studied smallpox virus as a possible bio-weapon during the 1950s and '60s and the Soviet Union produced and stockpiled massive weaponized quantities of it for this use.

Endemic smallpox was declared eradicated in 1980 by the World Health Organization (WHO) after an immense vaccination effort.[1] Although two WHO-approved repositories of *Variola* virus remain at the Centers for Disease Control and Prevention (CDC) in Atlanta and at the Russian State Centre for Research on Virology and Biotechnology (Koltsovo, Novosibirsk Region) Russian Federation, the extent of clandestine stockpiles and misplaced samples in other parts of the world remains unknown.[6] The WHO Advisory Committee on *Variola* virus research has recommended repeatedly that all stocks of smallpox be destroyed. However, destruction has been deferred periodically since 1986 by the WHO Health Assembly due to concerns over the need for further study of the virus given its potential as a bio-agent.[3]

The US military ended routine smallpox vaccination in 1989, but began again in 2003 for troops deployed to Southwest Asia and the Republic of Korea. Routine civilian vaccination in the US was discontinued in 1972. Thus most of the American, and indeed the world, population is now susceptible to infection with *Variola* or any other orthopox virus.

The full-length sequences of several *Variola* strains have been published. Rapid advances in synthetic biology now make it at least theoretically possible to reconstruct *Variola* solely from fragments produced utilizing a DNA synthesizer. The construction of a *Mycoplasma* organism as well as a polio virus (the former with a genome three times larger than *Variola*) has demonstrated the feasibility of such an accomplishment. Thus, the old strategy of closely supervising existing stocks of *Variola* no longer ensures that a determined and sophisticated adversary could not produce and use a smallpox bio-weapon.[7, 8]

Clinical Features

The incubation period of naturally acquired smallpox averages 12 d, although it can range from 7 to 19 d after exposure. After the primary viremia, virus disseminates to other lymphoid tissues, spleen, liver, bone marrow, and lung and causes a secondary viremia. Clinical manifestations begin with malaise, high fever (to 104° F), rigors, vomiting, headache, backache, and prostration; 15% of patients develop delirium. Approximately 10% of light-skinned patients exhibit an erythematous rash during this phase. Two to 3 d later, an enanthem consisting of small, painful ulcerations of the tongue and oropharynx appears simultaneously with (or within 24 h of) a discrete rash about the face, hands, and forearms.[6, 9, 10]

After development of eruptions on the lower extremities, the rash spreads centrally to the trunk over the next week. The exanthem typically begins as small, erythematous macules which progress to 2 or 3 mm papules over 2 to 3 d, then to 2 to 5 mm vesicles within another 1 or 2 d. Four to 7 d after rash onset, the vesicles become 4 to 6 mm umbilicated pustules, often accompanied by a second, smaller fever spike. Lesions are more abundant on the extremities and face, and this "centrifugal" distribution is an important diagnostic feature. In distinct contrast to varicella, lesions on various segments of the body remain generally synchronous in their stages of development. Between 8 and 14 d after onset, the pustules form scabs that leave depressed depigmented scars after healing. Death, if it occurs, is usually during the second week of clinical disease. The precise cause of death is not entirely understood, but was historically attributed to "toxemia", with high levels of circulating immune complexes. Although *Variola* virus concentrations in the throat, conjunctiva, and urine diminish with time, the it can be readily recovered from scabs throughout convalescence. Therefore, patients should be isolated and considered infectious until all scabs have separated.[6, 10]

In the 20th century, two distinct types of smallpox were recognized. *Variola minor* was distinguished by milder systemic toxicity and more diminutive pox lesions, and caused a 1% case fatality rate (CFR) in unvaccinated victims. However, the prototypical disease caused by *Variola major* resulted in a CFR of about 3% and 30% in the vaccinated and unvaccinated, respectively. CFRs were higher in certain populations (e.g., Pacific islanders and Native Americans), at extremes of age, during pregnancy (average 65% for ordinary smallpox), and in people with immunodeficiencies. Greater fatalities were associated with higher concentrations of lesions, with confluence of lesions portending the worst prognosis. Smallpox during pregnancy resulted in an increased incidence of spontaneous abortions. Acute complications of smallpox included viral keratitis or secondary ocular infection (1%), encephalitis (<1%), and arthritis (up to 2% of children). Bronchopneumonia was also seen in severely ill patients.[1, 2]

Two other clinical forms of *Variola major* — termed flat-type and hemorrhagic-type smallpox — were notable for severe mortality. Flat-type smallpox occurred in 2 to 5% of all cases and was most common in children. Hemorrhagic smallpox occurred in 2 to 3% of all cases, was more common in pregnant women and the immunocompromised, and presented with both "early" and "late" forms. Early hemorrhagic disease had a shorter incubation period, often large areas of ecchymosis, and fulminant progression to death, sometimes before lesions had even formed. In the late form, the disease progression was typical, with discrete hemorrhagic areas forming at lesion sites. CFRs were approximately 95% in both flat and hemorrhagic forms in unvaccinated individuals. [2, 11]

Partially immune patients, especially those vaccinated several yrs before smallpox exposure, could develop less severe forms of disease. This modified smallpox is a clinical form characterized by fewer lesions which are more superficial, associated with a less pronounced fever and a more rapid resolution, often with lesion crusting within 10 d of onset. Some previously immune individuals or infants with maternal antibodies could develop a short-lived febrile syndrome without rash upon exposure to smallpox virus.[12]

Long-term sequelae in smallpox survivors include blindness from corneal scarring (1-4%), growth abnormalities in children, and disfiguring or even physically debilitating dermal scarring.[1]

Animal studies suggest that unnaturally large inhaled inocula of poxvirus may result in a significantly shortened incubation period (even as little as 3 to 5 d) and fulminant pulmonary disease with or without appearance of rash before death; the implications of these findings for human disease resulting from intentional smallpox aerosolization are unknown.[13]

Historically, smallpox tended to spread slowly through communities. Smallpox could become endemic in densely populated regions even in a population with up to 80% vaccination rates. Increased person-to-person spread of disease was associated with: 1) exposure to cases with confluent rash or severe enanthem; 2) exposure to cases with severe bronchiolitis and cough; 3) low humidity environment; 4) crowding (as in winter or rainy seasons). The average secondary attack rate of *Variola major* was 58.4% in unvaccinated household contacts and 3.8% in vaccinated household contacts.[1]

Monkeypox virus, a relative of *Variola*, occurs naturally in equatorial Africa. In 2003, an outbreak of 78 confirmed or suspected human cases occurred in the US due to exposure to exotic pets, some of which had been imported from Africa.[14] Descriptions of human monkeypox in Africa reveal a disease that could be clinically indistinguishable from smallpox with the exception of a generally lower CFR and notable cervical and inguinal lymphadenopathy appearing 1 to 2 d before the rash in 90% of cases.[15] The 2003 cases tended to be less severe, with often localized lesions only, no deaths, and no secondary transmission to other humans. (The west African strain involved, however, was apparently atypically less virulent than prototypical monkeypox disease in Africa.[16])

Diagnosis

Smallpox must be distinguished from other vesicular exanthems, such as chickenpox, erythema multiforme with bullae, allergic contact dermatitis and other orthopoxvirus infections. In a confirmed outbreak, smallpox would likely be a clinical diagnosis. Particularly problematic to the necessary infection control measures would be the failure to recognize relatively mild cases of smallpox in persons with partial immunity, or extremely severe cases in patients who "bypass" classical disease. Therefore, isolation of suspected cases, quarantine of potential exposures, and initiation of medical countermeasures should be promptly followed by an accurate laboratory diagnosis. Contact and airborne precautions should be implemented and providers who attend at bedside or collect or process specimens should be vaccinated. Specimens should be collected only upon the direction of public health officials, who will provide further guidance. Typical *Variola* specimens might include scrapings of skin lesions, lesion fluid, crusts, blood, or pharyngeal swabs. The CDC has prepared a useful poster and diagnostic algorithm[17] to assist in decision making.

A method of presumptive diagnosis is the demonstration of characteristic poxvirus virions on electron microscopy of vesicular scrapings. Under light microscopy, aggregations of *Variola* virus particles, called Guarnieri bodies, can be seen. Another rapid but relatively insensitive test for Guarnieri bodies in vesicular scrapings is Gispen's modified silver stain, in which cytoplasmic inclusions appear black. However, none of the above laboratory tests is capable of discriminating *Variola* from vaccinia, monkeypox, or cowpox.[3]

Identification of *Variola* has classically required isolation of the virus and characterization of its growth on chicken egg chorioallantoic membranes. Real-time PCR assays are now available and provide a rapid and specific diagnosis. Specific smallpox PCR diagnosis is presently available only at facilities participating in the Laboratory Response Network (LRN). A real-time PCR assay that detects all orthopoxviruses (including vaccinia) may be available from the 1st and 9th Army Medical Laboratories (AMLs), Aberdeen Proving Ground, MD, for a presumptive diagnosis.[18, 19]

Neutralizing antibodies to *Variola* form in the first week of illness and may persist for many yrs. Hemaglutination-inhibition antibodies are detectible by the 16th d of infection and complement fixation antibodies by the 18th, but both begin to decrease after 1 yr.[6]

Associated lab findings, including the complete blood counts (CBC) of patients with ordinary smallpox, often exhibited a neutropenia and lymphocytosis during the eruptive stage. Neutrophils could become elevated during the late pustular stage when secondary bacterial infections would occur. Mild thrombocytopenia was common. In hemorrhagic smallpox, thrombocytopenia was progressive and severe as disseminated intravascular coagulation developed.[1]

Medical Management

Medical personnel must be able to recognize a vesicular exanthem and consider the etiology as potentially *Variola*, and then quickly initiate appropriate isolation precautions and countermeasures. Any confirmed case of human smallpox should be considered an international emergency mandating immediate notification of public health authorities. Those exposed to known cases of smallpox should be monitored for a minimum of 17 d from the time of exposure regardless of their vaccination status; such individuals should be immediately isolated using contact and airborne precautions from the onset of fever. In a civilian setting, strict quarantine of asymptomatic contacts may prove to be impractical to enforce. A reasonable alternative would be to require contacts to remain at home and to check their temperatures daily. Any fever above 38°C (101°F) during the 17 d after exposure to a confirmed case would suggest the development of smallpox. The contact should then be isolated immediately, preferably at home, until smallpox is either confirmed or ruled out. Patients should be considered infectious until all scabs have separated and must remain in isolation until that time. Immediate vaccination or revaccination should also be undertaken for all personnel exposed to either weaponized *Variola* virus or a clinical case of smallpox. Caregivers should be vaccinated and continue to wear appropriate personal protective equipment regardless of vaccination status. Weaponized smallpox strains encountered in the future may be genetically altered to render the current vaccine ineffective, a possibility experimentally validated in animal models using similar poxviruses.[1, 6]

The potential for airborne spread to other than close contacts is controversial. In general, close person-to-person contact is required for transmission to reliably occur. Nevertheless, *Variola*'s potential for airborne spread in conditions of low relative humidity was demonstrated during two hospital outbreaks. Indirect transmission by contaminated bedding or by other fomites was infrequent. Some close contacts harbored virus in their throats without developing disease and hence might have served as a means of secondary transmission.[6]

Vaccination with a verified clinical "take" (vesicle with subsequent scar formation) within the past 3 yrs is considered to render a person immune to smallpox. However, given the difficulties and uncertainties under wartime conditions of verifying the adequacy of troops' prior vaccination, routine revaccination of all potentially exposed personnel would seem prudent if there exists a significant likelihood of smallpox exposure.[1, 20]

Antivirals for use against smallpox are under investigation. Cidofovir has had significant *in vitro* and *in vivo* activity in animal studies. Whether it would offer benefit beyond that of immediate post-exposure vaccination in humans has not been determined. While cidofovir is a licensed drug for IV administration, its use for treating smallpox is "off-label" and it should be administered as an IND (see Appendix J). Topical antivirals such as trifluridine or idoxuridine may be useful for treating smallpox ocular disease, but are difficult to obtain. Two new oral antivirals tecovirimat (*Arestvyr®*, ST-246) and CMX001 (a prodrug of cidofovir), are under investigation and have been utilized under "compassionate use" (i.e., "single use") IND requests to treat a limited number of severe cases of vaccinia-related adverse reactions. Data from monkey models of *Variola* and monkeypox have shown efficacy for tecovirimat and cidofovir. Tecovirimat is currently under development by SIGA Technologies, Inc., with funding provided from DHHS, Biomedical Advanced Research & Development Authority (BARDA). Although it is not yet approved by the FDA, tecovirimat is maintained in the Strategic National Stockpile (SNS).[4, 21, 22] (see Appendix I)

Supportive care is imperative for successful management of smallpox patients; measures include maintenance of hydration and nutrition, pain control, and management of secondary infections.[6]

Prophylaxis

Vaccine: Smallpox vaccine (made from vaccinia virus) is most often administered by percutaneous inoculation with 15 pricks (jabs) of a bifurcated needle, a process known as "scarification" because of the small, permanent scar that results. The current licensed smallpox vaccine is *ACAM2000* and, unlike previous smallpox vaccines, it is produced in cell culture. Vaccination after exposure to smallpox may prevent or ameliorate disease if given as soon as possible and preferably within 4 d of exposure. A vesicle typically appears at the vaccination site 5 to 7 d after inoculation, with associated erythema and induration. The lesion forms a scab and gradually heals over the next 1or 2 wks; the evolution of the lesion may be more rapid, with less severe symptoms, in those with previous immunity.[1, 6]

Smallpox vaccination side effects include low-grade fever and axillary lymphadenopathy. The attendant erythema and induration of the vaccination vesicle is frequently misdiagnosed as bacterial superinfection or cellulitis. More severe vaccine reactions (more common in primary vaccinees) include inadvertent ***autoinoculation*** of the virus to other sites such as the face, eyelid, or other persons (~ 6/10,000 vaccinees), and ***generalized vaccinia,*** which is a systemic spread of the virus to produce mucocutaneous lesions away from the primary vaccination site (~3/10,000 vaccinees). Approximately 1/10,000 primary vaccinees will experience a transient, acute ***myopericarditis.*** Rare, but often fatal, adverse reactions include ***eczema vaccinatum*** (generalized cutaneous spread of vaccinia in patients with eczema), ***progressive vaccinia*** (systemic spread of vaccinia in immunocompromised individuals), and ***post-vaccinia encephalitis.***[6, 24-26]

Vaccination is *contraindicated* in the following conditions unless a smallpox outbreak is documented: immunosuppression, HIV infection, history or evidence of eczema, other active severe skin disorders, pregnancy, or current household, sexual, or other close physical contact with person(s) possessing one of these conditions.[27] In addition, vaccination should not be performed in breastfeeding mothers, in individuals with serious cardiovascular disease or with three risk factors for cardiovascular disease, or individuals who are using topical steroid eye medications or who have had recent eye surgery. Despite these caveats, most authorities, including current CDC guidelines, state that, with the exception of significant impairment of systemic immunity, there are no *absolute* contraindications to post-exposure vaccination of a person who experiences *bona fide* exposure to *Variola*. However, concomitant vaccine immune globulin administration is recommended for pregnant and eczematous persons in such circumstances.[3, 6]

A second generation smallpox vaccine is currently made from a replication-defective "Modified Vaccinia Ankara" (MVA). Unlike conventional vaccinia, it cannot replicate in human cells. MVA was used in the 1960s in Germany during the later stages of global smallpox eradication. It was shown to be safe and immunogenic, but its protective efficacy in humans remained unknown. It was approved in Canada (*Imvamune*) and the European Union (*Imvanex*) in 2013. Although it is not licensed by the FDA as yet, it is maintained in the SNS.[28-30]

Passive Immunoprophylaxis: *Vaccinia Immune Globulin* (VIG) is indicated for some complications of the smallpox vaccine (*generalized vaccinia* with systemic illness, *ocular vaccinia* without keratitis, *eczema vaccinatum*, and *progressive vaccinia*), and should be available whenever administering vaccine. It is available as an IND through both DoD and the CDC in IM and IV formulations. A formulation of VIG-IV has been licensed, but is currently in very limited supply. The dose for prophylaxis or treatment is 100 mg/kg for the IV formulation (first line treatment). If VIG-IV is not available, cidofovir may be of use for treating vaccinia adverse events (second line). The intramuscular VIG formulation (VIG-IM) is dosed 0.6 ml/kg (third line). Due to the large volume of the IM formulation (42 ml in a 70 kg person), the dose would be given in multiple sites over 24 to 36 h. Limited data suggest that VIG may also be of value in post-exposure prophylaxis of smallpox when given within the first week after exposure, and concurrently with vaccination. Vaccination alone is recommended for those without contraindications to the vaccine. If greater than 1 wk has elapsed since exposure, administration of both products (vaccine and VIG), if available, is reasonable.[4, 6]

Equine Encephalitidies (VEE, EEE, & WEE)

Summary

Signs and symptoms: Incubation periods are 2 to 6 d (VEE), 5 to 15 d (EEE), and 5 to 10 d (WEE) in natural disease. These "encephalitides" all present as acute systemic febrile illnesses in which encephalitis actually develops in a variable percentage (4% of children; < 1% of adults for VEE; 4 to 5% for EEE; <1% in adults — but up to 100% in infants — for WEE). Symptoms include generalized malaise, spiking fevers, rigors, severe headache, photophobia, and myalgias. Nausea, vomiting, cough, sore throat, and diarrhea may follow. Full recovery from malaise and fatigue takes 1 or 2 wks. If encephalitis ensues, anticipate vomiting, stiff neck, drowsiness, paresis, impaired respiratory regulation, seizures, or coma. CNS disease could be much more common after a bio-warfare attack.

Diagnosis is clinical, based on epidemiology. Physical findings are nonspecific. Leukopenia with a striking lymphopenia is seen in VEE and leukocytosis with a neutrophilia in EEE and WEE. Virus may be isolated from serum, and in some cases throat or nasal swab specimens, in VEE. Virus isolation is typically not successful in EEE and WEE. Both neutralizing and IgG antibody in paired sera — or virus-specific IgM present in a single serum, or CSF, sample — indicates recent infection.

Treatment is supportive. Uncomplicated infections benefit from analgesics to relieve headache and myalgia. Patients who develop encephalitis may require anticonvulsants and intensive supportive care to maintain fluid and electrolyte balance, ensure adequate ventilation, and avoid complicating secondary bacterial infections.

Prophylaxis: A live, attenuated vaccine is available as an IND product for VEE. Another (formalin-inactivated, killed) IND vaccine is also available for boosting antibody titers in those initially receiving the live product. There are also formalin-inactivated, killed IND vaccines for EEE and WEE. There is, however, no accepted post-exposure prophylaxis (PEP). In experimental animals, α-interferon, and the interferon-inducer poly-ICLC, have proven highly effective as PEP for VEE.

Isolation and decontamination: Patient isolation and quarantine are not required. Standard precautions (augmented with vector control) while the patient is febrile is recommended for VEE. There is no evidence of direct human-to-human or horse-to-human transmission. The virus can be destroyed by heat (80° C for 30 min) and standard disinfectants.

Overview

Alphaviruses are single-stranded, enveloped, positive-sense ribonucleic acid (RNA) viruses that belong to the *Togaviridae* family. Currently, 29 species are in the *Alphavirus* genus, which can be classified into at least seven groups based on antigenic complex homolog.[1, 2] Although the alphaviruses have worldwide geographic distribution, members of this genus have classically been described as Old World or New World viruses based on their predominant distribution. The Old World viruses, found in Africa and Asia, primarily cause a rash and arthritis. Examples include chikungunya virus, O'nyong-nyong virus, and Ross River virus. The New World viruses, including Venezuelan equine encephalitis (VEE) virus , eastern equine encephalitis (EEE) virus, and western equine encephalitis (WEE) virus, are found in the Americas and cause encephalitis in equines (horses, donkeys, mules, burros), hence are often referred to as the equine encephalitic alphaviruses.[1]

The VEE virus (VEEV) complex consists of six closely related subtypes that differ in regard to ecology, epidemiology, and virulence for humans and equines. Subtypes IA/B and IC are known as the epizootic strains and are responsible for large-scale epidemics in North, Central, and South America. Subtypes ID, IE, and IF are the enzootic strains, which may cause disease in humans, but lack virulence for equines.[3, 4]

The EEE virus (EEEV) complex is divided into distinct lineages which vary in geographic, epidemiologic, phylogenetic, and pathogenic characteristics.[5, 6] North American EEEV strains are enzootic along the eastern seaboard and Gulf Coast of North America and the Caribbean and are responsible for the majority of human cases, with significant mortality rates in humans and equines. The South American EEEV strains are enzootic in Central America and South America and primarily result in equine disease.[2, 5] Recently, it has been recommended that all South American EEEV strains be revised into a new species called Madariaga virus (MADV).[5]

The WEE virus (WEEV) complex includes several viruses that differ in their ecology and virulence; however, only WEEV strain causes encephalic disease in humans.[1]

Alphaviruses cycle between invertebrate insect vectors and vertebrate reservoir hosts. For many alphaviruses, the insect vectors are mosquitoes and the vertebrate hosts are birds or small mammals.[1] In most cases, humans and equines are incidental hosts and become infected during outbreaks in the late summer and early fall, especially after periods of heavy rainfall. Unlike VEEV, in which there are often massive epizootics in horses and spillover epidemics in humans, EEEV and WEEV usually result in either individual cases or limited outbreaks in both horses and humans.[1, 7, 8]

Alphaviruses are also highly infectious by aerosol. In fact, VEEV, EEEV, and WEEV possess many of the required characteristics for strategic or tactical weapon development, including ease of large-scale production, virus stability, potential for aerosolization, and virulence.[3] VEEV is of particular concern because it produces overt disease in nearly all human infections and can produce a self-sustaining natural outbreak since equines are amplifying hosts. However, there is no evidence of direct human-to-human or horse-to-human transmission. Natural aerosol transmission is not known to occur. Alphaviruses are not considered stable in the environment, and are thus not as persistent as the bacteria responsible for Q fever, tularemia, or anthrax. Heat and standard disinfectants can easily kill VEEV, EEEV, and WEEV.

VEEV is better characterized than EEEV or WEEV, primarily because it was tested as a bio-warfare agent during the US offensive biological weapons program in the 1950s and '60s, as well as by the USSR in the same period and later. In compliance with President Nixon's November 1969 directive mandating the destruction of all existing stocks of US biological and chemical weapons, all VEEV weapon stocks under US control were destroyed under supervision.[9]

History and Epidemology

Although the first recorded epidemic of equine encephalitis occurred in the 1830s, it was not until 100 years later that three distinct, but antigenically related, virus complexes were recovered from horses with severe equine encephalitis: WEEV complex was isolated in the San Joaquin Valley in California in 1930[10], while EEEV was isolated in Virginia and New Jersey in 1933[11-14], and VEEV complex in Venezuela in 1938.[15]

Since its initial isolation, VEEV has caused several major epizootics/epidemics, primarily in Central and South America, involving hundreds of thousands of human cases and even more in equines.[2,4] Equines, especially horses, are very susceptible to epizootic VEEV, leading to high morbidity and mortality. Importantly, horses are also amplifying hosts for epizootic VEEV, meaning the resulting viremia permits mosquito transmission and therefore fuels epizootics. Epidemics are the consequence of spillover during epizootics: humans become infected by mosquitoes that previously fed on infected horses.[4,7] Infected humans can shed high levels of VEEV in their nasal secretions; however, direct human-to-human transmission has never been documented.[16] Additionally, human viremia following endemic VEEV infection is sufficient to infect potential vectors; however, extensive human disease has never been documented in the absence of equine amplification or enzootic vectors.[17] The most recent significant outbreak occurred in Venezuela and Columbia in 1995, resulting in over 75,000 human cases and 300 deaths. The total number of equine cases was not reported, but was probably similar in magnitude to human numbers.[18] Epizootic VEEV has not been isolated in the US since 1971. However, since its initial isolation and prior to more stringent personal protective measures, at least 150 symptomatic laboratory-acquired infections have been reported, most of which were known or thought to be aerosol infection.[19]

North American EEEV is endemic along the eastern seaboard, Great Lakes, and Gulf Coast regions of the US, and typically results in a low number of human cases annually. On average, six human cases with neuro-invasive disease are attributed to EEE each year. However, in 2010, there were ten human cases, including five deaths, and over 200 equine cases, most fatal. Outbreaks in humans occur in the late summer or early fall, are usually associated with heavy rainfall and warmer water temperatures, and are frequently preceded by cases of equine encephalitis. Humans, horses, and other mammals are considered dead-end hosts.[1]

Historically, WEEV has caused epizootics and epidemics in the western US; however, few cases have been reported in recent years. Several states in the US had human and/or equine outbreaks during the 1930s, '40s, and '50s, with equine epizootics being more severe than the human epidemics.[20, 21] There were an average of 34 human cases of neuroinvasive disease attributed to WEEV per year in the US from 1955 to 1984, but those numbers have declined rapidly since then with the last known case occurring in 1999.[1, 22, 23] Similar to EEEV, humans and equines are considered dead-end hosts.

Natural human epidemics are almost always preceded by epizootics, characterized by severe and often fatal (30-90%) encephalitic outbreaks in equids. However, a biowarfare attack with virus intentionally disseminated as an aerosol would most likely cause human disease as a primary event or simultaneously with equids. Occasionally during natural epidemics, illness or death in wild or free-ranging equines may not be recognized before the onset of human disease, therefore a natural epidemic could be confused with a bio-warfare event, and data on the onset of disease should be considered with caution. A more reliable method for determining the likelihood of an intentional event would be the presence of any of these alphaviruses outside of their natural geographic range. A bio-warfare attack in a region populated by equines and appropriate mosquito vectors could initiate an epizootic/epidemic in the case of VEEV.

Clinical Features

VEEV, EEEV, and WEEV cause similar nonspecific prodromal syndromes in humans; however, the consequences vary by virus complex. VEE epidemics are explosive, often resulting in thousands of cases, but VEEV is the least neuroinvasive of the encephalitic alphaviruses. While human susceptibility to VEEV is high (90-100%), and nearly 100% of those infected develop overt illness, the vast majority present as undifferentiated "flu-like" illness[24], with < 1% of adults and < 4% of children developing encephalitis.[25] The overall case fatality rate (CFR) for VEE is < 1%; however it is somewhat higher in those that develop encephalitis and may be as high as 35% in children and 10% in adults who develop VEE.[26] Recovery from an infection results in excellent short-term and long-term immunity to the infective strain, but may not protect against other strains of the virus.

VEEV primarily results in an acute, incapacitating, febrile illness with most infections being mild and self-limiting (in contrast to clinically apparent EEEV and WEEV infection, in which encephalitis occurs with increased frequency). After an incubation period as short as 28 h but typically 2 to 6 d, onset of prostration is usually sudden. This acute phase of illness is often manifested by generalized malaise, chills, spiking high fevers (38° C–40.5° C), rigors, severe headache, photophobia, and myalgias. Nausea, vomiting, and diarrhea are also common. Physical signs may include tachycardia, conjunctival injection, erythematous pharynx, and muscle tenderness. Severe symptoms generally subside within 2 to 4 d, followed by asthenia (malaise and fatigue) lasting another 1or 2 wks before full recovery. A biphasic illness, with recurrence of the acute symptoms 4 to 8 d after initial onset of disease, has been described infrequently.[27] Mild CNS findings include lethargy, somnolence, photophobia or mild confusion, with or without nuchal rigidity. Seizures, ataxia, paralysis, or coma follow more severe CNS involvement. Generally, about 10% of patients in natural epidemics will be ill enough to require hospitalization.[26] Experimental aerosol challenges in animals suggest that the incidence of CNS disease and associated morbidity and mortality could be much higher after a bio-warfare attack, as the virus may travel along the olfactory nerve and spread directly to the CNS and result in acute neurological signs.[7, 28-33] School-age children may be more susceptible to a fulminant form of the disease characterized by depletion of lymphoid tissues, encephalitis, interstitial pneumonitis, and hepatitis, which follows a lethal course over 48 to 72 h.[34] For those who survive encephalitic involvement, neurological recovery is usually complete, although one report documented motor disorders and an increased incidence of seizures in children following VEE outbreaks.[35] VEEV infection during pregnancy may cause encephalitis in the fetus, placental damage, spontaneous abortion, or severe congenital neuroanatomical anomalies.[16, 36] EEE outbreaks are usually more limited due to a low incidence of human infection (< 3% of the population at risk). Additionally, the neurological attack rate in one outbreak was estimated at 1 in every 23 cases of human infection.[37, 38] Therefore, of those who develop clinical symptoms, only about 4 or 5% will go on to develop encephalitis (full-blown EEE); however, it is the most severe of the alphavirus encephalitides, with CFRs ranging from 30 to 70%, with severe neurologic sequelae in those that survive.[37, 39]

The initial clinical presentation of EEEV infection is indistinguishable from that of VEEV or WEEV, with patients presenting with "flu-like" symptoms; however, the incubation period is slightly longer, ranging from 5 to 15 d. Adults typically exhibit a febrile prodrome for up to 11 d before the onset of neurological disease[40]; however, illness in children has a more sudden onset. The nonspecific prodrome is followed by severe headache, high fevers, lethargy, and seizures, often with rapid progression to coma and death.[39, 41, 42] In a recent retrospective study of 15 cases of EEE in children, fever, headache, and seizures were the most common clinical findings, with 87% of the patients becoming stuporous or comatose during the first 3 d of hospitalization. Radiographic lesions were noted in the basal ganglia, thalami, and cerebral cortex. Importantly, this study found an association between a short prodrome (i.e., the time between initial nonspecific symptoms and the first major neurologic symptom) and an increased risk of death or severe disease. The 8 patients which had a poor outcome all had a prodrome of 2 d or less, and all 4 deaths occurred in this group.[43]

Similarly, the initial clinical presentation of WEEV infection is indistinguishable from that of VEEV or EEEV. However, infection with WEEV results in encephalitis (full-blown WEE) less often; CFRs in natural epidemics range from 8 to 15%[3, 20], while that associated with lab accidents involving aerosol exposure has been closer to 40%.[44] The incubation period is 5 to 10 d for natural infection. In lab monkeys exposed by aerosol, the incubation period is 4 or 5 d.[45] A large percentage of patients with vector-borne infections are either asymptomatic or present with a nonspecific febrile illness or aseptic meningitis. The ratio of encephalitis cases per infection has been estimated to vary from 1:1,150 in adults, 1:58 in children to 1:1 in infants.[46] However, the severity of the syndrome and the incidence of inapparent infection almost certainly depend on the strain and dose of virus and the route of infection.

Patients with the most severe infections usually die within the 7 d of clinical illness, while other patients begin a gradual convalescence after the first week of encephalitic symptoms. Most adults recover completely, but may take mos to yrs to recuperate from fatigability, recurrent headaches, emotional lability and impaired concentration.[47] Some patients have neurologic sequalae such as motor weakness, cognitive deficits, or a seizure disorder. Similar to VEEV and EEEV, children carry a higher incidence of neurological sequelae, ranging from < 1% in those older than 1 yr, to > 50% in newborns. Congenital infection in the last trimester of pregnancy has been described, with resultant encephalitis in the infants.[48]

Diagnosis

A diagnosis of VEE, EEE, or WEE is suspected on clinical and epidemiological grounds, but confirmed by virus isolation for VEEV, or by serology, electrochemiluminescence (ECL), or PCR for VEEV, EEEV, or WEEV. A variety of serological tests are applicable, including IgM, ELISA, indirect fluorescent antibody, hemagglutination inhibition, complement-fixation, and IgG. For persons without prior known exposure to alphaviruses, a presumptive diagnosis may be made by identifying IgM antibody in a single serum sample taken 5 to7 d after onset of illness. PCR procedures are available for confirmation, but are generally available only as a rear echelon laboratory capability.

Samples suitable for performing diagnostic tests include blood culture for VEEV, or acute and convalescent sera, and CSF for VEEV, EEEV, or WEEV. Viremia during the acute phase of the illness—but not during encephalitis—is generally high enough to allow detection by antigen-capture ELISA or ECL for VEEV. Virus isolation is time consuming, but may be performed from serum and throat or nasal swab specimens collected in the first 3 d of illness by inoculation of cell cultures or suckling mice (a gold standard identification assay for VEEV). VEEV, EEEV, and WEEV should be isolated only in a BSL-3 laboratory.

In the cases of VEEV infection, the WBC count is often normal at the onset of symptoms and then usually shows a leukopenia with a striking lymphopenia, and sometimes a mild thrombocytopenia by the second to third day of illness. Each of these abnormalities will usually resolve over the ensuing 1 or 2 wks. In EEE, there may be an initial leukopenia, which then becomes a leukocytosis characterized by a neutrophilia. Temporary, mild elevations of LDH, AST, and ALP may also be present. In patients with encephalitis, CSF pressure may be increased and contain up to 1,000 WBCs/mm^3 (mostly mononuclear cells, unless very early in infection) and a mildly elevated protein concentration.

On purely clinical grounds, an alphavirus outbreak may be difficult to distinguish from one caused by influenza. Clues might include the appearance of a small proportion of neurological cases, lack of person-to-person spread, or concurrent encephalitis in equines. A bio-warfare aerosol attack could lead to an epidemic of febrile meningoencephalitis featuring seizures and coma. In a bio-warfare context, the differential diagnosis would include other causes of aseptic meningitis and meningoencephalitis.

Medical Management

No specific antiviral therapy exists; hence treatment is supportive only. Patients with uncomplicated alphaviral infection may be treated with analgesics to relieve headache and myalgia. Nausea and emesis can lead to dehydration and necessitate IV fluids in some cases. Patients who develop encephalitis may require anticonvulsants and intensive supportive care to maintain fluid and electrolyte balance, ensure adequate ventilation, and avoid complicating secondary bacterial infections. In the presence of mosquito vectors, patients should be housed in a screened room or in quarters treated with a residual insecticide for > 5 d after onset, or until afebrile, as human cases of VEE may be infectious for mosquitoes for > 72 h. Patient isolation and quarantine are otherwise not required; sufficient contagion control is provided by implementing standard precautions augmented with vector control while the patient is febrile. Patient-to-patient transmission by means of respiratory droplet infection has not been shown to occur. The virus can be destroyed by heat (80° C for 30 min) and standard disinfectants.

Prophylaxis

Vaccine: There are two Investigational New Drug (IND) VEE vaccines that have been administered to humans. The first, designated TC-83, was developed in the 1960s and is a live, attenuated cell-culture-propagated product of the Salk Institute. TC-83 is not effective against all VEEV complex serotypes. It has been used to protect several thousand persons against lab infections and is presently licensed for use in equines (it was used in the 1970-71 Texas epizootic in horses), but remains investigational for humans. It is given as a single 0.5-ml SQ dose. Fever, malaise, and headache occur in about 20% of vaccinees, and may be moderate to severe in 10% of those, necessitating bed rest for 1or 2 d. Another 18% fail to develop detectable neutralizing antibodies, but it is unknown whether they are susceptible to later infection. Contraindications for use include a concurrent viral infection or pregnancy. Individuals with diabetes mellitus, or with a close family history of it, should not receive TC-83.

The second IND vaccine, designated C-84, has also been tested, but not licensed, in humans and is prepared by formalin-inactivation of the TC-83 strain. C-84 is not used for primary vaccination, but rather to boost non-responders to TC-83. Administer 0.5 ml SQ at 2 to 4 wk intervals for up to 3 inoculations or until an antibody response is measured. Periodic boosters are required. (C-84 alone does not protect rodents against experimental aerosol challenge. Therefore, it is used only as a booster immunogen for TC-83.)

There are also IND vaccines for EEE and WEE, both of which are formalin-inactivated. The PE-6 strain of EEEV was passed in primary chick-embryo cell cultures and then was formalin-treated and lyophilized to make the currently available EEE product. Mild reactions to this vaccine were observed, and immunogenicity was demonstrated in initial clinical trials. A long-term follow-up study of 573 recipients indicated a 58% response rate after the primary series, and a 25% chance of failing to maintain adequate titers for 1 yr. Response rates and persistence of titers increased with the administration of additional booster doses.[49]

The WEE vaccine was similarly prepared using the B-11 or CM-4884 virus strain, which was serially passed and then formalin-inactivated. This vaccine caused only mild clinical reactions when administered to WEE-naive individuals. Long-term follow-up studies have indicated in a 50% response rate (neutralization titer > 1:40) after the primary series. However, only 20% maintain a titer for 1 yr, although this level can be increased to about 60 or 70% with additional boosters.[50] (Currently this product is not offered through the Special Immunizations Program at USAMRIID, due to its lot-to-lot variability in immunogenicity.)

As with all vaccines, the degree of protection afforded by these products depends upon the magnitude of the challenge dose; vaccine-induced protection could be overwhelmed by extremely high pathogen inocula. Research is underway to produce improved, second-generation VEE, EEE, and WEE vaccines.

Immunoprophylaxis: At present, there is no licensed pre- or post-exposure immunoprophylactic for the equine encephalidities. In animal models, protection from SQ and aerosolized VEEV has been demonstrated by passive transfer of neutralizing monoclonal antibodies administered 24 h pre- or 24 h post-infection.

Chemoprophylaxis: In experimental animals, α-interferon and the interferon-inducer poly-ICLC have proven highly effective for post-exposure chemoprophylaxis of VEE.[51] There are, however, no clinical data by which to assess efficacy of these products in humans.

Viral Hemorrhagic Fevers (VHFs)

Summary

Signs and symptoms: Viral hemorrhagic fevers (VHFs) are illnesses characterized by fever and bleeding diathesis. Manifestations often include flushing of the face and chest, petechiae, frank bleeding, edema, hypotension, and shock. Malaise, myalgias, headache, vomiting, and diarrhea occur frequently.

Diagnosis: Definitive diagnosis is usually made at a reference laboratory with advanced bio-containment (BSL-4) capability. However, early clinical diagnosis is crucial for appropriate management and to minimize potential nosocomial spread. Any patient with compatible signs and symptoms should suggest the possibility of a VHF.

Treatment: Intensive supportive care may be required. Antiviral therapy (IV ribavirin) may be useful in *Bunyaviridae* and *Arenaviridae* infections (specifically Lassa fever, Crimean-Congo hemorrhagic fever, and hemorrhagic fever with renal syndrome due to Old World hantavirus infection) and should be used only under an Investigational New Drug (IND) protocol. Convalescent plasma may be effective in Argentine or Bolivian hemorrhagic fevers; it is available only as an IND.

Prophylaxis: The only licensed VHF vaccine is the 17D yellow fever vaccine. Experimental vaccines for other VHFs are not readily available. Prophylactic ribavirin may be effective for some *Bunyaviridae* and *Arenaviridae* infections (again, available only as an IND).

Isolation and decontamination: Strict contact precautions (hand hygiene, double gloves, gowns, shoe and leg coverings & face shield or goggles) and droplet precautions (private room or cohorting, surgical mask within 3 feet) are mandatory. Airborne precautions (negative-pressure isolation room with 6 to 12 air exchanges per h) should also be instituted to the maximum extent possible and especially for procedures that induce aerosols (e.g., bronchoscopy). At a minimum, a fit-tested, HEPA filter-equipped respirator (e.g., an N-95 mask) should be used, but a battery-powered, air-purifying respirator (PAPR) or a positive pressure-supplied air respirator should be considered for personnel sharing an enclosed space with, or coming within 6 feet of, the patient. Multiple patients should be cohorted in a separate ward or building with a dedicated air-handling system when feasible. Environmental decontamination is accomplished with hypochlorite or phenolic disinfectants.

Overview

The VHFs are a diverse group of illnesses caused by lipid-enveloped, single-stranded RNA viruses from four viral families: *Arenaviridae, Bunyaviridae, Filoviridae,* and *Flaviviridae.* They are unified by their potential to present as severe febrile illness accompanied by shock and a hemorrhagic diathesis. The *Arenaviridae* include the etiologic agents of Lassa fever and Argentine (Junin), Bolivian (Machupo), and Venezuelan (Sabia) hemorrhagic fevers. The *Bunyaviridae* include the members of the *Hantavirus* genus that cause hemorrhagic fever with renal syndrome (HFRS); the Congo-Crimean hemorrhagic fever virus from the *Nairovirus* genus; and the Rift Valley fever virus from the *Phlebovirus* genus. The *Filoviridae* include Ebola and Marburg viruses. Finally, the *Flaviviridae* include dengue, yellow fever, and two viruses in the tick-borne encephalitis group that cause VHF—Omsk hemorrhagic fever (OHF) virus and Kyasanur Forest disease (KFD) virus. These viruses are spread in a variety of ways, frequently through blood/body fluid exposure, and most have zoonotic potential (transmission from animals to humans by a vector, inhalation, or ingestion of excretions/secretions of rodents); some may be transmitted person-to-person through a respiratory portal of entry. The Soviet Union was known to have weaponized both Ebola and Marburg viruses[1]; other VHF viruses are included in this handbook because of their *potential* for aerosol dissemination, weaponization, or likelihood for confusion with similar agents that might be weaponized.

History & Significance

Because these viruses are so diverse and occur in different endemic geographic locations, a comprehensive discussion is beyond the scope of this handbook. However, each viral infection possesses a number of different features that may provide insight into their possible importance as bio-agents.

Arenaviridae: **Lassa virus** causes Lassa fever in West Africa, where endemic transmission is related to exposure to the reservoirs: rodents of the *Mastomys* genus.[6] These animals are very common there and are often found nesting in human homes.[7] Over 5,000 deaths in West Africa are attributed to Lassa each year, with between 100,000 and 300,000 annual infections.[6,7] Argentine hemorrhagic fever (AHF) is caused by **Junin virus** and was first described in 1955 among corn harvestors[2]. Typically, 300 to 600 cases per yr occur in areas of the Argentine pampas. Bolivian, Brazilian, and Venezuelan hemorrhagic fevers are caused by the related **Machupo, Sabia**, and **Guanarito viruses**, respectively. Arenaviruses are transmitted from rodents to humans through inhalation of dusts contaminated with rodent excreta. Nosocomial transmission is probably possible with all arenavirus infections, but is certainly a problem with Lassa fever.[3,6,7] Lassa infection of healthcare workers has been attributed to parenteral exposures, contact with body fluids, and aerosols generated by patients.[7]

Bunyaviridae: **Crimean-Congo hemorrhagic fever** (CCHF) is a tick-borne disease with a widespread distribution from Africa through southeastern Europe, Central Asia and the Indian sub-continent. It may also be spread by contact with the body fluids or slaughtered meat of infected animals and in health-care settings.[7] The 2009 death of a US soldier who was infected with CCHF while stationed in Afghanistan was a reminder of the ongoing endemic disease risk in certain parts of the world. **Rift Valley fever** (RVF) is a mosquito-borne disease that occurs in Central and East Africa but can also be transmitted by handling infected tissues (animal slaughter), and by aerosol (particularly lab workers).[9] In 2000, a large outbreak occurred outside Africa in Yemen and Saudi Arabia.[9] RVF virus is not only on the DHHS Select Agent list, like most VHFs, but is also listed on the USDA Select Agent list as deleteriously affecting animals of agricultural significance.[10] The hantaviruses are rodent-borne viruses with a wide geographic distribution. **Hantaan** and closely related Old World hantaviruses cause hemorrhagic fever with renal syndrome (HFRS). Hantaan virus infection—also known as Korean hemorrhagic fever or epidemic hemorrhagic fever—is the most common human disease due to hantaviruses. It was described before WW II in Manchuria along the Amur River, among UN troops during the Korean conflict, and subsequently in Japan, China, and in the Russian Far East.[2,11] Severe disease from other hantaviruses also occurs in some Balkan states, including Bosnia, Serbia, and Greece. *Nephropathia epidemica,* a milder disease that occurs in Scandinavia and other parts of Europe, is caused by the **Puumala virus** carried by bank voles (*Microtus* and related genera).[12] New World hantaviruses (i.e., **Sin Nombre virus, Andes virus**) cause hantavirus pulmonary syndrome (HPS) in the Americas. However, HPS generally leads to respiratory and cardiovascular failure rather than hemorrhagic fever. Like the arenaviruses, hantaviruses are most commonly transmitted to humans via inhalation of dusts contaminated with rodent excreta.[11]

Filoviridae: Five species of **Ebola virus** (Tai Forest, Reston, Sudan, Zaire, and Bundibugyo) have been identified. *Ebola-Zaire* and *Ebola-Sudan* cause severe disease with high case fatality rates (CFRs).[13] Ebola hemorrhagic fever (EHF) was first recognized in Sudan (Ebola-Sudan) and a nearby region of Zaire (Ebola-Zaire) in 1976. In 1995, a single index case resulted in a large outbreak (316 cases) in Kikwit, Zaire.[14] Subsequent epidemics of Ebola-Zaire and Ebola-Sudan have occurred in Gabon, Ivory Coast, Uganda, Democratic Republic of Congo (former Zaire), and Sudan. In February 2014, the largest EHF outbreak to date began in Guinea and quickly spread to neighboring Liberia and Sierra Leone causing over 1,000 infections and more than 600 deaths at the time of writing. It was likely caused by a Zaire-Ebola lineage that spread from Central Africa into Guinea and West Africa in recent decades. *Ebola-Reston* was isolated from monkeys imported into the US from the Philippines in 1989. Infected monkeys developed hemorrhagic fever, and since this initial outbreak there have been other outbreaks in primate facilities in both the US and EU. After exposure to Ebola-Reston, several animal handlers sero-converted, but did not manifest clinical disease. Therefore, Ebola-Reston has not been recognized as a human pathogen.[2] In 2008, pigs were identified in the Philippines to be co-infected with Ebola-Reston and a porcine-specific virus. Again, some pig handlers sero-converted without clinical disease.[16] The role of pigs, if any, in the natural ecology of this disease remains unclear. In 1994, chimpanzees with lesions similar to those seen in humans infected with Ebola virus during the 1976 outbreaks were identified in the Taï Forest in Côte d'Ivoire, Africa. A scientist contracted the lab-confirmed *Ebola-Taï Forest* virus after working with post-mortem tissues and became ill. She made a full recovery.[17] In 2007, a VHF outbreak occurred in Bundibugyo District in western Uganda (149 cases, 25% CFR). Laboratory analysis confirmed the newest and fifth species of Ebola virus.[18] Recent data implicate bats as the reservoir, although the link to humans and ecology of these diseases remain murky.[2] It is not known why this disease appears intermittently.

Only a single species of Marburg virus (Lake Victoria) has been recognized. The first recognized outbreak occurred in Marburg, Germany, and in Yugoslavia, among people exposed to African green monkeys in 1967. It resulted in 37 cases with seven deaths.[2,19] Since then, Marburg epidemics have been sporadic and mostly in Africa. In 2005, an outbreak in Angola resulted in 356 deaths with most fatalities in children.[19] The Egyptian fruit bat (*Rousettus aegyptiacus*), found throughout Africa, is thought to be the reservoir.[20]

Filoviruses may be spread from human to human by direct contact with infected blood, secretions, organs, or semen.[2] Lab monkeys have been infected via airborne transmission experimentally, although the significance of this for human outbreaks remains unknown.[21]

Flaviviridae: Yellow fever and dengue are two mosquito-borne viruses that have had great importance in the history of military campaigns and military medicine. Tick-borne flaviruses include the agents of Kyasanur Forest disease in India, and Omsk hemorrhagic fever in Siberia.[2]

All of the VHF agents (except dengue) are lab infection hazards by aerosol (and even dengue has been nosocomially transmitted by blood splash). The aerosol infectivity for many of them has been studied and measured in experimental animal models. VHF agents cause severe disease and many have extremely high fatality rates. For these reasons, they are considered a significant potential biowarfare and bio-terrorism threat.[2]

Clinical Features

Hemorrhagic fever viruses can cause illnesses with diverse clinical presentations. In their most severe form, these manifest as the "VHF syndrome", with capillary leak, bleeding diathesis, and hemodynamic compromise leading to shock. Early symptoms of VHF are nondescript in most cases, consisting of fever and constitutional symptoms such as malaise, myalgias, and headache. This constellation of findings is difficult to distinguish from any number of viral, bacterial, or parasitic diseases.[2,22]

Diversity of clinical features among the VHFs probably stems from varying mechanisms of pathogenesis. For example, an immunopathogenic mechanism has been identified for dengue hemorrhagic fever, which usually occurs among patients previously infected with a heterologous dengue serotype. (A prominent theory explaining this phenomenon is called "antibody-dependent enhancement.")

Disseminated intravascular coagulation (DIC) is thought to underlie the hemorrhagic features of Rift Valley, Marburg, and Ebola fevers, but in most VHFs, the etiology of the coagulopathy is multifactorial (e.g., hepatic damage, consumptive coagulopathy, and primary marrow dysfunction) and the exact pathogenesis is still being elucidated for many of the VHFs.[2]

Why some infected persons develop full-blown VHF while others do not remains an unresolved issue. Virulence of the specific infecting agent clearly plays a large role. The VHF syndrome occurs in a majority of patients manifesting disease from filoviruses, CCHF, and the South American hemorrhagic fever (SAHF) viruses, while it occurs in a small minority of patients with dengue, RVF, and Lassa fever. The reasons for variation among patients infected with the same virus are still unknown, but probably stem from a complex system of virus-host interactions.

Differentiating the various VHFs before laboratory diagnosis may be difficult. Epidemiological context will be helpful in this regard, especially discerning the proportion of cases with mild or moderate disease as compared to the proportion with severe disease, or knowledge of recent travel to known endemic areas. Astute clinicians who are familiar with the clinical presentations of the various VHF diseases may be able to pick out unique features that implicate one disease over the others. Clinical manifestations of the various VHFs are discussed below. Table 1 provides a summary of disease characteristics.

Arenaviridae: The clinical features of the SAHFs are quite similar, but they differ significantly from those of Lassa fever. Onset of the SAHFs is insidious, resulting in high unremitting fever and constitutional symptoms. A petechial or vesicular enanthem involving the palate and tonsillar pillars is quite common, as is conjunctival injection and flushing of the upper torso and face. Patients frequently have associated neurologic disease, with initial hyporeflexia followed by gait abnormalities and cerebellar dysfunction. Seizures portend a grave prognosis. Fatality rates from the SAHFs are high, ranging from 15% to over 30%.[3,23]

In contrast, it is estimated that 80% of most natural infections with Lassa virus are mild or non-apparent.[7] The other 20% of infections result in severe disease, with a 15-20% CFR in hospitalized patients. The overall CFR for Lassa virus infection is around 1%, but wide disparities in reporting makes this a rough estimate. Patients frequently have retrosternal chest pain, a sore throat and proteinuria. Syndromes with features of encephalitis and/or meningitis are sometimes present, as are convalescent cerebellar syndromes. Serum AST levels in the hundreds or thousands of U/L are indicative of a poor prognosis. A common sequela of Lassa fever is deafness, and this occurs in up to 5,000 afflicted patients per yr. It may be transient or permanent.[7,23]

Bunyaviridae: CCHF is generally a severe, hemorrhagic disease. Onset is abrupt and GI and meningeal symptoms occur frequently. Petechiae and ecchymoses are common, as is mucosal bleeding. Hepatitis and jaundice probably results from direct viral cytotoxicity. Thrombocytopenia can be profound. CFRs range from 20% to 50%.[24,25]

RVF is usually a self-limiting, nondescript febrile illness. The most common sequela of an RVF infection is retinitis, and up to 10% of these patients have some residual vision loss. Only 1% develop hemorrhagic manifestations or severe hepatic disease, usually occurring as a second febrile phase after defervescence from an initial febrile phase of 3 to 7 d. A small minority of patients develop encephalitis after the initial febrile illness.[9,25]

The severity of hemorrhagic fever with renal syndrome (HFRS) depends largely on the infecting hantavirus. Puumala virus, common in northern Europe and Russia, causes a relatively mild form of disease (*nephropathica endemica*) that is associated with rare fatalities. The most severe form of HFRS is caused by Hantaan virus, and disease progession can be split into four phases. In the initial febrile phase, disease onset is usually abrupt and consists of fever, malaise, myalgia, headache, and lassitude. Some characteristic features are flushing of the face and neck, conjunctival and pharyngeal injection, cutaneous and mucosal petechiae (occurring by day 4 or 5), and profound lower back pain. In the second, hypotensive phase, mild DIC, thrombocytopenia, and capillary leak syndrome may ensue leading to hypovolemic shock. In the oliguric phase, renal dysfunction is pathognomonic, frequently progressing to oliguric renal failure. The final diuretic phase often accompanies convalescence, and here fluid management may be a significant challenge. Death occurs in 5% to 15% of Hantaan infections.[11,25]

Filoviridae: Ebola and Marburg infections present similarly. Onset is abrupt with fever, constitutional symptoms, nausea, vomiting, diarrhea, abdominal pain, lymphadenopathy, pharyngitis, conjuctival injection, and pancreatitis. A large number of patients develop a maculopapular rash around day 5, but this may be difficult to appreciate in dark-skinned persons. Elevated liver enzymes, increased blood urea nitrogen and creatinine, increased clotting times, and elevated d-dimers, but decreased fibrinogen, are typical clinical pathology findings. Delirium, obtundation, and coma are common. Hemorrhagic features develop as the disease progresses. Death occurs at the beginning of the second week of illness. Fatality rates from 25% (Bundibugyo) to over 80% (Marburg/Ebola Zaire) have been observed.[2,21]

Flaviviridae: Yellow fever is classically described as a severe biphasic illness, but it is apparent that a large number of infections are mild or subclinical. The initial phase of illness lasts about a week and consists of fever, constitutional symptoms, GI symptoms and other undifferentiated features. Objective findings are unimpressive except for the frequent appearance of relative bradycardia (Faget's sign) and leukopenia. Facial flushing and conjuctival injection may also be present. After a period of clinical improvement and defervescence (hours to days) some patients develop a second febrile phase. This so called "period of intoxication" is characterized by high fever, severe constitutional symptoms, obtundation, skin and mucous membrane hemorrhages, severe hepatitis and profound jaundice. Liver enzyme elevation occurs in a pattern consistent with hepatocellular damage, and bilirubin may be quite high.

Proteinuria is almost universal and is an excellent diagnostic clue. As severe disease progresses, renal failure consistent with hepatorenal syndrome may ensue. Death may occur in over 50% of patients with the hemorrhagic form of yellow fever.[2,26,27]

The two members of the tick-borne encephalitis complex causing hemorrhagic disease (Kyasanur Forest and Omsk) have similar clinical syndromes and are often biphasic. The first phase is a febrile syndrome of varying severity, associated with conjunctival suffusion, facial flushing, lymphadenopathy, and splenomegaly. In its most severe form, this syndrome may be accompanied by diffuse mucosal hemorrhaging and petechiae. Hemorrhagic pulmonary edema is a relatively common and distinct feature. A second phase of illness may occur 1-3 wks after remission. This second phase involves mainly neurologic disease. Fatality ranges from < 3% (Omsk) up to 10% (Kyasanur Forest). Survivors may experience neurologic complications after the initial acute clinical phase has passed.[2,28,29]

Dengue virus has not typically been considered a potential biological weapon agent, as it has not been shown in the laboratory to infect by aerosol. However, as noted, blood splashes in hospitals have spread the disease.

Table 1: Comparison of VHF agents and diseases

Family	Virus	Disease	Endemic area	Fatality	Nosocomial transmission	Characteristic features	Countermeasures
Flavivirus	Yellow fever virus	Yellow fever	Africa, South America	Overall 3-12%, 20-50% if severe second phase develops	No	Often biphasic, severe second phase with bleeding, very high bilirubin and transaminases, jaundice, renal failure	17-D live attenuated vaccine very effective in prevention, no postexposure countermeasure available
	KFD virus	Kyasanur Forest disease	Southern India	3-5%	No	Flu-like syndrome with addition of cough, GI symptoms, hemorrhage, bradycardia	Formalin-inactivated vaccine available in India
	OHF virus	Omsk hemorrhagic fever	Siberia	0.2-3%	No	Frequent sequelae of hearing loss, neuropsych complaints, alopecia	TBE vaccines (not avail. in US) may offer some cross-protection
Filoviruses	Ebola virus	Ebola hemorrhagic fever	Africa, Philippines (Ebola Reston)	50-90% for Sudan/Zaire	Common	Severe illness, maculopapular rash, profuse bleeding and DIC	Anecdotal success with immune serum transfusion
	Marburg virus	Marburg hemorrhagic fever	Africa	23-70%	Yes		

Bunyaviruses	CCHF	Crimean-Congo hemorrhagic fever	Africa, SE Europe, Central Asia, India	30%	Yes	Often prominent petechial/ecchymotic rash	Anecdotal success with ribavirin
	RVF	Rift valley fever	Africa	<0.5%	No	Hemorrhagic disease rare, classically associated with retinitis and encephalitis , Significant threat to livestock – epidemics of abortion and death of young	Effective livestock vaccines in Africa Human killed vaccine – DOD IND, live attenuated vaccine in clinical trials
	Hantavirus (Hantaan, Dobrava, Seoul, Puumala)	Hemorrhagic fever with renal syndrome (HFRS)	Europe, Asia, South America (rare)	5% for Asian HFRS	No	Prominent renal disease, marked polyuric phase during recovery, usually elevated WBC	Effective locally produced vaccines in Asia (not avail in US). Experimental vaccine at USAMRIID. Ribavirin effective in randomized, controlled clinical trial
Arenaviruses	Lassa virus	Lassa fever	West Africa	1-2%	Yes	Frequent unapparent/mild infection, hearing loss in convalescence common	Ribavirin effective in clinical trial with non-randomized controls
	Junin	Argentine hemorrhagic fever	Argentinean pampas	30%	Rare	Prominent GI complaints, late neurologic syndrome	Immune plasma, Ribavirin effective Candid 1 vaccine protective but not avail. in US
	Machupo	Bolivian hemorrhagic	Bolivia	25-35%	Rare	Similar to AHF	Immune plasma effective, ribavirin probably effective, Candid 1 vaccine protects monkeys

Diagnosis

A VHF should be considered in any patient presenting with a severe, acute febrile illness and evidence of vascular instability (postural hypotension, petechiae, easy bleeding, flushing of face and chest, non-dependent edema). Symptoms and signs suggesting additional organ system involvement are common (headache, photophobia, pharyngitis, cough, nausea or vomiting, diarrhea, constipation, abdominal pain, hyperesthesia, dizziness, confusion, tremor) but usually do not dominate the picture, with the exceptions listed above under "Clinical Features." A positive tourniquet test has been particularly useful in dengue hemorrhagic fever, but should be sought in other hemorrhagic fevers as well.[2,22]

A detailed travel history and a high index of suspicion are essential in making the diagnosis of VHF. Patients with arenavirus or hantavirus infections often recall proximity to rodents or their droppings; but as the viruses are spread to humans by aerosolized excreta or environmental contamination, direct contact with the infected rodents is not necessary. Large mosquito populations are common during RVF, yellow fever, or dengue transmission, but a history of mosquito bite is too common to be of diagnostic significance. Tick bites or nosocomial exposure are of some significance in suspecting CCHF. Large numbers of military personnel presenting with VHF manifestations in the same geographic area over a short time period should be considered a "red flag." A large natural outbreak is possible in an endemic setting, but a large number of cases should also prompt concern of a bio-agent attack.[2,22]

The clinical laboratory can be very helpful in presumptive diagnosis of VHF. Thrombocytopenia (exception: Lassa) and leukopenia (exceptions: Lassa, Hantaan, and CCHF) are the rule. Proteinuria and/or hematuria are common, and their presence is characteristic of AHF, BHF, and HFRS. High AST elevation is nonspecific for, but correlates with, severity of Lassa fever, and jaundice is a poor prognostic sign in yellow fever. Higher viral loads, renal failure, a high AST/ALT ratio (7-12 times higher AST), and low calcium (<6 mg/dl) appear to be poor prognostic factors for filoviral disease.[2,22,30]

In most geographic areas, the major consideration in the differential diagnosis is malaria. In such regions, bear in mind that parasitemia alone in patients partially immune to malaria does not prove that symptoms are due to malaria. Other diseases in the differential diagnosis should include typhoid fever, non-typhoidal salmonellosis, leptospirosis, rickettsial infections, shigellosis, relapsing fever, fulminant hepatitis, and meningococcemia. Non-infectious illnesses that could mimic VHF include acute leukemia, lupus erythematosus, idiopathic or thrombotic thrombocytopenic purpura, hemolytic uremic syndrome, and the multiple causes of DIC.[2]

Definitive diagnosis in an individual case rests on specific virology diagnosis. Most patients have readily detectable viremia at presentation (exception: hantavirus infections). Rapid enzyme immunoassays can detect viral antigens in acute sera from patients with AHF, Lassa fever, RVF, CCHF, and yellow fever. Lassa- and Hantaan-specific IgM often are detectable during the acute illness. Lack of antibody production in response to filoviral infection is a poor prognostic sign. Diagnosis by virus replication and identification requires 3 to 10 d or longer. PCR assays have been developed at USAMRIID and the CDC, and they may be helpful in making a presumptive diagnosis. With the exception of dengue, specialized microbiological containment is required for safe handling of these viruses. Appropriate precautions should be observed in collection, handling, shipping, and processing of diagnostic samples. Both the CDC (Atlanta, Georgia) and USAMRIID (Frederick, Maryland) have diagnostic laboratories functioning at the highest (BSL-4 or P-4) containment level.[2,30]

Medical Management

General principles of supportive care apply to managing the hemodynamic, hematologic, pulmonary, and neurologic aspects of VHFs, regardless of the specific etiologic agent. Intensive care is required for the most severely ill patients. Healthcare providers employing vigorous fluid resuscitation of hypotensive patients must be mindful of the propensity of some VHFs (e.g., HFRS) for pulmonary capillary leak. Vasoactive or inotropic agents are frequently required. The benefits of intravascular devices and invasive hemodynamic monitoring must be carefully weighed against the significant risk of hemorrhage. Restlessness, confusion, myalgia, and hyperesthesia should be managed by conservative measures, including the judicious use of sedatives and analgesics. Mechanical ventilation, renal dialysis, and anti-seizure therapy may be required. Secondary infections may occur as with any patient managed with invasive procedures and devices.[2]

Management of the hemorrhagic component of VHFs is controversial, but if attempted the approach mirrors that for any patient with a systemic coagulopathy. Aggressive treatment of mild bleeding in the absence of a definitive diagnosis of VHF is contraindicated. In cases of severe bleeding, red blood cells, platelets, and clotting factors should be replaced, guided by clinical indication and coagulation parameters. IM injections, aspirin, and other anticoagulant drugs should be avoided. Steroids are not indicated.[2]

The antiviral drug ribavirin is available for therapy of Lassa fever, HFRS, and CCHF under an IND protocol. A controlled clinical trial has clearly indicated that parenteral ribavirin reduces morbidity in HFRS. Several trials have suggested that it lowers both the morbidity and mortality of Lassa fever. In the HFRS field trials, treatment was effective if begun within the first 4 d of fever, and continued for a 10 d course. Both the CDC and DoD (USAMRIID) have IND protocols for the treatment of VHFs with IV ribavirin. Because the supply of IV ribavirin is limited, oral ribavirin may be required in a mass-casualty situation. Oral ribavirin is licensed for the treatment of hepatitis C infection and is commercially available in the US. Because it is not approved for use in VHFs, it should only be used under an IND protocol or EUA. Dosing recommendations for IV and PO ribavirin are in Table 2. Side effects include modest reversible hemolytic anemia and bone marrow suppression. Ribavirin is teratogenic in lab animals, but no human data exist. Potential risks to the fetus must be weighed against the potential life-saving benefit in pregnant women with grave illness. Safety in infants and children has not been established for IV ribavirin, but inhaled ribavirin has been used extensively in the treatment of respiratory syncytial virus infection in infants. Ribavirin has poor *in vitro* and *in vivo* activity against the filoviruses (Ebola and Marburg) and the flaviviruses (dengue, yellow fever, OHF and KFD).[2]

AHF responds to therapy with two or more units of convalescent plasma containing adequate amounts of neutralizing antibody and given within 8 d of onset. BHF appears to respond to passive immune therapy as well. Convalescent serum or immune globulin for SAHFs is not readily available in the US. This therapy is investigational and should be given only in consultation with experts.[2]

Table 2: Recommended ribavirin dosing for treatment of VHFs*

		Intravenous	Oral
Adults	Loading dose	30 mg/kg IV (max 2 g) once	2,000 mg PO once
	Maintenance dose	Day 1-4: 16 mg/kg IV (max 1 g) q6 h for 4 d Day 5-7: 8 mg/kg IV (max 500 mg) q8 h for 6 d	Wt > 75 kg: 600 mg PO bid for 10 d Wt < 75 kg: 400 mg PO in AM, 600 mg PO in PM for 10 d
Children	Loading dose	Same as adult	30 mg/kg PO once
	Maintenance dose	Same as adult	7.5 mg/kg PO bid for 10 d

*For confirmed or suspected arenavirus or bunyavirus or VHF of unknown etiology.[30]

Prophylaxis

The 17D live attenuated yellow fever vaccine is the only licensed vaccine available for any of the hemorrhagic fever viruses. The *Candid 1 vaccine* for AHF is a live, attenuated, investigational vaccine developed at USAMRIID. It was highly efficacious in a randomized, controlled trial in Argentine agricultural workers and it appears to protect against BHF in monkeys. Unfortunately, *Candid 1* is no longer manufactured and is not available in the US. Both inactivated and live-attenuated RVF vaccines are currently under investigation. The inactivated version continues to be administered to at-risk lab workers. There are presently no vaccines for the other VHF agents available for human use in the US. Several local vaccines for OHF, KFD, HFRS, and CCHF are used in their respective endemic areas, but these have not been rigorously studied.[2]

Persons with percutaneous or mucocutaneous exposure to blood, body fluids, secretions, or excretions from a patient with suspected VHF should immediately wash the exposed skin surfaces with soap and water and irrigate mucous membranes with copious amounts of water or saline solution.

Close personal contacts or indeed anyone, including medical personnel, exposed to blood or secretions from VHF patients (particularly Lassa fever, CCHF, and filoviral diseases) should be monitored for symptoms (fever and other signs) for the established incubation period. After a presumed bio-agent attack with an unknown VHF virus, any fever of 101°F or greater should prompt evaluation and consideration for immediate treatment with IV ribavirin until the particular agent is determined. However, the utility of post-exposure, pre-symptomatic ribavirin prophylaxis is questionable. The DoD IND protocol for ribavirin therapy of CCHF and Lassa fever may allow for prophylactic treatment of exposed personnel, in consultation with protocol investigators. Most patients will tolerate this regimen well, but should be under surveillance for breakthrough disease (especially after drug cessation) or adverse drug effects (principally anemia).[2,22]

Isolation & Decontamination

These viruses pose special challenges for hospital infection control. With the exception of dengue and hantaviruses, VHF patients harbor significant levels of potentially infectious virus in blood, body fluids, or secretions. Special caution must be exercised in handling hypodermic needles and other sharps that could result in parenteral exposure. Strict adherence to standard and contact precautions will prevent nosocomial transmission in most cases.[2] Droplet precautions were added as mandatory by the CDC in July 2014.[32] (See Appendix H, "Patient Isolation Precautions".)

Lassa, CCHF, Ebola and Marburg viruses may be particularly prone to nosocomial spread due to periods of high viremia corresponding with bleeding propensity. In several instances, secondary infections among contacts and medical personnel without direct body fluid exposure have been documented. These instances have prompted concern of an atypical aerosol transmission of infection. Therefore, when a VHF is suspected, additional infection control measures are indicated. The patient should be isolated in a private room with an adjoining anteroom to be used for donning and doffing protective barrier garments, storage of supplies, and decon of lab specimen containers. A negative-pressure room, with 6 to 12 air exchanges per h, is ideal for any VHF patient and is strongly advised for those with significant cough, hemorrhage, or diarrhea. All persons entering the room should use standard and contact precautions (i.e., double gloves, impermeable gowns with leg/shoe coverings, eye protection) as well as HEPA (e.g., N-95) masks or powered, air-purifying respirators (PAPRs). Note, however, that person-to-person aerosol transmission of these viruses, if it occurs, is a rare phenomenon.[4,5,22]

In the absence of a large, fixed MTF, or in the event of an overwhelming number of casualties, isolation rooms may not be available for all casualties. At a minimum, VHF patients should stay together in a separate building, or ward, with an air-handling system separate from the rest of the facility when feasible. Access should be restricted to those required to care for the patients. Personnel should undergo an external decon procedure at the point of leaving the contaminated patient-care area. A building, room or other dedicated area that is separated from the patient-care area should be established for donning and doffing protective gear. All waste (including linens) leaving the patient-care area should be decon'ed with bleach or quaternary ammonium compounds and double-bagged in clearly labeled biohazard waste bags. Ideally, this waste will be autoclaved or incinerated.[4,5,22]

Clinical specimens should be double-bagged, and the exterior of the outer bag should be decon'ed before transport to the lab. Excreta and other contaminated materials should be autoclaved or decon'ed by the liberal application of appropriate disinfectants. Clinical lab personnel are at significant risk for exposure and should employ a biosafety cabinet (if available) with barrier and respiratory precautions when handling specimens. Clinical specimens should be handled in a designated, isolated space within the lab. Access to this space should be limited and thorough decon of the space and equipment should be routine.[4,22]

No carrier state has been observed for any VHF, but excretion of virus in urine or semen may occur for some time during convalescence. Survivors should avoid sexual contact for > 3 mos after recovery. In fatal cases, there should be minimal handling of the remains, which should ideally be sealed in leak-proof material for prompt burial or cremation.[4,22]

BIOLOGICAL TOXINS

Toxins are poisonous substances produced by living organisms (animals, plants, or microbes). They are distinguished from chemical agents—such as VX, cyanide, or mustard—by the facts that they are (1) not man-made, (2) non-volatile (pose no vapor hazard), (3) usually not dermally active (mycotoxins are the exception), and (4) may be much more toxic (by weight). Toxins are similar to chemical agents, however, in that they will likely have a more rapid onset of symptoms after exposure (in hours, rather than days) compared to the progagating bio-agents discussed elsewhere in this book. A toxin's lack of volatility is an important property as it makes it unlikely to produce either secondary or person-to-person exposures, or to create a persistent environmental hazard.

A toxin's utility as an aerosol weapon is determined by its magnitude of toxicity, stability, and ease of production. The bacterial toxins, such as botulinum neurotoxins, are the most toxic substances (by weight) known (see Appendix F). Less toxic compounds, such as the mycotoxins, are thousands of times less toxic than botulinum toxins, and have limited aerosol potential. The relationship between aerosol toxicity and the quantity of toxin required for an effective open-air exposure is shown in Appendix G, which demonstrates that for some agents such as the mycotoxins and ricin, very large (ton) quantities would be needed for an effective open-air attack in a dispersed tactical environment. Stability limits the open-air potential of some toxins. For example, botulinum and tetanus toxins are large-molecular-weight proteins that are easily denatured by environmental factors (heat, desiccation, or UV light), thus limiting the downwind threat. However, one important consideration is that some toxins (e.g., certain botulinum serotypes) may be effective terrorist weapons when delivered by contamination of the food supply. Finally, some toxins (e.g., saxitoxin), might be both stable and highly toxic, but are so difficult to extract from natural sources that they can only feasibly be produced in minute quantities.

As with all bio-agents, the potential to cause incapacitation as well as lethality characterize the threat. Depending on the goals of an adversary, incapacitating agents may be more effective than lethal agents. Large numbers of ill patients might overwhelm the medical and evacuation infrastructure, will require specific medical treatment not normally available in hospitals on a large scale (e.g., ventilator assistance), and will assuredly create panic and disruption in the affected community. Several toxins, such as staphylococcal enteroxin B (SEB), pose a significant incapacitating threat by causing illness at doses much lower than those required for lethality.

A number of toxins have been weaponized by major state bio-weapons programs in the past. During the Cold War, the former US, UK, and USSR bio-warfare programs weaponized both botulinum toxins and SEB. In Iraq, in the 1980s, Saddam Hussein expended great effort to weaponize botulinum and aflatoxin. The four toxins considered most likely to be used as bio-agents today are botulinum toxins, ricin, SEB, and T-2 mycotoxins; these are therefore the ones discussed here.

Botulinum

Summary

Signs and symptoms: Symptoms usually begin with cranial nerve palsies, including ptosis (drooping eyelids), blurred vision, diplopia (double vision), dry mouth and throat, dysphagia (difficulty swallowing), and dysphonia (voice impairment). These findings are followed by symmetrical descending flaccid paralysis, with generalized weakness and progression to respiratory failure. Symptoms are dose-dependent and may begin as early as 12 to 36 h after inhalation, but can take several days to develop after exposure to low doses of toxin.

Diagnosis: Primarily clinical. Bio-agent attack should be suspected if multiple casualties simultaneously present with progressive descending flaccid paralysis. Laboratory confirmation can be obtained by bioassay (mouse neutralization) of the patient's serum. This bioassay is the accepted "gold standard" and a widely used method for detecting botulinum neurotoxin (BoNT), but can take up to 4 d for completion. Nerve conduction studies and electromyography can prove useful for differential diagnosis. Other assays that may be used for environmental or clinical samples, but lack formal accreditation and/or standardization, include immunoassays for bacterial antigen, polymerase chain reaction (PCR) for bacterial DNA, and reverse transcriptase-PCR (RT-PCR) for mRNA to detect active synthesis of toxin.

Treatment: Early administration of *Heptavalent Botulism AntiToxin (HBAT)* may prevent or decrease progression to respiratory failure and hasten recovery after exposure to all serotypes of BoNT. Intubation and ventilatory assistance are needed for respiratory failure. Tracheostomy may be required for long-term airway maintenance.

Prophylaxis: The pentavalent toxoid vaccine (previously used for protection against types A, B, C, D, and E; but not F or G) is no longer available as of 2011. No replacement vaccine is currently available.

Isolation and decontamination: Standard precautions are recommended for healthcare workers. BoNT is not dermally active and secondary aerosols are not a hazard from patients. Decontaminate with soap and water. BoNTs are inactivated by sunlight in 1 to 3 h. Heat (80°C for 30 min, 100°C for several min) and chlorine (>99.7% inactivation by 3 mg/L free available chlorine [FAC] in 20 min) also destroy BoNTs.

Overview

The botulinum neurotoxins (BoNTs) are a group of seven related proteins produced by the spore-forming bacillus *Clostridium botulinum* (Types A through G) and three other *Clostridum* species (*C. butyricum* [Type E], *C. baratii* [Type F], and *C. argentinense* [Type G]). A new serotype (H) has been tentatively identified from a case of infant botulism, but has not yet been fully investigated. These toxins are the most potent neurotoxins known; paradoxically, they have been used therapeutically to treat spastic conditions (strabismus, blepharospasm, torticollis, tetanus) and cosmetically to efface wrinkles. The spores are ubiquitous; they germinate into vegetative bacteria that produce toxins during anaerobic incubation. Industrial-scale fermentation can potentially produce large quantities of toxin for use as a bio-agent. There are three epidemiologic forms of naturally occurring botulism—foodborne, intestinal (infant or adult intestinal), and wound botulism. BoNT could be delivered via aerosol or used to contaminate food or water supplies. When inhaled, these toxins produce a clinical picture very similar to that of foodborne intoxication. The clinical syndrome (regardless of route of intoxication) produced by all these toxins is known as "botulism." Natural human botulism is primarily caused by BoNTs A, B, and E.

History & Significance

BoNTs have caused numerous cases of botulism when ingested in improperly prepared or canned foods. Many deaths have occurred from such incidents. It is theoretically possible, although difficult, to deliver BoNTs as an aerosolized biological weapon. Several countries and terrorist groups have weaponized BoNTs in the past. BoNTs were weaponized by Imperial Japan (1930s), the US (1940s-50s) in its now defunct offensive biowarfare program, and by the USSR. Evidence obtained by the UN in 1995 revealed that Iraq had filled and deployed over 100 munitions with nearly 10,000 liters of botulinum toxin. In the 1990s, the Aum Shinrikyo cult in Japan sought to weaponize and disseminate botulinum toxin on multiple occasions in Tokyo, although they failed to injure anyone in each case.

Toxin Characteristics

BoNTs are proteins with a molecular mass of about 150,000 daltons. Each of the seven toxin serotypes act to inhibit presynaptic acetylcholine release. The toxins produce similar effects when inhaled or ingested, although the time course may vary depending on the route of exposure and the dose received. BoNT could theoretically be used to sabotage food supplies.

These large proteins are readily denatured by environmental conditions. They are detoxified in open air within 12 h. Sunlight inactivates the toxins in 1 to 3 h. Heat destroys the toxins in 30 min at 80°C and in several min at 100°C. In water, the toxins are >99.7% inactivated by 20 min of exposure to 3 mg/L free available chlorine (FAC) similar to the military disinfection procedures; and 84% inactivated by 20 min at 0.4% mg/L FAC, similar to municipal water treatment procedures.

Mechanism of Toxicity

BoNT consists of two polypeptide subunits (A and B chains). The B chain binds to receptors on the axons of motor neurons. The whole toxin is transported into the axon, where the chains separate and the A chain exerts its cytotoxic effect by preventing release of acetylcholine (ACh) and blocking neuromuscular transmission (pre-synaptic inhibition). Recovery follows only after the neuron develops new axonal sprouts, a process which can take mos. The presynaptic inhibition affects both autonomic (muscarinic) and motor (nicotinic) cholinergic receptors. This interruption of neurotransmission may affect cranial nerves and nerves innervating skeletal muscle (resulting in paralysis) and the autonomic nervous system (nonreactive and dilated pupils, constipation, dry mouth, orthostatic hypotension).

Unlike the situation with nerve agent intoxication, where there is too much ACh due to inhibition of acetylcholinesterase, the problem in botulism is lack of the neurotransmitter in the synapse. Thus, pharmacologic measures such as atropine are *not* indicated in botulism and could exacerbate symptoms (see Appendix E).

Clinical Features

The onset of symptoms of inhalation botulism usually occurs between 12 and 36 h after exposure, but this is very dose dependent. Recent primate studies indicate that the signs and symptoms may not appear for several days when a low dose of the toxin is inhaled as against a mere matter of hours after ingestion or inhalation of higher doses.

Descending paralysis leads to cranial nerve palsies that are prominent early, with eye symptoms such as blurred vision due to mydriasis (dilated pupils), diplopia, ptosis, and photophobia, in addition to other cranial nerve signs such as dysarthria, dysphonia, and dysphagia. Flaccid skeletal muscle paralysis follows, in a symmetrical, descending, and progressive manner. Collapse and obstruction of the upper airway may occur due to weakness of the oropharyngeal musculature. As the descending motor weakness involves the diaphragm and accessory muscles of respiration, respiratory failure may occur abruptly. Progression from onset of symptoms to respiratory failure has occurred in as little as 24 h in cases of severe food-borne botulism.

The autonomic effects of botulism are manifested by typical anticholinergic signs and symptoms: dry mouth, ileus, constipation, and urinary retention. Nausea and vomiting may occur as nonspecific sequelae of an ileus. Mydriasis is seen in approximately 50% of cases.

Sensory symptoms usually do not occur. BoNT does not cross the blood/brain barrier and does not cause CNS disease. However, the psychological sequelae of botulism may be severe and require specific intervention.

Physical examination usually reveals an afebrile, alert, and oriented patient, although the paralysis may limit the patient's ability to respond. Postural hypotension may be present. Mucous membranes may be dry and crusted and the patient may complain of dry mouth or sore throat. There may be difficulty with speaking and swallowing. Gag reflex may be absent. Pupils may be dilated and even fixed. Ptosis and extraocular muscle palsies may also be present. Variable degrees of skeletal muscle weakness may be observed depending on the degree of progression in an individual patient. Deep tendon reflexes may be diminished or absent. With severe respiratory muscle paralysis, the patient may become cyanotic or exhibit narcosis from CO_2 retention.

Diagnosis

The occurrence of an epidemic of afebrile patients with progressive symmetrical descending flaccid paralysis would strongly suggest botulinum intoxication. Food-borne outbreaks have most often occurred in small clusters. Higher numbers of confirmed cases in a theater of operations should at least raise the consideration of a bio-agent attack with BoNTs.

Individual cases might be confused clinically with other neuromuscular disorders such as Guillain-Barre syndrome, myasthenia gravis, or tick paralysis. The edrophonium or *Tensilon*® test may be transiently positive in botulism, so it may not distinguish botulinum intoxication from myasthenia. The CSF in botulism is normal and the paralysis is generally symmetrical, which distinguishes it from enteroviral myelitis. Mental status changes generally seen in viral encephalitis should not occur with botulinum intoxication.

It may become necessary to distinguish nerve agent and/or atropine poisoning from botulinum intoxication. Nerve agent poisoning produces copious respiratory secretions, miotic pupils, convulsions, and muscle twitching, whereas normal secretions, mydriasis, difficulty swallowing, and progressive muscle paralysis is more likely in botulinum intoxication. Atropine overdose is distinguished from botulism by its CNS excitation (hallucinations and delirium) even though the mucous membranes are dry and mydriasis is present. The clinical differences between botulinum intoxication and nerve agent poisoning are depicted in Appendix E.

Laboratory testing is generally not critical to the diagnosis of botulism. Botulism is foremost a clinical diagnosis, and lab results can be inconclusive. Mouse neutralization (bioassay) remains the "gold standard" test. Therefore, serum samples should be drawn and sent to a laboratory capable of performing this assay. Other tests lack formal accreditation and/or standardization. PCR might detect *C. botulinum* genes in clinical specimens or environmental samples, but it must only be used in conjunction with the mouse bioassay, as PCR is not accredited for this purpose. Detecting toxin in clinical or environmental samples is possible on various immunoassay platforms. Clinical samples can include serum, gastric aspirates, stool, and respiratory secretions. Survivors do not usually develop an antibody response due to the very small amount of toxin necessary to produce clinical symptoms. Exposure does not confer immunity.

Medical Management

Supportive care, including prompt respiratory support, can be lifesaving. Respiratory failure due to paralysis of respiratory muscles is the most serious effect and, generally, the cause of death. Botulism cases reported before 1950 had a case fatality rate (CFR) of 60%. With the intervention, as appropriate, of tracheotomy or endotracheal intubation, ventilatory assistance, coupled with administration of botulinum immunoglobulin, CFRs are less than 5% today. However, initially unrecognized cases may have a higher fatality. Preventing nosocomial infections is a primary concern, along with hydration, nasogastric suctioning for ileus, bowel and bladder care, and preventing decubitus ulcers and deep venous thromboses. Intensive and prolonged nursing care may be required for recovery, which may take up to 3 mos for initial signs of improvement, and up to a year for complete resolution of symptoms.

Antitoxins: Early administration of botulinum antitoxin is critical, as it neutralizes the circulating toxin in patients with symptoms that will continue to progress without it. The antitoxin has no effect on toxin already bound to the nerve terminals. However, antitoxin is *never* withheld from the patient, even when treatment has been delayed.

Two different antitoxin preparations are available in the US. A bivalent human IV antiserum (types A and B, *BabyBIG*) was licensed in 2003 by the FDA and is available from the California Department of Health Services for treating infant botulism. This purified immunoglobulin is derived from pooled adult plasma from persons who were vaccinated with pentavalent botulinum toxoid (see below) and selected for their high titers of neutralizing antibody against botulinum neurotoxins type A and B. With the current absence of an approved vaccine, however, supplies of *BabyBIG* are limited.

A "despeciated" equine heptavalent antitoxin preparation against all seven serotypes has been prepared by cleaving the Fc fragments from horse IgG molecules, leaving $F(ab)_2$ fragments. The original product was developed by USAMRIID. In 2010, as an IND product—*Heptavalent Botulinum AntiToxin* (*HBAT*, Cangene Corporation)—it became the only botulinum antitoxin available in the US (at the CDC) for treatment of non-infant botulism. It was approved and licensed for commercial marketing by the FDA in March 2013. One vial (20 mL) of *HBAT* is administered to a patient as an IV infusion. It must be diluted with 0.9% sodium chloride in a 1:10 ratio before use. A volumetric infusion pump is used for slow administration (0.5 mL/min for the initial 30 min) to minimize the possibility of allergic reactions. If no reactions are noted, the rate is increased to 1 mL/min for another 30 min, and then if still no reaction is evident, to 2 mL/min for the remainder of the procedure.

Botulinum Antitoxin, Heptavalent, Equine, Types A, B, C, D, E, F, and G (*HE-BAT*) is also still available to the military under IND protocols. Use requires compliance with the experimental protocol. Administration requires skin testing with escalating dose challenges to assess the degree of an individual's sensitivity to horse serum before full-dose administration. Skin scratch tests should always precede intradermal tests.

Skin testing is performed by injecting 0.1 ml of a 1:10 dilution (in sterile physiological saline) of antitoxin intra-dermally in the patient's forearm with a 26 or 27 gauge needle. The injection site is monitored and the patient is observed for allergic reaction for 20 min. The skin test is positive if any of these allergic reactions occur: hyperemic areola at the site of the injection > 0.5 cm; fever or chills; hypotension with decrease of blood pressure > 20 mm Hg for systolic and diastolic pressures; skin rash; respiratory difficulty; nausea or vomiting; generalized itching. Equine-derived botulinum $F(ab')_2$ antitoxin is *not* administered if the skin test is positive. If no allergic symptoms are observed, the antitoxin is administered as a single IV dose in a normal saline solution, 10 ml over 20 min.

With a positive skin test, desensitization can be attempted by administering 0.01–0.1 ml of antitoxin SQ, doubling the previous dose every 20 min until 1.0–2.0 ml can be sustained without any marked reaction. Ideally, desensitization would be performed by an experienced allergist. Medical personnel administering *HE-BAT* should ensure ready IV access and be prepared to treat anaphylaxis with epinephrine and intubation, if necessary.

Prophylaxis

Vaccine: The pentavalent toxoid (PBT) of *C. botulinum* toxin types A, B, C, D, and E which was previously administered as an IND for pre-exposure prophylaxis was discontinued on 30 November 2011 due to declining efficacy and an increasing rate of adverse events. A recombinant A/B vaccine (Dyneport Vaccine Corporation) is currently undergoing human clinical trials, but is not yet licensed by the FDA and no Emergency Use Authorization (EAU) is in place. Thus, no approved vaccine is available at this time.

Antitoxin: There is no official indication at present for using a botulinum antitoxin as a prophylactic modality, except under extremely specialized circumstances. Post-exposure prophylaxis, using a heptavalent antitoxin, has been demonstrated effective in animal studies; however, as human data are not available, it is generally not recommended. This usage of heptavalent antitoxin may be considered after a known high-risk exposure to BoNT has occurred (e.g., a high-risk laboratory mishap) for all exposed, as an extraordinary measure.

Ricin

Summary

Signs and symptoms: Fever, chest tightness, cough, dyspnea, nausea, abdominal pain, anuria, dilation of pupils, headache and arthralgias occur 4 to 8 h after inhalational exposure. Airway necrosis and pulmonary capillary leak resulting in pulmonary edema may occur within 18 to 24 h, followed by severe respiratory distress and death from hypoxemia in 36 to 72 h.

Diagnosis: Acute lung injury in large numbers of geographically clustered patients may suggest exposure to aerosolized ricin. Nonspecific lab and x-ray findings include leukocytosis and bilateral interstitial infiltrates. The short time to severe symptoms and death would be unusual for infectious agents. Serum and respiratory secretions should be submitted for antigen detection by ELISA, but for metabolites only (due to the very short half-life of ricin). Acute and convalescent sera (circulating anti-ricin antibodies) allow retrospective diagnosis of survivors after about 2 wks.

Treatment is supportive and includes management of pulmonary edema. Gastric lavage and cathartics are indicated for ricin ingestion, but charcoal is of little value for such large molecules. Anti-ricin antibodies can be useful in the early stages of intoxication. Administration of IV fluids is for any route of exposure; positive–pressure ventilation may be needed after aerosol exposure. NSAIDs can be used to suppress the indiscriminate cell death cascades associated with the toxin, as well as the symptoms of intoxication.

Prophylaxis: Use of a mask is currently the best protection against inhalation. There is currently no licensed vaccine or prophylactic anti-toxin available for human use. However, there are two IND vaccines in development. A mutant recombinant RTA chain, *RiVax*, has been shown safe and immunogenic in humans in a phase 1 trial. A second clinical trial is underway. The second vaccine candidate is another recombinant RTA chain, *RVEc*, which has shown promise in animal models. It has undergone two phase 1 trials to date.

Isolation and decontamination: Standard precautions are recommended for healthcare workers. Ricin is non-volatile and secondary aerosols are not expected to be a hazard. Decon with soap and water. Hypochlorite solution (0.1% sodium hypochlorite) inactivates ricin.

Overview

Ricin is a potent protein cytotoxin derived from the beans of the castor plant (*Ricinus communis*). Castor beans are ubiquitous worldwide, and the toxin is fairly easy to extract. About two million metric tons of castor seeds are possessed annually in the production of castor oil. The waste mash from this process is 3 to 5% ricin by weight;

thus ricin is widely available. It is quite stable and extremely toxic by several routes of exposure, including the respiratory route. When inhaled as a small-particle aerosol, it may produce pathologic changes within 8 h and severe respiratory symptoms followed by acute hypoxic respiratory failure in 36 to 72 h.[1] The severity of intoxication by aerosolization is dependent on the particle size of the toxin.[2] The smaller the particle size, the further the toxin can travel into the lungs causing damage to alveoli resulting in reduced blood oxygenation. When ingested, ricin causes severe GI symptoms followed by vascular collapse, but rarely results in death.[3] IM injection causes induration and necrosis locally and, depending on dose, may cause fever, nausea, vomiting, tachycardia, hypotension, leukocytosis, lymphoid necrosis, renal failure, hematemesis, liver failure, and cardiac arrest.[3,4] This toxin also causes disseminated intravascular coagulation, microcirculatory failure, and multiple organ failure when given IV in lab animals.

History & Significance

Ricin toxin's significance as a potential bio-agent relates in part to its wide availability. During both World Wars, ricin was investigated as a potential bio-weapon. During WWI, ricin dust clouds were considered as one method of dissemination while "W bombs" were produced, but never used, during WWII.[5] Ricin was apparently used in the assassination of Bulgarian exile Georgi Markov in London in 1978. Markov was attacked with a specially engineered weapon disguised as an umbrella, which implanted an estimated 500 μg ricin pellet into his body.[4,5] This technique was used in at least six other assassination attempts in the late 1970s and early '80s. In 1994 and '95, four men from a tax-protest group known as the "Minnesota Patriots Council," were convicted of possessing ricin and conspiring to use it (by mixing it with the solvent dimethylsulfoxide) to murder law enforcement officials. In 1995, a Kansas City oncologist, Deborah Green, attempted to murder her husband by ricin food contamination. In 1997, a Wisconsin resident, Thomas Leahy, was arrested and charged with possession with intent to use ricin as a weapon. In 2003, ricin powder was discovered in a South Carolina incident[6] and in 2004 in the mail room of a United States senator. Lab analysis of samples from the South Carolina incident revealed no ricin contamination. No confirmed cases of ricin-associated illness were identified. In April 2013, three letters were sent to Mississippi Senator Roger Wicker, Mississippi judge Sadie Holland, and President Barack Obama. All three letters tested positive for ricin. James Everett Dutschke of Tupelo, Mississippi, was arrested and charged with the attempted use of a biological weapon. Two of the three letters were intercepted, while the one sent to Judge Holland was received by her, but she was not harmed. One month later, Texan actress Shannon Guess Richardson sent two more letters containing ricin to New York City mayor Michael Bloomberg and President Barack Obama. She pled guilty to possession and production of a biological toxin. In addition to its ready availability and ease of extraction, these incidents have added to ricin's media notoriety and may have increased its appeal to would-be bio-terrorists.

Toxin Characteristics

Ricin is a type II ribosome inactivating protein (RIP). It consists of two hemagglutinins and two toxins.[7] The toxins, RCL III and RCL IV, are dimers with molecular masses of about 66,000 daltons. They are made up of two polypeptide chains, an A chain and a B chain, which are joined by a disulfide bond.[7] Large quantities of ricin can be produced relatively easily and inexpensively by a simple technology. Ricin can be prepared in liquid or crystalline form, or it can be lyophilized to make a dry powder. It can be disseminated as an aerosol, injected into a victim, or used to contaminate food or water. Ricin is stable under typical ambient conditions, but is detoxified by heat (80°C for 10 min or 50°C for about an h at pH 7.8) and chlorine (>99.4% inactivation by 100 mg/L free available chlorine [FAC] in 20 min). Low chlorine concentrations (e.g., 10 mg/L FAC), as well as iodine at up to 16 mg/L, have no effect on ricin. Aerosolization of ricin would not be the most lethal method for mass dissemination when compared to other potential bioweapons. Ricin's toxicity (LD_{50}) is marginal compared to other toxins, such as botulinum and SEB (incapacitating dose). Estimates suggest that eight metric tons of ricin could only achieve a 50% casualty rate over an area of 100 km^2[2, 8]. An enemy would thus need to produce it in very large quantities to cover a significant area on a battlefield, a fact which limits its utility.

Mechanism of Toxicity

Ricin's cytotoxicity is due to inhibition of protein synthesis. The B chain binds to cell-surface receptors containing β-1,4-linked galactose residues and the toxin-receptor complex is taken into the cell by endocytosis.[9] The A chain has endonuclease activity and even very low concentrations will inhibit DNA replication and protein synthesis. In rodents, the histopathology of aerosol exposure is characterized by necrosis of upper and lower respiratory epithelium, causing tracheitis, bronchitis, bronchiolitis, and interstitial pneumonia with perivascular and alveolar edema.[10] There is a latent period of 8 h after inhalational exposure before histologic lesions are observed in animal models. In rodents, ricin is more toxic by the aerosol route than by other routes.

Clinical Features

The clinical picture depends on the route of exposure. After aerosol exposure, signs and symptoms depend on the dose inhaled. Accidental sublethal aerosol exposures, which occurred in humans in the 1940s, were characterized by onset of fever, chest tightness, cough, dyspnea, nausea, and arthralgias within 4 to 8 h[4, 11]. The onset of profuse sweating some hours later was commonly coincided with termination of most of the symptoms. Although lethal human aerosol exposures have not been described, the severe pathophysiologic changes seen in the animal respiratory tract, including necrosis and severe alveolar flooding, were sufficient to cause death from acute respiratory distress syndrome (ARDS) and respiratory failure. Time to death in experimental animals is dose dependent, occurring 36 to 72 h after inhalation.[12] Exposed humans can be expected to develop severe lung inflammation with progressive cough, dyspnea, cyanosis, and pulmonary edema.

By other routes of exposure, ricin is not a direct lung irritant; however, IV injection can cause minimal pulmonary perivascular edema due to vascular endothelial injury. Ingestion causes necrosis of the GI epithelium, local hemorrhage, and hepatic, splenic, and renal necrosis. Only 13 deaths have been recorded since the late 1880s out of 875 reported cases.[13] (Most of the deaths were attributed to the injection of the toxin.) Ingestion of ricin is rarely lethal due to the degradation of the toxin by the low pH of the stomach acid. IM injection causes severe local necrosis of muscle and regional lymph nodes with moderate visceral organ involvement.

Diagnosis

An attack with aerosolized ricin would be primarily diagnosed by observation of the clinical features in the appropriate epidemiological context. Acute lung injury affecting a large number of geographically clustered cases should raise suspicion of an attack with a pulmonary irritant such as ricin, although other pulmonary agents could present with similar signs and symptoms. Other biological threats, such as SEB, Q fever, tularemia, plague, and some chemical warfare agents like phosgene, need to be included in the differential diagnosis. Ricin-induced pulmonary edema would be expected to occur much later (1 to 3 d post-exposure) compared to that induced by SEB (about 12 h post-exposure) or phosgene (about 6 h post-exposure). Ricin intoxication will progress despite treatment with antibiotics, in contrast to an infectious process. Ricin intoxication does not cause mediastinitis as with inhalational anthrax. Ricin patients do not plateau clinically as with SEB intoxication. Additional supportive clinical or diagnostic features after aerosol exposure to ricin include the following: bilateral infiltrates on CXR, arterial hypoxemia, neutrophilic leukocytosis, and a bronchial aspirate rich in protein compared to plasma, which is characteristic of high-permeability pulmonary edema.

Specific ELISA and ECL tests of serum and respiratory secretions, or immunohistochemical stains of tissue may be used where available to confirm the diagnosis. Due to the rapid cellular uptake and distribution of ricin, early detection is critical to patient care and survival.[14] Ricin has a biphasic half-life, an alpha and beta phase, limiting detection to 24 h post-intoxication.[15] Several biochemical methods and platforms are used for ricin detection using labeled, antibody-bound magnetic beads (M1M ECL-based ricin immunoassay and Luminex MAGPIX), capture and detection antibodies (Handheld Assay Detection Devices and MSD PR2 model 1900), or by liquid chromatography/mass spectrometry (LC/MS).[4] Since the toxin has such a short half-life, additional methods need to be developed to identify other metabolites of the toxin.

PCR can be used to detect castor bean DNA in most ricin preparations.

Ricin is an extremely immunogenic toxin, and paired acute and convalescent sera should be obtained from survivors to measure antibody response for retrospective confirmation.

Medical Management

Management of ricin-intoxicated patients varies according to the exposure route. Patients with pulmonary intoxication are managed by the appropriate level of respiratory support (oxygen, intubation, ventilation, positive end-expiratory pressure [PEEP], and hemodynamic monitoring) and treatment for pulmonary edema, as indicated.

GI intoxication is best managed by vigorous gastric lavage, followed by use of cathartics, such as magnesium citrate. Superactivated charcoal administration to the patient is of little value for large molecules such as ricin. Volume replacement of GI fluid losses is important. Anti-ricin antibodies may mitigate the damage caused by ricin if implemented during the early stages of intoxication.[1,16] NSAIDs can be used to suppress the indiscriminate cell death cascades associated with the toxin, as well as the symptoms of intoxication.[17]

In percutaneous exposures, treatment is primarily supportive.

Prophylaxis

The M-40 protective mask is effective in preventing aerosol exposure. Although a vaccine is not currently available, candidate vaccines are under development. USAMRIID currently has a ricin toxin A (RTA) chain vaccine, *RVEc*™, in clinical trials with the Final Clinical Study Report anticipated for mid-2014. This vaccine is well tolerated and immunogenic conferring protection against lethal aerosol exposures in animals.[18] The second vaccine candidate is another recombinant RTA chain, *RVEc*, which has shown promise in animal models and has undergone a phase 1 trial (2011-2013).[19] Pre-exposure prophylaxis with such vaccines is currently the most promising anticipated defense against a bio-warfare attack with ricin.

Staphylococcal Enterotoxin B (SEB)

Summary

Signs and symptoms of SEB intoxication via ingestion begin 1 to 6 h (range: 1 to 12 h) and are manifested by nausea, vomiting, abdominal cramps, and/ or diarrhea that resolve within 24 to 48 h. In contrast, aerosol exposure (after a latent period of 3 to 12 h; range: 1.5 to 18 h) is manifested by a sudden onset of high fever, chills, headache, malaise, myalgia, and nonproductive cough. Some may develop shortness of breath and retrosternal chest pain. Symptoms tend to plateau soon at a fairly stable clinical state. Fever generally lasts 2 to 5 d, after which the other symptoms resolve except that cough may persist up to 4 wks. Pulmonary edema or ARDS may occur in severe cases, and delivery of high doses may result in toxic shock and death. Aerosol exposed patients may also present with nausea, vomiting, and diarrhea, as well as upper respiratory tract symptoms (sore throat/hyperemic pharynx, rhinorrhea and/or sinus congestion), or conjunctival injection. GI symptoms are likely to be more profound if toxin is swallowed. Conjunctivitis, localized periocular swelling, and GI symptoms may occur after direct ocular exposure.

Diagnosis is clinical, informed by epidemiological features. After aerosol exposure, patients present with a febrile illness and respiratory symptoms, but CXR is usually normal. Large numbers of patients presenting in a short time with typical symptoms and signs of SEB aerosol exposure suggest an intentional attack with this toxin. (Foodborne intoxication would be suggested by several individuals presenting with GI symptoms within 1 to 6 h after ingestion of a common source food.)

Treatment: Supportive. Artificial ventilation may be needed for very severe cases, and attention to fluid management is essential.

Prophylaxis: Protective mask. There is currently no human vaccine available.

Isolation and decontamination: Standard precautions are recommended for healthcare workers. Secondary aerosols are not a hazard. Ocular exposure to SEB (i.e., direct eye contact from contaminated hands) has resulted in SEB intoxication (conjunctivitis, local swelling, GI symptoms). Dermal exposure to concentrated SEB solutions may cause dermatitis. Soap and water are recommended for decon of skin. SEB contaminated food should be destroyed. Direct sunlight likely accelerates decay of SEB, but the specific persistence (duration in hours/days) on surfaces is unknown.

Overview

Staphylococcus aureus produces a number of exotoxins, one of which is staphylococcal enterotoxin B (SEB).[1-5] Such toxins are referred to as exotoxins since they are excreted from the organism. These toxins (a common cause of food poisoning due to improperly handled food) are also known as enterotoxins as they exert their effects mainly on the intestines if ingested.[6,7] SEB has been identified as a potential weapon of bio-terrorism as it is one of the more potent staphylococcal enterotoxins, and may result in significant morbidity after inhalation of low (nanogram) doses.[7] Inhalational SEB intoxication is manifested as a nonspecific febrile illness (sudden onset of high fevers, chills, myalgia, malaise, and cough) that may be associated with significant respiratory symptoms and result in incapacitation of most military personnel for 1 to 2 wks.[8-10]

History & Significance

Staphylococcal enterotoxins have been a common cause of food poisoning outbreaks.[11] These accidental intoxications often occur in a group setting such as a church picnic or other community event, and are due to improperly handled food and temperature holding, combined with ingestion of a common contaminated food source. Although an aerosolized SEB weapon would not likely produce significant fatalities, it could render most exposed personnel clinically ill and unable to perform their mission for 1 or 2 wks.[10] The resulting demand on medical and logistical systems could be overwhelming. For these reasons, SEB was one of the seven bio-agents weaponized and stockpiled by the US during its offensive bio-weapons program (1943-1969). SEB toxin could also be used to sabotage food or small-volume water supplies.

Toxin Characteristics

Staphylococcal enterotoxins are proteins ranging between 22 and 38 kilo-daltons molecular mass (SEB is 28,494 daltons).[6] They are extracellular products of coagulase-positive staphylococci. Up to 50% of clinical isolates of *S. aureus* produce exotoxins. They are produced in culture media and also in foods when there is overgrowth of the bacterium. Related toxins include toxic-shock syndrome toxin-1 (TSST-1) and exfoliative toxins. SEB is one of several identified classes of antigenically distinct enterotoxins.[1-3,6,12] These toxins are moderately stable. They are resistant to inactivation by proteolytic enzymes in the GI tract, such as pepsin.[5] Staphylococcal enterotoxins are heat stable (may be heat resistant under various conditions of pH, salt concentration, media, and toxin purity).[5,9,13,14] SEB causes symptoms when inhaled at even very low (nanogram) doses in humans: a dose of several logs lower ($\geq$ 100 times less) than the lethal inhalational dose would be sufficient to incapacitate 50% of those exposed.[9,10] GI symptoms from SEB ingestion may occur with doses as low as 50 μg.[7] Dermal exposure to SEB (dose as low as 1 $\mu g/cm^2$) may cause dermatitis.[8,15,16] Persons exposed to SEB should decontaminate skin using soap and water for $\geq$ 15 min (irrigate eyes for 15 min with water for ocular exposures). While sunlight may result in decay of SEB, the specific persistence (duration in hours or days) is unknown.[17]

Mechanism of Toxicity

Staphylococcal enterotoxins belong to a class of potent immune stimulants known as bacterial superantigens. Superantigens bind to major histocompatibility complex type II receptors on antigen-presenting cells, leading to the direct stimulation of large populations of T-helper cells while bypassing the usual antigen processing and presentation. This induces a brisk cascade of pro-inflammatory cytokines (such as tumor necrosis factor, interferon, interleukin-1 and interleukin-2), with recruitment of other immune effector cells, and relatively deficient activation of counter-regulatory negative feedback loops. This results in an intense inflammatory response that injures host tissues. Released cytokines are thought to mediate many of the toxic effects of SEB.[6,12,18-22]

Clinical Features

Symptoms of SEB intoxication begin after a latent period of 3 to 12 h (range 1.5 to 18 h) after inhalation, or 1 to 6 h (range: 1 to 12 h) after ingestion.[7,8] Symptoms depend upon the route of exposure. Ingestion results in predominantly GI symptoms: nausea, vomiting, abdominal cramps, and diarrhea.[6,7,11] Inhalation results in a non-specific febrile illness, characterized by the sudden onset of high fever (range: 103° to 105° F), chills, headache, malaise, myalgia, and cough.[8] Some patients may develop retrosternal chest pain and dyspnea. Pulmonary edema or ARDS may occur in severe cases (attributed to activation of pro-inflammatory cytokine cascades in the lungs that leads to pulmonary capillary leak and pulmonary edema).[23] GI symptoms may also accompany respiratory exposure due to inadvertent swallowing of the toxin after normal mucocilliary clearance, or simply as a systemic manifestation. Upper respiratory symptoms (sore throat, rhinorrhea, sinus congestion, profuse postnasal drip) and conjunctival injection may develop in some patients.[8,16] Ocular exposure may result in localized purulent conjunctivitis, periorbital edema, and GI symptoms (even in the absence of toxin ingestion).[8,15] Dermal exposure to concentrated SEB solutions (including dermal patch tests containing SEB) may cause dermatitis (erythema, induration, and fine scaling of the skin).[8,15,16]

Symptoms from ingestion of SEB generally resolve in 24 to 48 h. Fever, chills and prostration, and other symptoms due to inhalation generally last from 2 to 5 d, but a cough may persist for up to 4 wks[8]; patients may not be able to return to duty for 2 wks.[20,24] Symptoms from ocular exposure generally resolve in 3 to 5 d.[8]

Physical examination in patients with SEB intoxication is often unremarkable. In inhalational intoxication, conjunctival injection or hyperemia of the pharynx may be present, and postural hypotension may develop due to fluid losses. Chest examination is unremarkable except in the unusual case where pulmonary edema develops. CXR is usually normal, but severe cases may exhibit increased interstitial markings, atelectasis, and occasionally pulmonary edema or acute respiratory distress syndrome (ARDS). Leukocytosis is common, with WBC counts often ≥10,000 cells/mm^3 (range: 8,000 to 29,000 cells/mm^3) according to the experience of laboratory-acquired inhalational cases in the former US biological warfare program.[8,20] Liver functions tests are usually normal.[20]

Diagnosis

Diagnosis of SEB intoxication is based on clinical and epidemiologic features. Because the symptoms of inhalational SEB intoxication may be similar to several respiratory pathogens including influenza, adenovirus, and mycoplasma, the diagnosis may initially be unclear. All of these illnesses might present with fever, nonproductive cough, myalgia, and headache. The presence of leukocytosis and upper respiratory tract findings in SEB intoxication may further contribute to misdiagnosis as an infectious process.[8] An SEB attack would result in an onset of illness in most cases within a single 24 h period. Influenza or community-acquired pneumonia should involve patients presenting over a more prolonged interval. Symptoms of SEB intoxication tends to plateau rapidly to a fairly stable clinical state, whereas inhalational anthrax, tularemia pneumonia, or pneumonic plague would all continue to progress if left untreated. Tularemia, plague, and Q fever (unlike SEB intoxication) are infections that are often associated with infiltrates on CXR. The initial differential diagnosis may also include hantavirus pulmonary syndrome or inhalation of various chemical agents (mustard, phosgene) or other bio-toxins. Naturally occurring staphylococcal food poisoning does not present with pulmonary symptoms.

Lab confirmation of SEB intoxication includes immunological antigen detection assays (immunochromatographic lateral flow assays [hand-held devices], enzyme-linked immunosorbent assays [ELISA], electrochemiluminescence [ECL] assays, and time-resolved fluorescence [TRF] assays) on environmental and clinical samples, and gene amplification (PCR, to detect staphylococcal genes) on environmental samples.[25-37] SEB has also been detected using reverse passive latex agglutination assays, radioimmunoassays, immunoblotting, mass spectrometry, macroarray systems, and biosensor-based techniques (i.e., surface plasmon resonance detection).[38-46] While it has been detected in the serum of four ICU patients (assay detection limit was 5 pg/ml), successful detection in the serum is uncommon.[47] Studies in mice have detected low levels (range: 45 to 100 ng/ml) in the serum within 2 h after intranasal challenge and up to 36 h post-challenge.[32] The toxin was cleared rapidly from the serum, and was detected in the urine for several h post-exposure.[32] Therefore, serum and urine specimens to assess for SEB should be obtained as early as possible after inhalational SEB exposure. Respiratory secretions and nasal swabs (within 24 h of exposure) to assess for SEB may also be obtained. Acute and convalescent sera may retrospectively help support a diagnosis of SEB intoxication (4-fold increase in titers should be demonstrated as antibodies to staphylococcal superantigens may be present in the healthy population — particularly individuals colonized with *S. aureus*).[48]

Medical Management

Currently, therapy is limited to supportive care. Individuals with inhalational exposure to SEB should be closely monitored for signs of respiratory compromise or hypotension. Oxygen supplementation should be provided, if clinically indicated. Mechanical ventilation or vasopressors may be required in severe cases.[20] Fluid support may be required in SEB intoxication with severe GI symptoms (nausea, vomiting, diarrhea) or shock. Acetaminophen (for fever and myalgias), cough suppressants, and anti-emetics should be employed, as needed. The value of treatment with steroids, if any, is unknown. Most patients with SEB inhalational intoxication improve within 5 d after the onset of illness, but will likely be unfit for duty for 1 to 2 wks.

Prophylaxis

There is currently no approved human vaccine to prevent SEB intoxication. In animal studies, however, vaccine candidates have demonstrated protection against SEB challenge. A recombinant attenuated mutant SEB vaccine candidate is currently in advanced development for safety and immunogenicity testing in humans (phase I study initiated in 2013).[6,20,49-52] Experimentally, passive immunotherapy can reduce fatalities in animals, but only if given within 4 to 8 h after inhalation or immediately post-challenge to within 4 h after intra-peritoneal challenge.[53-57] Because of the rapidity of SEB binding with MHC Class II receptors (<5 min *in vitro*), active vaccination is considered the most practical defense. Interestingly, many healthy persons may have detectable antibody titers to SEB and other staphylococcal superantigens through natural exposure. While these antibodies may possibly provide some protection during *S. aureus* septicemia, it is not known if these naturally-acquired antibodies would provide any protective effect against aerosol SEB exposure.[32, 48, 58]

T-2 Mycotoxins

Summary

Signs and symptoms: Exposure causes skin pain, pruritus, redness, vesiculation, necrosis, and sloughing of the epidermis. Effects on the airway include nose and throat pain, nasal discharge, itching and sneezing, cough, dyspnea, wheezing, chest pain, and hemoptysis. Similar effects occur after ingestion or eye contact. Severe intoxication results in weakness, ataxia, collapse, prostration, shock, and death.

Diagnosis: Suspect mycotoxin if an aerosol attack occurs in the form of "yellow rain" with droplets of variously pigmented oily fluids contaminating clothes and the environment, especially if field tests for vesicant chemical agent are negative. No rapid diagnostic test for mycotoxins is available for clinical field use. Confirmation requires lab-based testing of blood, tissue, or environmental samples.

Treatment: No specific antidote; treatment is supportive. Soap and water washing, even 4-6 h after exposure, can significantly reduce dermal toxicity; washing within 1 h may prevent toxicity entirely. M291 skin decontamination kit should be used if available. Superactivated charcoal should be given orally if the toxin is swallowed.

Prophylaxis: The only defense is to prevent exposure by wearing a protective mask and clothing (or topical skin protectant) during an attack. No specific immunotherapy or chemotherapy is available for use in the field.

Isolation and decontamination: Outer clothing should be removed and exposed skin decon'ed with soap and water. Eye exposure should be treated with copious saline irrigation. Secondary aerosols are not a hazard; however, direct contact with contaminated skin or clothing can produce secondary dermal exposures. Contact precautions are warranted until decon is completed. After decon, standard precautions are recommended for healthcare workers. A 3-5% solution of sodium hypochlorite should be used for environmental decon.

Overview

Mycotoxins are metabolites of fungi produced through secondary biochemical pathways. *Trichothecene* compounds are one of a number of different classes of mycotoxins, which also include the aflatoxins, rubratoxins, ochratoxins, and fumonisins. Trichothecenes are a very large family of chemically related metabolites produced by a variety of molds and are important for their effect on crops. *T-2 mycotoxins* are trichothecenes also produced by a number of mold species; they are low-molecular-weight compounds that are resistant to heat and UV light thus rendering them extremely stable in the environment. Unlike other biological toxins—and unlike the propagating bio-agents—T-2 mycotoxins are potent dermal irritants.[1] Delivered in a sufficient dose, they can cause severe skin, and potentially systemic, reactions. In an intoxicated human or animal, they are rapidly metabolized to HT-2, T2-triol, and T-2 tetraol within hours of exposure. Possible dermal, ocular, respiratory, and GI exposures, and their characteristic signs and symptoms, should be anticipated after an aerosol attack with mycotoxins.[2-4]

History & Significance

The potential for T-2 mycotoxin use as a weapon was suggested to bioweaponeers during and after World War II by an event in Orenburg, Russia: over 10% of the civilian population there was affected when they ingested bread made with wheat flour unintentionally contaminated with the common mild *Fusarium*.[5] Some developed a protracted, ultimately fatal, illness christened as "alimentary toxic aleukia" (ATA) and characterized initially by abdominal pain, diarrhea, vomiting, prostration, and within days, fever, chills, myalgias and bone marrow depression with granulocytopenia and secondary sepsis. Survival beyond this point was accompanied by the development of painful pharyngo-laryngeal ulcerations and diffuse bleeding into the skin (petechiae, then ecchymoses), melena, hematochezia, hematuria, hematemesis, epistaxis, and vaginal bleeding. Pancytopenia and GI ulceration/erosion developed secondary to the profound depression of bone marrow and mucosal protein synthesis and to cell-cycle progression through DNA replication.

Owing to their environmental stability and dissemination potential, it was understood that the T-2 mycotoxins could be weaponized. Controversy still prevails over the "yellow rain" incidents where mycotoxins allegedly were released from aircraft by the Soviet Union and its allies during the conflicts in Laos (1975-81), Cambodia (1979-81), and Afghanistan (1979-81).[6] It was estimated that there resulted more than 6,300, 1,000, and 3,042 deaths in those three countries, respectively.[7] The victims included both unarmed civilians and guerrilla forces. These groups were not protected with gas masks or chemical protective clothing and had little ability to defend against the attacking enemy aircraft. The attacks supposedly occurred in remote jungle areas, which made definitive confirmation of reports and recovery of agent extremely difficult. Some authorities have asserted that the "yellow clouds" were, in fact, bee feces produced by swarms of the migrating insects.[8] This theory failed to account for the reported deaths and injuries. Much of the debate centered upon the veracity of eyewitness and victim accounts, but there is evidence for serious consideration of these allegations of biological (or chemical) weapon use.[9-12] A recent history of the Soviet biological weapons program concludes that there is evidence of Soviet-era offensive mycotoxin weapons research and development.[13]

In Iraq, according to UNSCOM, Saddam Hussein is known to have produced, weaponized, and stockpiled the mycotoxin known as aflatoxin by the end of the 1980s.[14,15]

Trichothecene mycotoxin exposures in the developed world have typically involved accidental ingestion of contaminated foodstuffs. Fatal pulmonary hemorrhages in infants occuring in the US state of Ohio about 20 years ago raised suspicion that the cause may have been due to such exposure in homes secondary to mold overgrowth.[16] Cases of sudden infant death syndrome (SIDS) have been attributed to *Stachybotrys* mycotoxin exposure in homes secondary to mold overgrowth resulting from flooding.[17]

Toxin Characteristics

The trichothecene mycotoxins are low-molecular-mass (250-500 daltons) non-volatile compounds produced by filamentous fungi (molds). The structures of approximately 150 trichothecene derivatives have been described and are produced by more than 350 species, most notably of the genera *Fusarium, Myrotecium, Trichoderma,* and *Stachybotrys.*[18] These substances are relatively insoluble in water, but are highly soluble in organic solvents such as acetone, ethanol, methanol and propylene glycol. Trichothecenes can vaporize when heated in organic solvents. Extraction of these mycotoxins from fungal cultures yields a yellow-brown liquid that evaporates into a yellow greasy crystalline product (some believe this to be the substance found in "yellow rain"). T-2 mycotoxin is unique among the bio-agents in that systemic toxicity can result from any of the major routes of exposure—transdermal, oral, or inhalational.

The trichothecenes are extremely stable and resistant to heat and UV light inactivation. They retain their bioactivity even when autoclaved; heating to 900° F for 10 min or 500°F for 30 min is required for inactivation. A 3-5% solution of sodium hypochlorite is effective for inactivating T-2 mycotoxins and the efficacy can be further enhanced with the addition of small amounts of alkali.[19] The US Army's decontaminating agents DS-2 and Supertropical bleach inactivate T-2 toxin within 30 to 60 min. In lab animals, washing contaminated skin with soap and water within 4 to 6 h removed 80-98% of the toxin, which prevented dermal lesions and death.

Mechanism of Toxicity

Trichothecenes are potent inhibitors of protein synthesis and have a pronounced effect on actively proliferating cells, such as those found in the skin, GI tract, and bone marrow. Because this cytotoxic effect mimics the hematopoietic and lymphoid effects of radiation sickness, the mycotoxins are referred to as "radiomimetic agents." T-2 mycotoxins interfere with peptidyl transferase activity and inhibit either the initiation or elongation of process of translation. The mycotoxins also alter cell membrane structure and function, inhibit mitochondrial respiration, and inactivate certain enzymes. Recent molecular studies suggest that T-2 mycotoxins also induce apoptosis (programmed cell death) through a reactive oxygen species–mediated mitochondrial pathway.[20] It is estimated that T-2 mycotoxin is about 400 times more potent in producing skin injury than mustard.[21]

Clinical Features

Clinical signs, symptoms, and severity will vary depending on the route of exposure, duration of exposure (acute, subacute, chronic), toxin concentration, and total dose. In a bio-warfare attack, the toxin or toxins could adhere to and penetrate the skin, be inhaled, or be ingested. In the alleged yellow rain incidents, symptoms of exposure from all three routes seemed to coexist. Contaminated clothing may serve as a reservoir for further (secondary) toxin exposure. Early symptoms beginning within minutes of exposure include burning skin pain, redness, tenderness, blistering, and progression to skin necrosis with eventual leathery blackening and sloughing of large areas of skin. Upper respiratory exposure may result in nasal itching, pain, sneezing, epistaxis, and rhinorrhea. Pulmonary and trachea-bronchial toxicity would produce dyspnea, wheezing, and cough. Mouth and throat exposure could cause pain and blood-tinged saliva and sputum. Anorexia, nausea, vomiting, and watery or bloody diarrhea with cramps and abdominal pain will likely occur with ingestion. Eye pain, tearing, redness, foreign body sensation, and blurred vision may follow ocular exposure. Skin symptoms occur in minutes to hours and eye symptoms in minutes. Systemic toxicity can occur via any route of exposure, and results in weakness, prostration, dizziness, ataxia, and loss of coordination. Tachycardia, hypothermia, and hypotension follow in severe cases. Death may occur in minutes, hours, or days. The most common symptoms are vomiting, diarrhea, skin involvement with burning pain, redness and pruritus, rash or blisters, bleeding, and dyspnea. A late effect of systemic absorption is pancytopenia, predisposing to bleeding and sepsis.

No human mortality or morbidity data have been reported for T-2 mycotoxin use as a bio-weapon. Information regarding fatalities from the few instances of accidental ingestion of contaminated food is quite varied, with 10 to 60% case fatality rates reported in Russia's Orenburg district in the 1940s.

Diagnosis

Clinical and epidemiological findings provide clues to the diagnosis. High attack rates, dead animals of multiple species, along with physical evidence such as yellow, red, green, or other pigmented oily liquids, suggest mycotoxin exposure. Rapid onset of symptoms in minutes to hours supports a diagnosis of a chemical or toxin attack. In addition, the coexistence of cutaneous, ocular, respiratory, and GI symptoms may support the suspicion of mycotoxin exposure. Mustard and other vesicant agents must be considered, especially if there is a distinctive odor and visible residue; rapid detection of these is by a field chemical test (M8 paper, M256 kit). Symptoms of mustard toxicity are also delayed for several hours after exposure. Inhalation of SEB or ricin aerosols can cause fever, cough, dyspnea, and wheezing, but does not affect the skin.

There are several commercial immunoassay kits on the market that detect trichothecene mycotoxins in grain and feed. (However, no data exist to differentiate the expected environmental background levels of these substances from potential toxic and/or intentional contamination.) Unfortunately, no rapid diagnostic test is currently available for field clinical use. Serum and urine should be collected and sent to a reference laboratory for antigen detection. The mycotoxins and their metabolites are eliminated in urine and feces; 50-75% is eliminated within 24 h; however, metabolites can be detected as late as 28 d after exposure. Pathologic specimens yielding diagnosis may include blood, urine, lung, liver, and stomach contents. Environmental and clinical samples can be tested using gas liquid chromatography (GLC), a high-performance liquid chromatography (HPLC)-mass spectrometry (MS) combination technique, or various ELISA techniques. GLC–MS and HPLC–MS are the best and most sensitive methods for detecting mycotoxins. This system can detect as little as 0.1-1.0 parts per billion of T-2, which is sensitive enough to measure T-2 levels in the plasma of toxin victims.

Medical Management

No specific antidote or therapeutic regimen is currently available. All therapy is supportive. If a soldier is unprotected during an attack, the outer uniform should be removed as soon as possible. The skin should be thoroughly washed with soap and water. This may reduce dermal toxicity, even if delayed for 4 to 6 h after exposure.[22] (Contaminated clothing as well as wash waste from the decon process should be exposed to bleach [5% sodium hypochlorite] for 6 h or more to neutralize any residual myxotoxin.) The M291 skin decontamination kit can also be used to remove skin-adherent T-2. XE-556 resin, which is similar to the XE-555 resin in the M291 kit, was shown to be effective in the physical removal of T-2 toxin from the skin in animal studies.

Treatment for cutaneous involvement will resemble standard burn care. The eyes should be irrigated copiously with normal saline or water to remove toxin if eye pain or tearing is apparent. Standard therapy for poison ingestion, including the use of superactivated charcoal to absorb swallowed T-2 toxin, should be administered to victims of an unprotected aerosol attack. (Some have advocated activated charcoal use even after inhalational exposure as the toxin that is adherent to the oral mucosa may thus be bound.[23]) Respiratory support may be necessary. Serial lymphocyte count may identify patients who will become immunocompromised. For systemic intoxication, some survival benefit was seen with administration of dexamethasone, diphenhydramine, naloxone, methylthiazolidine-4-carboxylate, metoclopramide, magenesium sulfate, and sodium bicarbonate in animal studies. No similar studies have been conducted in humans. Likewise, the utility of administering colony-stimulating factors to patients presenting with bone marrow suppression in this context is purely theoretical.

Prophylaxis

Physical barrier protection of the skin, mucous membranes, and airway (use of HAZMAT suits or chemical protective mask and clothing, such as MOPP gear) are the only practically effective methods of protection during an attack. The Skin Exposure Reduction Paste Against Chemical Warfare Agents (SERPACWA), has been shown to block dermal irritation in animal studies and can be applied at closure points of chemical over-garments as well as to any skin-exposed areas.[24] It is FDA-approved for use against dermally active toxins. Also available to the DoD and many NATO forces is the Reactive Skin Decontamination Lotion (RSDL). This product acts by a combination of physical removal and nucleophilic breakdown, which renders the original toxic substance (chemical or biological) non-toxic.[25]

Candidate immunologic products (vaccines and monoclonal antibodies), and chemo-protective pre-treatments, are being studied in animal models, but are not available for field use.

EMERGING THREATS: NOVEL INFECTIOUS DISEASES & NEW POTENTIAL BIO-WEAPONS

Emerging Infectious Diseases

Emerging infectious diseases were defined in a landmark report by the Institute of Medicine in 1992[1] and include those infectious diseases that are: (1) newly recognized as occurring in humans (or animals or plants), (2) newly occurring in a different population or geographic region, (3) affecting greater numbers of individuals, or (4) evolving important new attributes (e.g., antimicrobial drug resistance or increased virulence). Even though some "emerging" diseases have been recognized for more than 30 years (e.g., AIDS, Lyme disease, Ebola virus disease, Legionnaire's disease), their importance has not diminished, and the factors associated with their emergence are still relevant.

Many factors contribute to the emergence of new infectious diseases, most notably environmental (including climate) change, increased global travel and trade, social and political upheaval (including military conflicts), and genetic changes in microbial agents, hosts, or vector populations. Once a new disease is introduced into a susceptible human population, it may spread rapidly and could challenge the medical and public health infrastructures. If the disease is severe, it may lead to social disruption and cause severe economic impact. It should be noted that these effects could be seen not only with a new human disease, but also with diseases of crops and/or food production animals. Outbreaks of novel infectious agents such as Ebola virus, the Middle East respiratory syndrome (MERS) virus and novel influenza viruses appear to be occurring with increasing frequency and with a greater potential for serious consequences. In addition, there is increasing instances of viruses appearing in new geographic regions, as with the case of West Nile virus in the United States in 1999, chikungunya virus in the Caribbean in 2013 and Ebola virus in West Africa in December 2013.

In a 2008 study funded by the National Science Foundation (NSF) and published in *Nature*, about two-thirds of emerging infections were found to be zoonotic (animal in origin) and the majority of those came from wild animals (e.g., monkey-pox, coronaviruses, Ebola virus).[2] Important geographic areas of emergence include Sub-Saharan Africa, India and China, and South America. New pathogens may be transmitted directly by hunting or accidental contact with wildlife, while others may be transmitted from wildlife to livestock to people (e.g., Malaysia's Nipah virus or Australia's Hendra virus). Humans have evolved little resistance to zoonotic diseases, so the diseases can be extraordinarily lethal.

About 20% of known emerging infections are caused by multidrug-resistant strains of previously known pathogens, such as *Mycobacterium tuberculosis*. Wealthier nations' increasing dependence on, and misuse of, antibiotics amplifies the proliferation of such dangerous variants of common bacteria. An example is enterotoxigenic *Escherichia coli*, now spread widely and with great speed because products like raw vegetables are processed in huge, centralized facilities, and hastily packaged for rapid onward shipment and consumption.

Emergence of pandemic influenza, Ebola virus, Marburg virus, MERS-CoV, anthrax, West Nile virus, prion diseases, multidrug-resistant tuberculosis (MDR-TB), and scores of other "new" diseases remind clinicians and public health officials to remain ever vigilant for outbreaks of novel or unexplained diseases. These emerging infections have a potential to become future biological threats on a large scale, as indeed some of them have already. Natural emerging disease outbreaks may be difficult to distinguish from the intentional introduction of infectious diseases for nefarious purposes; hence, consideration must also be given to this possibility before any question of etiology is considered settled.

Because emerging infectious diseases are so diverse, exotic, and vary enormously according to geographic location, their complete description is beyond the scope of this handbook. Summaries of a few recent emerging infections follow, but one should be mindful that the most worrisome pathogen may well be the one not yet recognized.

Pandemic Influenza

The threat for pandemic spread of human influenza is substantial. The pathogenicity of influenza viruses is directly related to their ability to rapidly alter their eight viral RNA segments. New antigenic variation results in the formation of new hemagglutinin (HA) or neuraminidase (NA) surface glycoproteins, which may go unrecognized by an immune system primed against heterologous strains.

Two distinct phenomena contribute to a renewed susceptibility to influenza infection among persons previously infected. Clinically significant variants of influenza A viruses may result from mutations in the HA and NA genes, expressed as minor structural changes in the viral surface proteins. As few as four amino acid substitutions in any two antigenic sites can cause a clinically significant variation. These minor changes result in an altered virus able to circumvent host immunity. Additionally, genetic reassortment between avian and human, or avian and porcine, influenza viruses may lead to major changes in HA or NA surface proteins known as "antigenic shift." In contrast to the gradual evolution of strains subject to "antigenic drift", antigenic shift occurs when an influenza virus with a completely novel HA or NA formation moves into humans from other host species. Global pandemics such as the one in 2009 have resulted from such antigenic shifts.

Influenza causes more than 30,000 deaths and more than 100,000 hospitalizations annually in the US. Pandemic influenza viruses have emerged regularly in 10- to 50-yr cycles for the last several centuries. During the 20th century, influenza pandemics occurred four times: 1918 (Spanish influenza, a H1N1 virus), 1957 (Asian influenza, an H2N2 subtype strain), in 1968 (Hong Kong influenza, an H3N2 variant), and most recently, in 2009 (California H1N1 influenza).

The 1918 influenza pandemic illustrates a worst-case public health scenario: it caused 675,000 deaths in the US and 20-40 million deaths worldwide. Morbidity in most affected communities was between 25 and 40%; case fatality rates (CFRs) averaged about 2.5%, compared with the 0.1% in more typical flu outbreaks (a 25-fold increase). A re-emergent 1918-like influenza virus would have devastating societal effects, even in the event that anti-viral medications proved effective.

The 1957-58 pandemic caused 66,000 excess deaths, and the 1968 pandemic caused 34,000 excess deaths in the United States.

In April 2009, an outbreak of influenza-like illness occurred in Mexico and the US; the CDC reported seven cases of a novel A/H1N1 influenza virus. The disease then spread very rapidly, with the number of confirmed cases rising to 2,099 by May 7, 2009, despite aggressive measures taken by the Mexican government. On June 11, 2009, the World Health Organization (WHO) declared an H1N1 pandemic (pandemic alert phase 6), the first global influenza pandemic since the 1968 Hong Kong flu. Fortunately, the 2009 H1N1 virus was fatal in 0.01–0.03% of those infected, making it considerably less lethal than previous pandemic strains (1918 virus was 100 times more lethal). However, incidence and CFRs for the 2009 pandemic varied by age. Children (5-14 yrs old) had the highest estimated incidence rate and the lowest CFR (0.01%), whereas elders ≥65 yrs old) had the lowest estimated incidence rate and highest CFR (0.98%).

The emergence of the pandemic 2009 influenza virus reaffirmed the world's susceptibility to reemerging infections. The 1918 virus was thought to have emerged from birds, then, almost simultaneously, moved into humans and swine. In contrast to the 1918 virus, the 2009 flu virus contained genes from five different flu viruses: North American swine influenza, North American avian influenza, human influenza, and two swine influenza viruses typically found in Asia and Europe.[3]

Wild aquatic birds are the reservoirs of all subtypes of influenza A virus, where they generally cause no harm. Transmission from aquatic birds to humans was originally hypothesized to require infection of an intermediate, such as a pig, that has both human-specific and avian-specific receptors on its respiratory epithelium.

Now scientists understand that influenza A viruses can transmit directly from birds to humans. But pigs remain a natural "mixing vessel" for flu because they can be infected both by avian and human strains allowing for the reassortment before the microbe moves on. When pigs become simultaneously infected with more than one virus, the viruses can swap genes, producing new variants which can pass to humans and sometimes spread among them. In 2010, scientists from Hong Kong determined that the 2009 pandemic virus was a reassortment of viruses previously found in pigs, forming a new hybrid swine flu virus.

Avian Influenza

"Avian influenza virus" usually refers to influenza A viruses primarily found in birds. However, occasional confirmed cases of human infection with several subtypes of avian influenza virus have been reported since 1997. Most human cases of avian flu have resulted from direct contact with infected poultry (e.g., domestic chickens, ducks, and turkeys) or surfaces contaminated with secretion/excretions from these birds. The spread of avian influenza viruses from an ill person to another person has been reported only very rarely, and transmission has been limited, inefficient, and unsustained.

An epizootic of highly pathogenic avian influenza virus (HPAI H5N1) emerged in Southeast Asia in 2003 before spreading to other continents, mostly in animals (poultry, aquatic birds), but also in humans. By January 2011, over 6,780 animal outbreaks of HPAI H5N1 had been reported in 51 countries. Several countries (e.g., Egypt, Indonesia) suspended animal surveillance for HPAI H5N1 several years earlier even though they had accounted for 20% of the world's animal outbreaks. In July 2013, the WHO announced a total of 630 confirmed human cases, which resulted in the deaths of 375 people since 2003.[4] Disease caused by another avian flu virus (H7N9) was first reported in March 2013 in China. By May of that year, 37 people had died from the infection. As of April 2014, the virus has infected 419 people, leading to 127 deaths.[5]

Avian influenza in humans presents like other types of influenza: usually beginning with fever, chills, headaches and myalgias, and often involving the upper and lower respiratory tract with development of cough, dyspnea, and, in severe cases, acute respiratory distress syndrome (ARDS). Laboratory findings may include pancytopenia, lymphopenia, elevated liver enzymes, hypoxia, positive RT-PCR and positive neutralization assay for the specific virus.

Novel Coronaviruses (SARS and MERS)

Another example of zoonotic spread of a new infectious disease was the emergence of severe acute respiratory syndrome (SARS) in Southeast Asia in 2003 due to a novel coronavirus that jumped the species barrier from animals to humans and rapidly spread to 29 countries in less than 90 days. Bats appear to be the natural reservoir of the virus, which ultimately infected a total of 8,273 individuals around the world and killed 775 people (CFR = 9.4%).[6] Fortunately, the spread of SARS has been fully contained with the last infected human case seen in June 2003 (disregarding a 2004 lab exposure).

In 2012, a new SARS-like illness emerged in Saudi Arabia.[7] A new species of coronavirus was isolated from sputum specimens of the index patient and given the name Middle Eastern respiratory syndrome (MERS)-coronavirus (CoV). Person-to-person transmission of MERS-CoV was confirmed in a cluster of over 30 hospitalized cases in the Al-Hasa governorate of Saudi Arabia. And by the end of 2013, there have been 163 confirmed cases of infection resulting in 71 deaths (CFR = 44%).[8] The majority of these cases were from Saudi Arabia, but France, Italy, Jordan, Qatar, Tunisia, the United Kingdom, and the United Arab Emirates have all reported cases as well. Cases outside of the Middle East all had recorded recent travel to the Middle East.

Prior to 2003, only two coronaviruses were known to infect humans, and those caused only mild respiratory disease. Now there are at least 6 coronaviruses known to infect humans and many more that cause disease in a variety of animals. Obvious parallels can be drawn between the recent MERS epidemic and the SARS epidemic of 2003. Although the reservoir for MERS-CoV has not been definitely identified, both viruses are thought to circulate in bats. SARS-like coronaviruses were identified in three species of bats, and several studies have shown the presence of MERS-CoV (or viral nucleic acid) in fecal samples of bats. However, there is no indication that MERS-CoV is jumping directly from bats into humans. One possibility is that MERS-CoV may move from bats through an intermediate host that has a closer association with humans. Serum surveys of livestock in Egypt, Oman, and Spain identified high levels of antibodies to MERS-CoV in dromedary camels.[9,10] Subsequently, MERS-CoV RNA was detected in 3 camels that had close association with two human cases.

Emerging foodborne disease–*Escherichia coli* O104:H4

In the summer of 2011, two separate outbreaks of bloody diarrhea and hemolytic-uremic syndrome (HUS) occurred in Europe.[11,12] One was centered in Germany and comprised 3,816 cases of bloody diarrhea, 845 cases of HUS and 54 deaths; whereas the other occurred in France and comprised 15 cases of bloody diarrhea, 9 of which progressed to HUS. These were not caused by *E. coli* O157:H7, the typical bacterial cause of HUS. Rather, these outbreaks were caused by a much more virulent form of Shiga toxin-producing *E. coli* called *E. coli* O104:H4 and represented the highest frequency of HUS and death recorded from such a bacterial strain. An epidemiological investigation determined that contaminated sprouts were the source of the outbreak and that this was a consequence of tainted seeds of fenugreek (a widely cultivated legume) from an exporter in Egypt who had obtained them from a German distributor supplying a German sprout farm. A portion of the original seed shipment was also sent to an English seed distributor, which repackaged the seeds and supplied them to French garden stores, leading to the outbreak in France.

Rapid whole genome sequencing was used to fully characterize the *E. coli* from the 2011 German outbreak in near real-time. This comprehensive analysis took place in the first days and weeks of the outbreak, rapidly enough to inform physicians treating infected patients and epidemiologists tracing the source of the pathogen. Only this kind of rapid whole-genome sequencing allowed investigators to determine that the outbreak strain was an extremely rare form of the bacterium that was a 'hybrid' of enteroaggregative *E. coli* and enterohemorrhagic *E. coli*. Researchers also determined that this was distinct from other *E. coli* O104:H4 strains because it contained a prophage encoding a Shiga toxin and a distinct set of other virulence and antibiotic-resistance factors.

Chikungunya virus in the Western Hemisphere

The first recorded outbreak of chikungunya occurred in the Newala District of Tanzania (former Tanganyika) in Africa in 1952. The infection manifested with a sudden onset of incapacitating joint pain and high fever, leading locals to call it *chikungunya* meaning "that which bends up" in the local Makonde language. The disease also often leads to the development of a maculopapular rash, anorexia, constipation, and arthralgia, which could last for months following the infection. In some patients, the joint pain is so severe even months after infection that they were unable to change position without help.

The chikungunya virus is an Old World alphavirus, transmitted by *Aedes* species mosquitoes that are found mainly in Africa and Southeast Asia. While there were numerous documented outbreaks of chikungunya throughout Africa and Asia in the 1960s and '70s, little disease activity was seen between 1980 and 2000. In 2000, however, the virus reemerged in a big way when an estimated 50,000 people were infected in Kinshasa, Democratic Republic of the Congo, the first reappearance of the virus there in 39 years.[13] In 2004, an outbreak occurred on Lamu Island off the coast of Kenya in which there were 1,300 reported cases out of a total population of 18,000 on the island. A seroprevalence study conducted after the epidemic found that 75% of the population had detectable antibodies to the virus, indicating that approximately 13,500 people had been infected. The virus further spread to Mombasa, Kenya, and then to the Comoros Islands, where an estimated 215,000 people contracted the disease.[14]

Additional outbreaks occurred on the Indian Ocean islands of Mauritius, the Seychelles, Madagascar, and Mayotte, culminating in a large outbreak on Reunion Island in 2005-2006 in which an estimated 255,000 people were infected.[15] The outbreak on Reunion Island was unusual because it appeared that the main vector responsible for transmission was *Aedes albopictus*, the Asian Tiger mosquito, and not *A. aegypti*, the virus' usual mosquito vector. Additionally, genetic characterization of the virus revealed that single amino acid change in the envelope glycoprotein enabled the virus to infect *A. albopictus* mosquitoes much more efficiently.[16,17] In December 2013, the WHO reported confirmed cases of chikungunya on the Caribbean Island of St. Martin. None of the cases reported recent travel outside of St. Martin, indicating that these are the first reported cases of local transmission of chikungunya virus in the

Western Hemisphere. As of February 2014, the virus has been found in 10 Caribbean countries resulting in nearly 3,000 confirmed cases and over 13,000 suspected cases.[18]

New Potential Biological Weapons

The evolving bio-warfare/bio-terrorism threat is becoming more complex because of increased bio-agent variety and the increasing ease of *in vitro* genetic modification. Although *Bacillus anthracis* (anthrax) will remain an attractive option for many state and non-state perpetrators, some groups may focus on new types of viral and bacterial agents. The availability of bio-warfare-relevant technologies, materials, information, and expertise has increased, as has publicity about potential vulnerabilities. Novel genetic engineering and other advances in biotechnology provide powerful capabilities to modify virtually any bio-agent, affecting characteristics such as enhanced virulence, increased environmental stability, resistance to medical countermeasures, and defeat of physical barriers, bio-detectors, and laboratory diagnostics.

While there are no simple solutions to the threat of emerging infectious disease and novel biological weapons, expansion of US national expertise and fostering of new international partnerships may greatly help create synergies for the detection and deterrence of biological threats. The type of situational awareness needed for a global pandemic overlaps with that needed to detect a major bio-terrorist campaign in its early stages. Along with the wider civilian community, the Department of Defense (DoD) has recognized that emerging infectious diseases represent an uncontrolled source of mayhem, which could be harnessed for nefarious purposes. The appearance of a new or reemerging infectious disease can have global implications. During the past 20 yrs, more than 30 novel lethal pathogens have been identified. In addition to the traditional bio-agents such as anthrax and plague, more familiar reemerging pathogens, such as influenza, represent significant future threats to both military and civilian populations. This is especially true since modern molecular biology techniques allow modified or completely new organisms to be made in the laboratory.

The DoD has placed increased emphasis on non-proliferation and emerging threats and recognize the challenge of developing countermeasures against non-traditional agents. Addressing these novel bio-agents is a central objective of the Homeland Security Presidential Directive (HSPD)-18, *Medical Countermeasures against Weapons of Mass Destruction* (2007), written in coordination with the Executive Office of the President, DoD, and Department of Health and Human Services (DHHS). As technological advances continue to evolve, our defensive capabilities should preferably include a twotiered approach for development and acquisition of medical countermeasures, which will balance the immediate need to provide a capability to mitigate the most catastrophic of the current chemical, biological, radiological and nuclear threats, with long-term requirements to develop more flexible, broader spectrum countermeasures to address future threats.

HSPD-18 frames the biological threat spectrum into four distinct categories, the last three of which concern non-traditional agents.

a. ***Traditional agents:*** naturally-occurring microorganisms or toxins with the potential to be disseminated to cause mass casualties (e.g., *Bacillus anthracis* [anthrax] and *Yersinia pestis* [plague]).

b. ***Enhanced agents:*** traditional agents that have been modified or selected to enhance their ability to harm human populations or circumvent current countermeasures, such as a bacterium that has been modified to be antibiotic resistant.

c. ***Emerging agents:*** previously unrecognized pathogens that might be naturally occurring and present a serious risk to human populations (e.g., MERS-coronavirus).

d. ***Advanced agents:*** novel pathogens or biologicals that have been artificially engineered in the laboratory to bypass traditional medical countermeasures or produce a more severe or otherwise enhanced spectrum of disease.

DoD's Chemical and Biological Defense Program (CBDP)

Enacted by Congress in 1993, Public Law 103-160 created the DoD Chemical and Biological Defense Program (CBDP). The Assistant to the Secretary of Defense for Nuclear and Chemical and Biological Defense Programs (ATSD [NCB]) is the principal advisor to the Secretary and Deputy Secretary of Defense, and the Under Secretary of Defense for Acquisition, Technology, and Logistics (USD [AT&L]) on nuclear energy, nuclear weapons, and chemical and biological defense and provides overall coordination, integration, and oversight of the CBDP.

Novel bio-agents and emerging infectious diseases present complex challenges for the nation and our warfighters. The CBDP has implemented steps to assess and mitigate risks associated with these emerging threats, including analysis of non-traditional agents and the expansion of the Transformational Medical Technologies (TMT) Initiative.

Transformational Medical Technologies (TMTs)

The DoD's TMT mission is to protect the warfighter from emerging and genetically engineered biological threats by providing a robust response capability ranging from identification of pathogens through to the development of medical countermeasures. TMT is pursuing technologies to characterize unknown pathogens and rapidly develop medical countermeasures to newly identified threats. The program intends to spur innovative research to develop broad-spectrum medical countermeasures that are peer-reviewed and FDA approved.

The TMT initiative is a vital part of the National Biodefense Strategy and the Integrated National Biodefense Medical Countermeasures Portfolio (INBDP), which is coordinated with the Executive Office of the President, DoD, and DHHS. This active interagency participation is essential to the development and implementation of an effective biodefense capability for the nation. The overarching goal of the TMT is to provide proof-of-process for development of platform technologies that allow for the rapid development of Medical Countermeasures (MCMs); determination of the genetic sequences for pertinent threats against which to screen, identify, and characterize potential biodefense threats; and development of needed broad-spectrum countermeasures for viral and intracellular bacterial (ICB) pathogens.

The TMT Initiative integrates the science and technology capabilities of the Defense Threat Reduction Agency (DTRA) with the acquisition capabilities of the DoD Joint Program Executive Office for Chemical and Biological Defense (JPEO–CBD) into a single process responsible for the end-to-end development and delivery of capabilities enabling rapid response to genetically engineered and emerging biological threats. The TMT initiative receives program oversight from the ATSD(NCB) and guidance from an executive office made up of senior leadership from both the JPEO–CBD and DTRA.

Defense Advanced Research Projects Agency (DARPA)

The CBDP has a memorandum of understanding with DARPA to manage the Advanced Manufacturing of Pharmaceuticals (AMP) program. The goal of this program is to create a rapid, flexible, and cost-effective production technology capable of producing millions of doses of protein for a new therapeutic monoclonal antibody or vaccine within 12 weeks of notification at low cost and with an unprecedented purity for any emerging infectious threat.

A second DARPA initiative to respond faster to unknown or emerging novel biothreat agents is their 7-day Biodefense Initiative. Under this effort, countermeasures could be developed for multiple unrelated infectious agents within 7 days. This two-phase program focused on preventing infection, sustaining survival until a curative response is available, providing transient immunity, and speeding the onset of adaptive immunity. The goal is to develop highly innovative approaches to counter any known, unknown, naturally occurring or engineered pathogen. Particular interest focuses on new approaches that obviate traditional and rate-limiting steps (e.g., pathogen isolation, culture, identification, antigen processing by the immune system, and onset of adaptive immunity).

Biological Threat Reduction Program (BTRP)

Former US Senators Richard Lugar (Rep., Indiana) and Sam Nunn (Dem., Georgia) produced the Nunn-Lugar Act in 1991, establishing the Cooperative Threat Reduction (CTR) program. The CTR program has helped the states of the former Soviet Union to safeguard and dismantle their enormous stockpiles of nuclear, chemical and biological weapons, related materials, and delivery systems. DTRA executes the CTR program and works in coordination with partner governments and other US Government agencies who administer related projects.

While the initial focus of the CTR program has been on the most pressing nuclear proliferation threats, funding was also directed toward improving the physical protection, safety and security of facilities that housed dangerous bio-agents under the cooperative Biological Threat Reduction program (BTRP). The BTRP helps build capacity in partner countries by improving detection, diagnostics, monitoring, and reporting of endemic and epidemic diseases whether naturally occurring or man-made.

The BTRP has developed cooperative disease surveillance programs with partner nation governments and has helped partners comply with the World Health Assembly (WHA) International Health Regulations (IHR) and reporting guidelines for the World Organization for Animal Health (OIE) and the UN's Food and Agricultural Organization (FAO). In 2009, the National Academy of Sciences (NAS) congressionally-mandated report, "*Global Security Engagement: A New Model for Cooperative Threat Reduction,*" recommended an expanded Nunn-Lugar model of global security engagement to counter the 21st century terrorist threats. Today, the Nunn-Lugar Global Cooperation Initiative gives a higher priority to global engagement and surveillance for biological threats.

Another primary mission of the BTRP is to help consolidate "Especially Dangerous Pathogen" (EDP) collections, including those on the US Select Agent List, into one or two safe and secure facilities per country. These actions have greatly helped to prevent the sale, theft, diversion, or accidental release of bio-weapons related materials, technology, and expertise.

While BTRP's activities since 1991 have been focused on former Soviet countries (Armenia, Azerbaijan, Georgia, Kazakhstan, Ukraine, Uzbekistan), there is now the organizational mandate for similar work in Afghanistan, Pakistan, and Sub-Saharan Africa under the rubric of the Cooperative Biological Engagement Program (CBEP).

The CBDP formally added emerging infectious diseases to the biodefense mission set in October 2009. Subsequently, DoD executed chemical and biodefense program funds for emerging infectious disease preparedness and response activities. The CBDP Fiscal Year 2012-2017 *Program Strategy Guidance* declared that "infectious diseases, either emerging or reemerging, must be a focus of DoD, and we must be ready to play an important role in responding to pandemics, whether naturally occurring (H1N1) or not (smallpox)."

Bioengineered Threats and Synthetic Biology

Without human intervention, the natural world has produced innumerable microbial threats that continue to emerge and cause new forms of disease. However, recently (in terms of human history), we have acquired the technical capacity to create microbial threats far more deadly than natural evolution could create. Genetic engineering, the intentional molecular manipulation of genes and/or genomes, has proven, like so many technologies, to have capacity for both good and ill. A few examples from the open scientific literature are mentioned here to illustrate the seriousness of the threat of genetically engineered microorganisms (GEMs).

Antibiotic resistant strains of *B. anthracis* have been derived, not only by biological selection, but also more directly by genetic engineering. Scientifically, the capacity to do so with any bacterial threat is easily available. Similarly, for anyone moderately skilled in microbiology, it is obvious that otherwise harmless bacteria may be engineered to synthesize toxins made by unrelated lethal strains of bacteria. Buffering the threat, unauthorized conduct of most such experimentation has become not only difficult but illegal – subject to fines and incarceration – in many countries including the US. In the US, federally funded research that many result in knowledge that could be used for nefarious purposes, so called "dual use research of concern," or DURC, is subject to review prior to initiation of research and also at the stage of submission of the data for publication.

Today, viral genomes can quite easily be manipulated in the laboratory and infectious viruses can be generated from plasmid DNA. The progression of this technology with human pathogens began some 20 years ago with the simpler viruses (positive sense, single-strand, small genomes) such as poliovirus, alphaviruses, and flaviviruses. It has grown to include negative-strand viruses (e.g., vesicular stomatitis virus, respiratory syncytial virus, Ebola virus, and Crimean-Congo hemorrhagic fever virus) and segmented viruses (e.g., influenza virus). The relatively large genome of vaccinia virus can be derived from DNA cloned into bacteria. Even the capacity to derive a human pathogenic virus (poliovirus) completely by chemical synthesis was demonstrated.[19] Even more controversial were the efforts to genetically resurrect the 1918 influenza virus that killed some 20 million persons before disappearing and the proposals to genetically manipulate smallpox virus.[20,21] Perhaps the most prominent example of DURC in recent years came in late 2011, when two independent research groups prepared to publish research studies in which mutations were introduced into highly pathogenic influenza H5N1 viruses that facilitated efficient transmission of the viruses in the ferret model, and thus presumably in humans as well.[22,23] The ensuing debate resulted in a self-imposed moratorium on such research by influenza scientists in the US and internationally. As a result, research proposals for this type of study submitted for US federal funding are subject to additional layers of review. It is expected that other countries will follow suit, if they do not already have such a framework in place.

Ultimately, the capacity to create deadly pathogens through genetic engineering is restrained in large part by technical knowledge and opportunity, and in the final analysis, by intent. That is, what is straightforward for skilled scientists is impossibly difficult for the untrained and unequipped. However, a determined person with the appropriate set of knowledge and skills may succeed in the creation of GEMs. Unfortunately, such organisms could also be created by well-intentioned scientists who underestimate the unexpected consequences of their work.

Bioregulators/Biomodulators

Bioregulators, or biomodulators, are biochemical compounds, such as peptides, that occur naturally in organisms. Advances in biotechnology have created the potential for the misuse of bioregulators as biological weapons. As bio-weapons, they could damage the nervous system, alter moods, trigger psychological changes, and kill. The potential military or terrorist use of bioregulators is somewhat similar to that of toxins. Many bioregulators can be used to cause illness, but only a few can threaten civilian populations on a large scale. If released upon a civilian population in sufficient quantity and concentration, they could pose significant challenges for public health and medical responses.

Biological response modifiers (BRMs) direct the myriad complex interactions of the human immune system. Examples of BRMs include erythropoietins, interferons, interleukins, colony-stimulating factors, stem cell growth factors, monoclonal antibodies, tumor necrosis factor inhibitors, and vaccines. A growing understanding of the structure and function of various BRMs has resulted in many novel compounds including synthetic analgesics, antioxidants, antiviral, and antibacterial substances. For example, BRMs are used to treat debilitating rheumatoid arthritis by targeting cytokines that contribute to the disease process, to reduce symptoms and decrease inflammation. Recently marketed BRM-based medications include etanercept (*Enbrel*) and infliximab (*Remicade*), both of which have been used to target the tumor necrosis factor alpha (TNF-α) cytokine, as well as anakinra (*Kineret*), which targets interleukin-1 (IL-1). More of these new drugs are currently in development. It can be easily imagined that research to develop various BRMs could be subverted to a malicious end. That is, instead of using BRMs to suppress cancer growth or disease susceptibility, such compounds could potentially be developed to have the opposite effect, causing illness and death to those exposed.

What countermeasures and solutions exist? Laws and regulations to preclude accidental or intentional creation of new deadly organisms, or possession of the deadly agents already existing in nature, have been implemented in the US (e.g., 7 CFR Part 331, 9 CFR Part 121, and 42 CFR Part 73), but these bounds are difficult, if not impossible, to enforce internationally. Also helpful are the myriad coordination meetings and rehearsals for public health responses to pandemic natural threats such as smallpox or a pandemic flu virus. In the case of the outbreak of a contagious GEM, classical methods of epidemiology and quarantine would likely be exceedingly helpful. Unfortunately, the development of specific medical countermeasures (vaccines, anti-infective drugs) for a previously unknown organism usually takes many years. Some regard this as impetus to redirect greater funding toward discovery of generic methods of boosting innate immunity in persons in a manner that would provide increased resistance to most, if not all infectious agents. A related approach is to target common cellular pathways used and shared by many unrelated agents, especially viruses. Still, as with conventional agents, great localized harm could be done and widespread panic produced by a GEM, even if medical countermeasures were nominally available.

Synthetic biology

Genome synthesis is no longer limited to the realm of viruses. In 2008, researchers described the complete chemical synthesis of all 582,970 nucleotides of the *Mycoplasma genitalium* genome.[24] The starting material for the synthesis was short oligonucleotides that can be purchased for $0.10 per base or less. Following closely on the heels of this achievement, the same group in 2010, reported the complete chemical synthesis of the 1.08 megabase-pair genome of *M. mycoides.*[25] This genome was synthesized in a manner similar to that of *M. genitalium,* but they went one step further. They transplanted the synthetic genome into the "husk" of a *M. capricolum* cell from which the normal genome had been removed. The cellular materials left behind after removing the normal genome were able to accept the new, synthetic genome and kick-start replication of the novel bacterium *M. mycoides* JCVI-syn1.0 (named after the J. Craig Venter Institute where the work was performed).

The concept of "genomic warfare" is highly speculative and beyond the scope of this handbook. Undoubtedly, as scientific understanding of this technology increases and becomes more widely available, the threat of the development and use of genomic weapons will increase as will the challenge to develop effective medical countermeasures. Ultimately, the capacity to create deadly new organisms through genetic engineering is restrained in large part by technical knowledge and opportunity. What may appear straightforward for skilled scientists can be impossibly difficult for the untrained and unequipped. However, a determined person with the appropriate knowledge, skills, or access to personnel with such skills may succeed in malevolent creation of GEMs. As scientists develop more sophisticated laboratory procedures and increase their understanding of molecular biology and the genomics of both the pathogens and of humans, the possibility of bioengineering virulent, antimicrobial-resistant, and vaccine-resistant bacteria and viruses (or other as yet unknown pathogens) for nefarious uses will increase.

PERSONAL PROTECTION

The DoD's currently fielded chemical protective equipment, which includes the protective mask, the Joint Services Lightweight Integrated Suit Technology (JSLIST) chemical protective overgarment (CPO)—which replaces the battle dress overgarment (BDO)—protective gloves; protective footwear covers, and multipurpose rain/snow/CW overboots (MULO) will effectively protect against a bio-agent attack.

The standard issue mask, the M40, is available in three sizes, and when worn correctly, will protect the face, eyes, and respiratory tract. The M40 employs a single, standard screw-on C2A1 filter element which incorporates two separate but complementary mechanisms: 1) impaction and adsorption of agent molecules onto ASC Whetlerite carbon filtration medium, and 2) static electrical attraction of particles which are able to pass carbon filtration medium on first pass. Proper maintenance and periodic replacement of the crucial filter elements is of utmost importance. The filter MUST be replaced when:

1. The elements become immersed in water, crushed, cut, or otherwise damaged.
2. Excessive breathing resistance is encountered.
3. The "ALL CLEAR" signal is given after exposure to a bio-agent.
4. Thirty days have elapsed in the combat theater of operations (also, the filters must be replaced every 30 d once opened).
5. Supply bulletins indicate lot number expiration.
6. So ordered by the unit commander.

The filter element must only be changed in an un-contaminated environment. Two styles of optical inserts for the protective mask are available for personnel requiring visual correction. The wire frame style is considered to be the safer of the two and is more easily fitted into the mask. A prong-type optical insert is also available. A drinking tube on the mask can be used while in a contaminated environment. Note that the wearer should disinfect the canteen and tube by wiping with a 5% hypochlorite solution before use.

The Joint Service General Protective Mask (JSGPM, US Army XM-50) is a lightweight protective mask incorporating state-of-the-art technology. It is composed of heavy rubber, has a chlorobutyl/silicone base with a polynomial spline eye lens, incorporates a hydration port, and has a 50% performance improvement over the M40, for Joint force protection requirements. It provides above-the-neck, head-eye-respiratory protection against CBRN threats, including toxic industrial chemicals. JSGPM is replacing the M40/M42 series of protective masks for the Army and Marines, and the MCU-2/P series of protective masks for the Air Force and Navy. It is intended to interface with Joint service vehicles, weapons, communication systems, individual clothing and protective equipment, and CBRN personal protective equipment. JSGPM production and fielding began in 2008, and will continue until the Service's requirements are filled.

The JSLIST is available seven sizes, woodland and desert patterns, and can be used for 45 d in an uncontaminated environment. Once opened it can be laundered up to six times and may be worn for 24 continuous h in a contaminated environment. The JSLIST is replaced by using the MOPP-gear exchange procedure described in the *Soldier's Manual of Common Tasks.* The discarded suit should be incinerated or buried. Chemical protective gloves and overboots come in various sizes and are both made from butyl rubber. They may be decontaminated and reissued. The gloves and overboots must be visually inspected and decon'ed as needed after every 12 h of exposure in a contaminated environment. While the protective equipment will protect against bio-agents, it is noteworthy that even standard uniform clothing of good quality affords a reasonable protection against dermal exposure of surfaces covered.

The BDO is a two-layer, two piece garment consisting of coat and trousers. A water-repellant treated nylon/cotton twill outer layer, with an inner layer of polyurethane foam/nylon tricot laminate impregnated with activated charcoal. Available in 8 sizes, the BDO is no longer in production, and is being replaced by the JSLIST.

Those casualties unable to continue wearing protective equipment should be held and/or transported within patient protective wraps designed to protect the patient against further chem/bio-agent exposure. These wraps consist of a charcoal lining similar to the BDO, with a bottom layer of impermeable rubber. HCWs transporting such patients may want to consider adding a filter blower unit to generate overpressure, and thereby enhance protection and provide cooling.

Collective protection by using either a hardened or unhardened shelter equipped with an air filtration unit providing overpressure can protect personnel in a biologically contaminated environment. An airlock ensures that no contamination will be brought into the shelter. In the absence of a dedicated structure, enhanced protection can be afforded within most buildings by sealing cracks and entry ports, and providing air filtration with HEPA filters within existing ventilation systems. The key problem is that availability of these shelters can be limited in military situations, costly to produce and maintain, and difficult to deploy. Personnel must be decon'ed before entering the collective protection unit.

The inhalational route is the most important route of exposure to bio-agents. Bio-agents can be dispersed as aerosols from point or line source disseminations. Unlike some chemical threats, aerosols of bio-agents disseminated by line source munitions (e.g., sprayed by low-flying aircraft or speedboats along the coast) do not leave hazardous environmental residue (although anthrax spores may persist and could pose a hazard near the dissemination line). In contrast, aerosols generated by point-source munitions (i.e., stationary aerosol generator, bomblets, etc.) are more apt to produce ground contamination, but only in the immediate vicinity of dissemination. Point-source munitions leave an obvious signature that may alert the field commander that a BW attack has occurred. Because point-source munitions always leave an agent residue, this evidence can be useful for detection and identification purposes.

Aerosol delivery systems for bio-agents most commonly generate invisible clouds with particles or droplets of $< 10\ \mu m$. They can remain suspended for extensive periods. The major risk in such an attack is pulmonary retention of inhaled particles. To a much lesser extent, some particles may adhere to an individual or his clothing, especially near the face. The effective area covered varies with many factors, including wind speed, humidity, and sunlight. In the absence of an effective real-time detection and alarm systems or direct observation of an attack, the first clue may be mass casualties fitting a clinical pattern compatible with one of the bio-agents. This may occur hours, days, or weeks after an attack.

Toxins may cause direct pulmonary effects or be absorbed and cause systemic toxicity. They are frequently more potent by inhalation than by any other route. A unique clinical feature may be seen which is not observed by other routes (e.g., pulmonary edema after SEB exposure). Mucous membranes, including conjunctivae, are also vulnerable to many bio-agents. Physical protection is then quite important and the use of full-face masks equipped with small-particle filters, like the chemical protective masks, assumes a high degree of importance.

With reference to force protection, other routes for delivering bio-agents are thought to be less significant than inhalation, but are nonetheless serious concerns. Contamination of food and water supplies, either deliberately or incidentally after an aerosol attack, represents a hazard for infection or intoxication by ingestion. Determination as to whether food and water supplies are free from contamination is always important, and should be made by appropriate preventive medicine authorities in the event of a bio-attack.

Intact skin provides an excellent barrier against almost all bio-agents—T-2 mycotoxins are the sole exception, due to their dermal activity. It is also important to consider that, mucous membranes and abrasions, or otherwise damaged integument, can allow for passage of some bio-agents, and should therefore be protected in the event of an attack.

FIELD DETECTION

Accurate and timely intelligence is required to develop an effective defense in biological warfare (BW) and bio-terrorism. Once an agent has been dispersed, detecting the bio-agent before its arrival over the target (and in time for personnel to don protective equipment), is referred to as "detect to warn". However, the concept of "detect to warn" is an ideal standard that to date has not been fully achievable. Interim systems for detecting dispersed bio-agents are just now being fielded in limited numbers. Until highly accurate reliable detectors become widely available, the first indication that a biological attack has occurred will most likely be ill patients or collateral effects on animals. Therefore, the timely monitoring of medical surveillance data resulting in "detection to treat" is critical for detecting a BW attack in time to potentially affect the outcome of those who may have been exposed, but who are not yet ill[1, 2].

The development of real-time detection capability for BW agents and pathogens of military significance has become one of the most challenging, high-priority areas of research within both the DoD and civilian sectors. Sensors fielded to date provide presumptive results only for a limited number of bio-agents. Several systems have been deployed and several more are in the technology demonstration stage of development; the following systems are highlighted here:

1. The Biological Integrated Detection System (BIDS) is a HMMWV (high mobility multi-purpose wheeled vehicle)-mounted system that concentrates aerosol particles from environmental air, then subjects the particle sample to antibody-based detection assays for selected bio-agents. It is presently capable of detecting eight BW agents within 45 min.[3]

2. The Interim Biological Agent Detection System (IBADS) is a semi-automatic version of the BIDS designed for shipboard use. It is capable of detecting the same eight bio-agents as the BIDS but within 25 min.[3]

3. Portal Shield is an independent aerosol collector capable of detecting up to eight bio-agents within 25 min using antibody-based detection. It is designed for fixed installations and can be networked and interfaced with chemical warfare sensors.[4,5]

4. The Joint Biological Point Detection System (JBPDS) is designed to detect ten bio-agents. Like the Portal Shield it can operate as part of a network. It is designed to have a process time of less than 18 min, to decrease to less than ten min in future versions. JBPDS is intended to be used on multiple platforms and by all military services.[3-5]

5. The Dry Filter Unit (DFU) represents a standardized point detection system for bio-agent surveillance and is designed to collect aerosolized bio-particulates from ambient air and then subject them for analysis by several complementary technologies including hand-held assays (HHAs), real-time polymerase chain reaction assays (RT-PCR), and other microbiological confirmatory techniques.[3-6] Samples may be processed at nearby labs or delivered to established high-volume laboratories set up specifically for such purposes. There is also a Biological Weapons Agent-Sampling (BWAS) kit designed for manual sampling and testing with the HHAs.

6. The Long-Range Biological Standoff Detection System (LRBSDS) is under development and is designed to provide a first-line biological standoff detection capability; that is a "detect to warn" capability.[3] It will employ an infrared laser to detect aerosol clouds at a standoff distance of up to 30 km. A second-generation system may extend the range to 100 km. This system will be available for fixed-site applications or may be deployable aboard rotary or fixed-winged aircraft. The Short-Range Biological Standoff Detection System (SRBSDS) is in the research and development phase. It will employ UV and laser-induced fluorescence to detect biological aerosol clouds at distances of up to 5 km. The information will be used to provide early warning, enhance contamination avoidance efforts, and as a cue for other detection capabilities. These systems do not identify the bio-agent but may indicate an approaching biological aerosol. The SRBSDS will be designed to differentiate biological aerosols from other non-biological aerosols. Confirmation of a live bio-agent or potent toxin could then be done using the BIDS or a BWAS Kit and a DFU.

7. Hand-held assays are simple one-time-use immunochromatographic devices very similar to urine test strips used for home pregnancy tests. These tests provide a "yes/no" response to the presence of 10 bio-agents within 15 min. A skilled user may derive a semi-quantitative measure of a bio-agent's presence by the degree of color change, but this is only related to presence/absence. HHAs are currently employed in virtually all fielded military biological detection systems (BIDS, portal shield, DFUs, JBPDS), and are also present in developmental systems. HHAs are versatile enough to be used in automated readers, as well as read manually. Although reliable, they are designed only for presumptive identification of agents. Samples must

subsequently undergo additional testing with complementary technologies before a definitive identification can be made.

8. The Joint Biological Agent Identification and Diagnostic System (JBAIDS), is similar to the Ruggedized Advanced Pathogen Identification Device (RAPID). Both systems that employ RT-PCR technology to identify bio-agents.[7-11] These are the current technologies utilized by DoD field laboratories and they are designed to be portable, reusable systems capable of field confirmatory or theater validation identification of bio-agents. The systems rely on technically advanced processes and critical reagents provided through each respective program.

9. FilmArray[R] is a multiplex RT-PCR "lab in a box" platform capable of providing diagnostic solutions within a few hours on raw, primary specimens.[12-14] The FilmArray[R] is configured so that each array/film offers diagnostic panels for different organisms associated with specific subjects and/or syndromes, such as respiratory illnesses or bio-defense. Unknown specimens are injected into a pouch at a specified volume and then inserted into the analyzer device. The analyzer extracts organism (viral or cellular) nucleic acid material, if necessary, reverse transcribes to cDNA, amplifies target groups based upon organism, re-amplifies targets to eliminate non-specific cross talk due to multiplexing, and then reads the array matrix to generate a diagnostic solution, all within a few hours.

10. MagPix[R] is a multiplex system that utilizes multi-colored carboxylated polystyrene microbeads, resulting in up to 500 different distinct beads.[15, 16] The microbeads can be attached to either antibodies, nucleic acid oligos, or other protein molecules with the objective to detect interaction with these attached molecules, such as protein detection, serology measurements of exposure, and amplified nucleic acid target detection. This technology utilizes LED sensors obviating past problems with delicate lasers. Also, the assays are quick and real time, allowing expeditious diagnostic results.

11. MSD[R]: Mesoscale Discovery utilizes antibody-coated wells within multiple well plates coupled to an electrode catalyst plate and MSD-Tag™ detection antibodies that are able detect antigens via electro-chemi-luminescence.[17] The antigen or antibody (in the case of plates absorbed with antigen) specimens are added to each well of a 24, 96, or 384 well plate and bind based upon their specific interaction with the capture agent. Detection antibodies are then added. If an interaction takes place between the capture agent and the analyte, the buffer solution undergoes a chemical reaction with the labeled detection antibody and light is produced. The instrument sensor then measures the amount of light produced.

The above systems provide only presumptive tests for a limited number of bio-agents and are still "detect-to-treat" systems rather than the desired "detect-to-warn" systems, but with a higher level of confidence than assays used in the past. There are many other systems under development by the DoD and others that employ innovative detection methods such as oligo arrays, various types of mass spectrometry, quick and efficient sequencing, and single or multiple complementary technologies. These are not standardized systems and have yet to be integrated into the DoD through the formal acquisitions process. Other government agencies are working on systems similar to Portal Shield that use antibody detection schemes to yield field presumptive results for both domestic and military use.

Eventually, planners hope to have a reliable "detect-to-warn" capability. In the meantime multiple services and agencies have developed improved tactics, techniques, and procedures to better provide a forward field confirmatory testing capability for both environmental samples and clinical specimens. Units like the Area Medical Laboratory (AML), Navy-FDPMU (Forward Deployed Preventive Medicine Unit), and the Air Force FFBAT (Biological Augmentation Team) have been equipped with RT-PCR instruments such as the JBAIDS to provide for genetic analysis of samples that have been collected and tested as presumptively positive. Additionally, these systems have also been installed in the medical laboratories onboard Navy carrier and amphibious ships.

The current Concept of Operations outlines four levels of testing; 1) presumptive, 2) field confirmatory, 3) theater validation, and 4) definitive.[3] A single positive test provides only a presumptive identification of a bio-agent since false positives are possible with nearly all laboratory tests. Field confirmation requires that at least two tests analyzed by detecting two different markers because the probability of two tests generating false positive results simultaneously is quite low. Theater validation tests examine two or more independent biomarkers with different technology. Definitive analysis requires that the sample be evaluated at a lab endorsed by a US-recognized accreditation body and that the confidence be greater than 99%.

Standoff bio-agent detection ("detect-to-warn") remains a challenging problem and is currently an area of intense research and development. Tomorrow's detectors promise to be faster, more sensitive, and more reliable than those fielded today. Until such detectors are developed and fielded, we must rely heavily on a layered system of defense to protect against biological attacks including timely and accurate intelligence, analysis of medical surveillance data, proper use of personal and collective physical protection equipment, use of medical countermeasures (vaccines and chemoprophylactic drugs), post-event deployment of antibiotics and antivirals, and well developed response protocols.

DECONTAMINATION

Biological contamination is the introduction of infectious agents to a body surface, food or water, or other inanimate object. In this context, *decontamination* (decon) involves either disinfection or sterilization to reduce microorganisms to a safe level on contaminated articles, thus rendering them suitable for use. *Disinfection* is the selective reduction of undesirable microbes to a level below that posing a transmission hazard. *Sterilization* is the elimination of all organisms.

Decon methods have always played an important role in the control of infectious diseases. However, the most effective means of rendering microbes harmless (e.g., toxic chemical sterilization) may be impractical, as these methods may pose a hazard to humans, or damage equipment. Bio-agents may be also be decon'ed by mechanical, chemical, and physical methods.

1. Mechanical decon involves measures to remove, but not necessarily neutralize, an agent. An example is drinking water filtration to remove certain water-borne pathogens (e.g., *Dracunculus medinensis, Naegleria fowleri*), or the use of an air filter to remove aerosolized anthrax spores, or soap and water to wash agent from the skin.

2. Chemical decon renders bio-agents harmless by the use of disinfectants that may be a liquid, gas, or aerosol. Factors impacting effectiveness include contact time, solution concentration, composition of the contaminated surface, and characteristics of the agent to be decon'ed. Some disinfectants are harmful to humans, animals, the environment, and/or materiel.

3. Physical processes (heat, ionizing radiation, UV light) are other methods that can be employed for decon'ing objects.

It is important that, given the characteristic incubation periods of bio-agents, significant time may have elapsed between the attack and the patients' presentation with illness due to the attack. During this time it is quite probable that external decon of any residual agent may have already occurred through natural means. Thus, it is only in rare circumstances that patients presenting with illness due to a biological attack will require purposeful external decon.

Dermal exposure to a suspected biological aerosol should be immediately and vigorously treated by soap and water washing. This removes nearly all the agent from the skin surface. Hypochlorite solutions, or other powerful disinfectants, are reserved for gross contamination (i.e., after the spill of solid or liquid agent from munitions directly onto the skin). In the absence of chemical agent or gross biological contamination, these disinfectants will confer no additional benefit, may be caustic, and may predispose patients to colonization and resistant superinfection by eliminating the normal skin flora. Grossly contaminated skin surfaces should be washed with a 0.5% sodium hypochlorite solution, if available, with a contact time of 10 to 20 min. Concentrations higher than 0.5% are *not* recommended. If reaerosolization of agent is a concern due to the presence of gross contaminant that has been removed from a victim, a damp cloth or towel should be placed directly over the material and a 5% solution of hypochlorite (or equivalent disinfectant) should be liberally applied to saturate it. The saturated fabric/bio-agent should then be properly disposed of IAW established protocol.

Ampules of calcium hypochlorite—$Ca(ClO)_2$—are currently fielded in the Chemical Agent Decon Set (CADS) for mixing hypochlorite solutions. The 0.5% solution can be made by adding one 6-ounce container of calcium hypochlorite to 5 gallons of water. The 5% solution can be made by adding eight 6-ounce ampoules of calcium hypochlorite to 5 gallons of water (eight ounces of hypochlorite to every one gallon of water). Commercial off-the-shelf bleach can be used when access to the CADS is not available. It is recommended that more recognizable brand names, such as *Clorox*, be used as they have been tested and found to be more consistent in quality. These solutions evaporate quickly at high temperatures. If made in advance, they should be stored in closed containers, preferably the containers should be made of plastic—but NOT metal, as the hypochlorite will cause the metal to corrode. Chlorine solutions should always be placed in distinctly marked containers, as without markings it is very difficult to tell the difference between the 5% chlorine solution and the 0.5% solution.

A 0.5% sodium hypochlorite—NaClO—solution is made of one part *Clorox* and nine parts water (1:9) as standard stock *Clorox* is a 5.25% sodium hypochlorite solution with an average pH about 12 which enables long term shelf storage. The solution is then applied with a cloth or swab. The solution should be made fresh daily with the pH adjusted to bring it into the acidic range. When specifically decon'ing for possible weaponized anthrax, a pH adjusted hypochlorite solution is preferred. At acidic pH values of 6.8 or lower, the hypochlorite solution will be 80 to 200 more times more antimicrobial than at the alkaline pH values at which it is manufactured and stored. A small amount of household vinegar is sufficient to lower the pH values to an acidic range.

Diluted hypochlorite at an alkaline pH is a relatively poor disinfectant, but acidified diluted hypochlorite will kill virtually anything in 10 to 20 min. Prepare the 5% hypochlorite solution as above with seven 6-ounce ampoules to four gallons of water and then add 32 ounces of household vinegar.

Generally, soap and water wash is the preferred method for bio-agent decon of contaminated persons. In a scenario in which a pH adjusted dilute ($\leq$ 0.5%) hypochlorite solution is to be used for decon of gross contamination of multiple personnel, it is recommended that a "bio-decontamination line" be employed so as to limit cross-contamination. Small, makeshift lines can be constructed by placing a tarpaulin on the ground and using wash basins (e.g., small children's pools, or even just large trash bags). Using such a linear method will keep suspected contamination in the basins/bags as personnel move through the line, from the "contaminated" end toward the "clean" end, and into the clean basins/bags, thereby leaving contaminated materials behind.

The following steps, correlated with the illustration, constitute one possible set-up for a bio-decon line for a small number of contaminated person (CPs).

Figure: Operation of a suggested bio-decontamination line:

1. Contaminated person (CP) steps into the first basin & removes outer garments & boots.
2. CP steps from the first basin to the wash basin.
3. CP is washed with pH adjusted hypochlorite solution (or wash yourself if required).
4. CP steps into the rinse basin & waits the recommended contact time (10-20 min).
5. Apply the solution to another CP while the first CP is waiting on contact time.
6. After 10-20 min, rinse the solution off the CP with water.
7. The CP may now step into, or beside, one of the bags & place remaining clothing (undergarments & footwear) or other PPE in a bag for disposal. The disposal bag should be sealed & marked so as to prevent cross-contamination.
8. Attendant will take the CP off line.

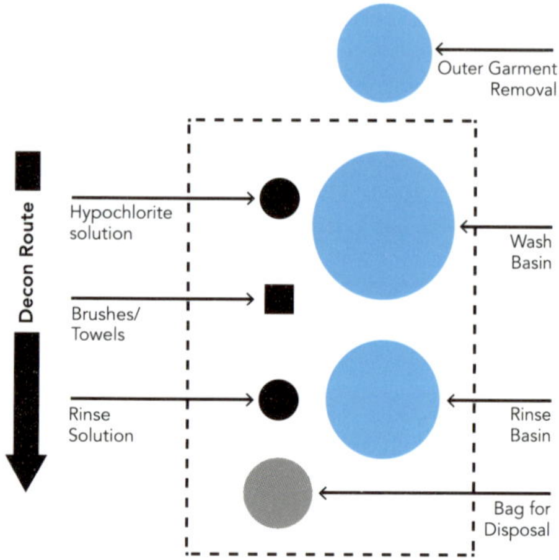

Chlorine solution must NOT be used in (1) open body-cavity wounds (as it may lead to the formation of adhesions), or (2) brain and spinal cord injuries. However, this solution (0.5% strength) may be instilled into non-cavity wounds and then removed by suction to an appropriate disposal container. Within about 5 min, this contaminated solution will be neutralized and non-hazardous. Copious irrigation with saline or other surgical solutions should be subsequently performed. Corneal opacities may result from chlorine solution being sprayed into the eyes.

For decon'ing fabric clothing or equipment, a 5% hypochlorite solution should be used, although many fabrics will be damaged with this concentration of hypochlorite. For decon'ing equipment, a contact time of 30 min before normal cleaning is required. This is corrosive to most metals and injurious to most fabrics, so rinse thoroughly and oil metal surfaces after completion.

Bio-agents may be rendered harmless through such physical means as heat and radiation. Agents are rendered completely harmless by sterilization with dry heat for 2 h at 160°C. If autoclaving with steam at 121°C and 1 atmosphere of overpressure (15 psi), the time may be reduced to 20 min, depending on volume. Solar UV radiation has a disinfectant effect, often in combination with drying. This is effective in certain environmental conditions but is hard to standardize for practical usage for decon purposes.

The health hazards of environmental contamination by bio-agents differ from those of persistent or volatile chemical agents. Aerosolized particles in the 1-5 μm size range will remain suspended by Brownian motion and can disseminate widely.

Suspended bio-agents would be eventually inactivated by solar UV light, desiccation, and oxidation. Little, if any environmental residues would remain. Possible exceptions include residue near the dissemination line or in the immediate area surrounding point-source munitions. Bio-agents deposited on the soil would be subject to degradation by environmental stressors and competing soil microflora. Simulant studies suggest that secondary reaerosolization would be difficult, but may pose a human health hazard. Environmental decon of terrain is costly and difficult. If grossly contaminated terrain, streets, or roads must be passed, the use of dust-binding spray to minimize reaerosolization may be considered. If it is necessary to decon these surfaces, chlorine-calcium or lye may be used. Otherwise, rely on the natural processes that, especially outdoors, lead to the decon of agent by drying and solar UV radiation. Rooms in fixed spaces are best decon'ed with aerosolized gases or liquids (e.g., formaldehyde). This is usually combined with surface disinfectants to ensure complete effectiveness.

For further information, see FM 3-5, *NBC Decontamination*; FM 4-02.7, *Health Service Support in a NBC Environment*; and Army FM 8-284, *Treatment of Biological Warfare Agent Casualties.*

Electronic copies of all DoD publications are available at the Defense Technical Information Center (DTIC), http://www.dtic.mil/ dtic.

APPENDIX A: GLOSSARY OF MEDICAL TERMS & ACRONYMS

This glossary is a list of medical terms and bio-defense acronyms used in this book. Some entries were adapted from: Stedman's Electronic Medical Dictionary *(Williams & Wilkins, Baltimore, MD, 2006) and Mandell et al,* Principles and Practice of Infectious Diseases *(7th Edition, Churchill Livingstone, 2009).*

Acetylcholine (ACH, Ach)–The neurotransmitter substance at cholinergic synapses, which causes cardiac inhibition, vasodilation, gastrointestinal peristalsis, and other parasympathetic effects. It is liberated from preganglionic and postganglionic endings of parasympathetic fibers and from preganglionic fibers of the sympathetic as a result of nerve injuries, whereupon it acts as a transmitter on the effector organ; it is hydrolyzed into choline and acetic acid by acetylcholinesterase before a second impulse may be transmitted.

ACIP–Advisory Committee on Immunization Practices; Overseen by the CDC.

Active vaccination -The act of artificially stimulating the body to develop antibodies against infectious disease by the administration of vaccines or toxoids.

Adenopathy–Swelling or morbid enlargement of the lymph nodes.

AFMAN–U.S. Air Force Manual.

AHF–Argentine hemorrhagic fever, a VHF.

AIDS–Acquired Immunodeficiency Syndrome.

AIGIV–Anthrax Immune Globulin, Intravenous.

Airborne precautions–*See* Transmission-based precautions.

Aleukia–Absence or extremely decreased number of leukocytes in the circulating blood.

ALP–Alkaline phosphatase.

ALT–Alanine aminotransferase, a liver enzyme.

AM–Morning (Latin, *ante meridiem*)

A.M.P.L.E.–Mneumonic for a bio-agent medical history: Allergies/Arthropods, Medications/MOPP status, Past medical history (travel, vaccine, occupational), Last meal, Expose (decon).

Analgesic–1. A compound capable of producing analgesia, i.e., one that relieves pain by altering perception of nociceptive stimuli without producing anesthesia or loss of consciousness. 2. Characterized by reduced response to painful stimuli.

Anaphylaxis–The term is commonly used to denote the immediate, transient kind of immunologic (allergic) reaction characterized by contraction of smooth muscle and dilation of capillaries due to release of pharmacologically active substances (histamine, bradykinin, serotonin, and slow-reacting substance), classically initiated by the combination of antigen (allergen) with mast cell-fixed, cytophilic antibody (chiefly IgE).

Anderson's Fallacy–Belief that only hummingbirds have rapid heart rates.

Anticonvulsant–An agent that prevents or arrests seizures.

Antigen–Any substance that, as a result of coming in contact with appropriate cells, induces a state of sensitivity or immune responsiveness and that reacts in a demonstrable way with antibodies or immune cells of the sensitized subject in vivo or in vitro.

Antitoxin–An antibody formed in response to and capable of neutralizing a biological poison; a serum prepared from animals vaccinated against a specific toxin.

AR–Army Regulation.

ARDS–Acute Respiratory Distress Syndrome.

Arthralgia–Severe pain in a joint, especially one not inflammatory in character.

ASAP–As soon as possible.

ASD(HA)–Assistant Secretary of Defense for Health Affairs.

AST–Aspartate aminotransferase, a liver enzyme.

Asthenia–Weakness or debility.

Ataxia–An inability to coordinate muscle activity during voluntary movement, so that smooth movements occur. Most often due to disorders of the cerebellum or the posterior columns of the spinal cord; may involve the limbs, head, or trunk.

Atelectasis–Decrease or loss of air in all or part of the lung, with resulting loss of lung volume itself.

ATLS–Advanced Trauma Life Support.

ATSD(NCB)–Assistant to the Secretary of Defense for Nuclear, Chemical, and Biological Defense Programs.

Atropine–An anticholinergic, with diverse effects (tachycardia, mydriasis, cycloplegia, constipation, urinary retention) attributable to reversible competitive blockade of acetylcholine at muscarinic type cholinergic receptors; used in the treatment of poisoning with organophosphate insecticides or nerve gases.

Augmentin–A formulation of ampicillin and clavulanic acid.

AVA–Anthrax Vaccine Adsorbed.

BDO–Battle dress overgarment.

BHF–Bolivian Hemorrhagic Fever, a VHF.

BID or bid- Twice each day.

BIDS–Biological Integrated Detection System.

Bilirubin–A yellow bile pigment formed from hemoglobin during normal and abnormal destruction of erythrocytes. Excess bilirubin is associated with jaundice.

Bio-agent–Biological agent (*q.v.*); biological threat agent.

Biocontainment–In laboratory biosafety, is the the physical containment of highly pathogenic organisms or agents (bacteria, viruses, and toxins), usually by isolation in environmentally and biologically secure cabinets or rooms, to prevent accidental infection of workers or release into the surrounding community during scientific research. Often confused with "isolation" and "quarantine".

Biological agent–A bacterium, virus, protozoan, parasite, fungus, or toxin that can be used purposefully as a weapon in bio-terrorism or biological warfare; biological threat agent, bio-weapon, or bio-agent.

Bio-toxin–See toxin.

Bio-surveillance–The gathering, analysis and interpretation of data related to disease activity and threats to human and animal health to achieve early warning, detection and situational awareness (DoD definition).

Blood agar–A mixture of blood and nutrient agar used for the cultivation of many medically important microorganisms.

BMR–Biological response modifier.

BoNT–Botulinum neurotoxin.

BRM–Biological response modifier.

Bronchiolitis–Inflammation of the bronchioles often associated with bronchopneumonia.

Bronchitis–Inflammation of the mucous membrane of the bronchi.

Brucella–A genus of encapsulated, nonmotile bacteria (family Brucellaceae) containing short, rod-shaped to coccoid, gram-negative cells. These organisms are parasitic, invading all animal tissues and causing infection of the genital organs, the mammary gland, and the respiratory and intestinal tracts, and are pathogenic for humans and various species of domestic animals. They do not produce gas from carbohydrates.

BSAT–Biological Select Agent or Toxin (see Appendix C).

BSL–Bio-safety level.

BSV–Bio-surveillance (*q.v.*).

BTRP–Biological Threat Reduction Program.

Bubo–Inflammatory swelling of one or more lymph nodes, usually in the groin; the confluent mass of nodes usually suppurates and drains pus.

Bulla, gen. and pl. bullae–A large blister greater than 1 cm in diameter appearing as a circumscribed area of separation of the epidermis from the subepidermal structure (subepidermal *bulla*) or as a circumscribed area of separation of epidermal cells (intraepidermal *bulla*) caused by the presence of serum, or occasionally by an injected substance.

BW–Biological warfare; bio-warfare (less commonly, biological weapons).

BWAS–Biological Weapons Agent Sampling [kit].

BWC–Biological Weapons Convention (1972, 1975).

C–Celsius or centigrade.

CA–California.

CADS–Chemical Agent Decon Set.

Carbuncle–Deep-seated pyogenic infection of the skin and subcutaneous tissues, usually arising in several contiguous hair follicles, with formation of connecting sinuses; often preceded or accompanied by fever, malaise, and prostration.

Case Fatality Rate (CFR)–The proportion or percentage of deaths within a designated population of people with a particular disease, over the course of the disease. (*Cf.* mortality rate.)

CBC–Complete blood count.

CBDP–The DoD's Chemical and Biological Defense Program.

CBEP–Cooperative Biological Engagement Program.

CBRN(E)–Chemical, biological, radiological, and nuclear (and explosives).

CCHF–Crimean-Congo hemorrhagic fever; a VHF.

CDC–U.S. Centers for Disease Control and Prevention, Atlanta, Georgia.

cDNA–complementary DNA; DNA synthesized from a messenger RNA (mRNA) template in a reaction catalysed by the enzyme reverse transcriptase.

Cerebrospinal–Relating to the brain and the spinal cord.

CF–Complement fixation.

Cf–Latin *confer*, meaning "compare" or "consult".

CFR–Case Fatality Rate (*q.v.*); also Code of Federal Regulations.

Chemoprophylaxis–Prevention of disease by the use of chemicals or drugs.

Cholinergic–Relating to nerve cells or fibers that employ acetylcholine as their neurotransmitter.

CJCS–Chairman of the Joint Chiefs of Staff.

Cipro–Ciprofloxicin, a flouroquinolone antibiotic.

Cm(s)–Centimeter(s).

CMV–Cytomegalovirus.

CNS–Central nervous system.

Coagulopathy–A disease affecting the coagulability of the blood.

Coccobacillus–A short, thick bacterial rod of the shape of an oval or slightly elongated coccus.

Conjunctiva, pl. conjunctivae–The mucous membrane investing the anterior surface of the eyeball and the posterior surface of the lids.

Contact precautions–*See* Transmission-based precautions.

CONUS–Continental United States.

CPO–Chemical protective overgarment.

CPT–Current Procedural Terminology; maintained by the American Medical Association.

CSF–Cerebrospinal fluid.

CT–Computed tomography.

CTR–DTRA's Cooperative Threat Reduction program.

Cutaneous–Relating to the skin.

CW–Chemical warfare.

CXR–Chest X-ray; chest radiograph.

Cyanosis–A dark bluish or purplish coloration of the skin and mucous membrane due to deficient oxygenation of the blood, evident when reduced hemoglobin in the blood exceeds 5 g per 100 ml.

D or d–Day(s).

DARPA–Defense Advanced Research Projects Agency.

Decon–Decontamination.

DEOC–The CDC Director's Emergency Operations Center.

DFA–Direct fluorescence antibody or direct immunofluorescence immunoassay (*see* Fluorescent antibody).

DFU–Dry filter unit.

DHHS–United States Department of Health and Human Services; Oversees FDA, CDC, etc.

DHS–United States Department of Homeland Security.

Diathesis -The constitutional or inborn state disposing to a disease, group of diseases, or metabolic or structural anomaly.

DIC–Disseminated intravascular coagulation.

Diplopia -The condition in which a single object is perceived as two objects. SYN: double vision.

Disinfection–Application of a **disinfectant** (antimicrobial chemical agent) to non-living objects to destroy surface microorganisms; does not necessarily constitute **sterilization** (*q.v.*), especially as resistant bacterial spores may survive.

Distal–Situated away from the center of the body, or from the point of origin; specifically applied to the extremity or distant part of a limb or organ.

DNA–Deoxyribonucleic acid.

DoD–United States Department of Defense.

DODI–DoD Instruction.

DODD–DoD Directive.

Doxy–The antibiotic doxycycline.

Droplet precautions–*See* Transmission-based precautions.

DTRA–The DoD's Defense Threat Reduction Agency.

DURC–Dual use research of concern.

DVD–Digital versatile disc (or digital videodisk)

Dysarthria–A disturbance of speech and language due to emotional stress, to brain injury, or to paralysis, incoordination, or spasticity of the muscles used for speaking.

Dysphagia, dysphagy–Difficulty in swallowing.

Dysphonia–Altered voice production.

Dyspnea–Shortness of breath, a subjective difficulty or distress in breathing, usually associated with disease of the heart or lungs; occurs normally during intense physical exertion or at high altitude.

Dystocia–Slow or difficult labor or delivery.

Ecchymosis–A purplish patch caused by extravasation of blood into the skin, differing from petechiae only in size (larger than 3 mm diameter).

ECG–Electocardiogram; electrocardiography.

Echo–Echocardiogram.

ECL–Electrochemiluminescence.

Eczema–Generic term for inflammatory conditions of the skin, particularly with vesiculation in the acute stage, typically erythematous, edematous, papular, and crusting; followed often by lichenification and scaling and occasionally by duskiness of the erythema and, infrequently, hyperpigmentation; often accompanied by sensations of itching and burning.

ED_{50}–Median effective dose; the dose that produces the desired effect; when followed by a subscript (generally "ED_{50}"), it denotes the dose having such an effect on a certain percentage (e.g., 50%) of the test animals.

Edema–An accumulation of an excessive amount of watery fluid in cells, tissues, or serous cavities.

EDP–Especially dangerous pathogen(s).

EEE or EEEV–Eastern Equine Encephalitis [virus].

EIND–Emergency IND (*q.v.*); See Appendix J.

Electrochemiluminescence–A method used to identify microorganisms. Similar in operation to ELISA, FA and sandwich antibody assays. A capture antibody bound to a magnetic bead captures the target microorganism. Another antibody labeled with a ruthenium tris-bipyridyl compound ($Ru(bpy)_3^{2+}$) is introduced. A magnet is used to pull the beads to an electrode which is used to excite the ruthenium compound which then emits light. The light is detected revealing the presences of the target organism. The method is easily automated and is generally faster than either ELISA or FA.

ELISA–Enzyme-linked immunosorbent assay (*q.v.*).

EM–Electron microscopy; electron microscope.

Enanthem, enanthema–A mucous membrane eruption, especially one occurring in connection with one of the exanthemas.

Encephalitis (*pl.* **encephalitides**)–Inflammation of the brain.

Endotoxemia–Presence in the blood of endotoxins.

Endotracheal intubation–Passage of a tube through the nose or mouth into the trachea for maintenance of the airway during anesthesia or for maintenance of an imperiled airway.

Enterotoxin–A cytotoxin specific for the cells of the intestinal mucosa.

Enzyme-Linked Immunosorbent Assay (ELISA)–A method used to detect a microbial antigen or an antibody to a microbial antigen. It works by chemically linking an enzyme to an antibody that recognizes and adheres to the desired antigen or antibody. Any unbound antibody-enzyme complex is removed. A chemical that is converted by the enzyme into a fluorescent compound is applied and allowed to react. The fluorescence is then detected to reveal the presence or absence of the antigen or antibody.

EO–Executive Order.

Epidemic–the rapid spread of infectious, or other, disease to a large number of people in a given population within a short period of time; a threshold number of cases within a specific time frame is often pre-designated by experts to trigger notification.

Epidemic curve–A pattern, often presented as a histogram, depicting an outbreak of disease; useful in identifying the transmission method or source, and in predicting the future rate of infection.

Epistaxis–Profuse bleeding from the nose.

Epizootic–1. Denoting a temporal pattern of disease occurrence in an animal population in which the disease occurs with a frequency clearly in excess of the expected frequency in that population during a given time interval. 2. An outbreak (epidemic) of disease in an animal population; often with the implication that it may also affect human populations.

Erythema–Redness of the skin due to capillary dilatation.

Erythema multiforme–An acute eruption of macules, papules, or subdermal vesicles presenting a multiform appearance, the characteristic lesion being the target or iris lesion over the dorsal aspect of the hands and forearms; its origin may be allergic, seasonal, or from drug sensitivity, and the eruption, although usually self-limited (e.g., multiforme minor), may be recurrent or may run a severe course, sometimes with fatal termination (e.g., multiforme major or Stevens-Johnson syndrome).

Erythrocyte–A mature red blood cell.

Erythropoiesis–The formation of red blood cells.

ESR–Erythrocyte sedimentation rate ("sed rate").

EU–European Union.

EUA–Emergency Use Authorization. (See Appendix J.)

Exanthema–A skin eruption occurring as a symptom of an acute viral or coccal disease, as in scarlet fever or measles.

Extracellular–Outside the cells.

Extraocular–Adjacent to but outside the eyeball.

F–Fahrenheit.

FA–Fluorescent antibody (*q.v.*).

FAC–free available chlorine.

Fasciculation–Involuntary contractions, or twitchings, of groups (fasciculi) of muscle fibers, a coarser form of muscular contraction than fibrillation.

FBI–US Federal Bureau of Investigation.

FDA–US Food and Drug Administration; Part of DHHS.

FD&C Act–Federal Food, Drug and Cosmetic Act (1938).

Febrile–Denoting or relating to fever.

FEMA–Federal Emergency Management Agency.

FHP–Force Health Protection.

FL–Florida.

FM–Field Manual.

Fomite–Objects, such as clothing, towels, and utensils that possibly harbor a disease agent and are capable of transmitting it.

Formalin–A 37% aqueous solution of formaldehyde.

Fluorescent antibody–A microbiological method to detect microorganisms, usually bacteria. An antibody with an attached fluorescent molecule is applied to a slide containing the bacteria and washed to remove unbound antibody. Under UV light the bacteria to which antibodies are bound will fluoresce, revealing their presence. An antibody may be applied *primarily* (DFA: direct fluorescence antibody, or direct immunofluorescence assay) or *secondarily*, using two antibodies (IFA: indirect fluorescence antibody, or indirect immunofluorescence assay).

Fulminant hepatitis–Severe, rapidly progressive loss of hepatic function due to viral infection or other cause of inflammatory destruction of liver tissue with associated coagulopathy and encephalopathy.

G-CSF–Granulocyte-colony stimulating factor.

GEM–Genetically engineered microorganisms.

Generalized vaccinia–Secondary lesions of the skin after vaccination, which may occur in subjects with previously healthy skin but are more common in the case of traumatized skin, especially in the case of eczema (eczema vaccinatum). In the latter instance, generalized vaccinia may result from mere contact with a vaccinated person. Secondary vaccinial lesions may also occur after transfer of virus from the vaccination to another site by means of the fingers (autoinnoculation).

GI–Gastrointestinal.

Glanders–A chronic debilitating disease of horses and other equids, as well as some members of the cat family, caused by *Pseudomonas mallei*; it is transmissible to humans. It attacks the mucous membranes of the nostrils of the horse, producing an increased and vitiated secretion and discharge of mucus, and enlargement and induration of the glands of the lower jaw.

GLC–Gas liquid chromatography.

G or g–Gram(s).

Granulocytopenia—Less than the normal number of granular leukocytes in the blood.

Guarnieri bodies–Intracytoplasmic acidophilic inclusion bodies observed in epithelial cells in variola (smallpox) and vaccinia infections, and which include aggregations of Paschen body's or virus particles.

H or h–Hour(s).

HA–Hemagglutination assay.

HBAT–*Heptavalent Botulinum Antitoxin.*

HCQ–Hydroxychloroquine.

HCW–Health care worker.

HE-BAT–*Botulism Antitoxin, Heptavalent, Equine* (A, B, C, D, E, F and G).

HEL–Human erythroleukemia.

Hemagglutination–The agglutination of red blood cells; may be immune as a result of specific antibody either for red blood cell antigens per se or other antigens that coat the red blood cells, or may be nonimmune, as in hemagglutination caused by viruses or other microbes.

Hemagglutinin–A substance, antibody or other, that causes hemagglutination.

Hematemesis–Vomiting of blood.

Hematuria–Any condition in which the urine contains blood or red blood cells.

Hemopoietic–Pertaining to or related to the formation of blood cells.

Hemodynamic–Relating to the physical aspects of the blood circulation.

Hemolysis–Alteration, dissolution, or destruction of red blood cells in such a manner that hemoglobin is liberated into the medium in which the cells are suspended, e.g., by specific complement-fixing antibodies, toxins, various chemical agents, tonicity, alteration of temperature.

Hemolytic Uremic Syndrome–Hemolytic anemia and thrombocytopenia occurring with acute renal failure.

Hemoptysis–The spitting of blood derived from the lungs or bronchial tubes as a result of pulmonary or bronchial hemorrhage.

HEPA–High-Efficiency Particulate Air [filter].

Hepatic–Relating to the liver.

Heterologous–1. Pertaining to cytologic or histologic elements occurring where they are not normally found. 2. Derived from an animal of a different species, as the serum of a horse is heterologous for a rabbit.

HFRS–Hemorrhagic fever with renal syndrome. A viral hemorrhagic fever syndrome caused by viruses of the genus *Hantavirus*, Bunyaviridae family, with renal impairment as the primary organ manifestation.

HHA–Hand held assay.

HHS–See DHHS.

Histogram–A graphical representation of the distribution of data. (See epidemic curve).

HPLC-MS–High-performance liquid chromatography-mass spectrometry.

HPS–Hantavirus pulmonary syndrome.

HQ–Headquarters.

HSPD–Homeland Security Presidential Directive.

HUS–Hemolytic-uremic syndrome.

Hyperemia–The presence of an increased amount of blood in a part or organ.

Hyperesthesia–Abnormal acuteness of sensitivity to touch, pain, or other sensory stimuli.

Hypotension–Subnormal arterial blood pressure.

Hypovolemia–A decreased amount of blood in the body.

Hypoxemia–Subnormal oxygenation of arterial blood, short of anoxia.

IA–Inhalational anthrax.

IATA–International Air Transport Association.

IAW–In accordance with.

ICB–intracellular bacterial [pathogen].

ICD–International Classification of Diseases; published by the WHO.

ICLC–Interstitial Cajal-like cells.

ICU–Intensive care unit.

ID–Infectious disease.

IDE–Investigational Device Exemption; similar to an IND.

Idiopathic–Denoting a disease of unknown cause.

IF–Immunofluorescence.

IFA–Indirect immunofluorescence assay, or indirect immunofluorescence antibody (*see* Fluorescent antibody).

Ig–Immunoglobulin.

IHR–International Health Regulations.

IM–Intramuscular; intramuscularly.

IMDG–International Maritime Organization Dangerous Goods [code].

Immunoassay–Detection and assay of substances by serological (immunological) methods; in most applications the substance in question serves as antigen, both in antibody production and in measurement of antibody by the test substance.

Incubation period–the period between exposure to a pathogen (bacterium, virus, fungus) and the first symptoms or signs of infection (*cf.* **latent period**).

IND–Investigational New Drug; FDA's terminology for an experimental drug or vaccine, not approved for general use.

Induration–1. The process of becoming extremely firm or hard, or having such physical features. 2. A focus or region of indurated tissue.

Inguinal–Relating to the groin.

Inoculation–Introduction into the body of the causative organism of a disease.

IRB–Institutional Review Board.

Isolation–Voluntary or compulsory separation and confinement of an individual known or suspected to be infected with a contagious disease agent (whether ill or not) to prevent further infections. In a system devised, and periodically revised, by the CDC, various levels comprise application of one or more "precaution" (e.g., contact, droplet, airborne). (*cf.* **biocontainment**, **quarantine**).

IV–Intravenous; intravenously.

In vitro–In an artificial environment, referring to a process or reaction occurring therein, as in a test tube or culture media.

In vivo–In the living body, referring to a process or reaction occurring therein.

JAMA–*Journal of the American Medical Association.*

JBPDS–Joint Biological Point Detection System.

JBAIDS–Joint Biological Agent Identification and Diagnostic System.

JPEO-CBD–The DoD's Joint Program Executive Office for Chemical and Biological Defense.

JSGPM–Joint Service General Protective Mask (US Army XM-50).

JSLIST–Joint Services Lightweight Integrated Suit Technology.

KFD–Kyasanur Forest disease [virus]; a tick-borne encephalitis.

Kg–Kilogram(s).

KGB–The USSR's "Committee for State Security" [*Komitet gosudarstvennoy bezopasnosti*].

Latent period–the period between exposure to a toxin and the first symptoms or signs of intoxication (*cf* **incubation period**).

LD_{50}–In toxicology, the LD_{50} of a particular substance is a measure of how much constitutes a lethal dose. In toxicological studies of substances, one test is to administer varying doses of the substance to populations of test animals; that dose administered which kills half the test population is referred to as the LD_{50}.

LDH–lactate dehydrogenase, a liver enzyme.

LED–light-emitting diode.

Leukopenia–The antithesis of leukocytosis; any situation in which the total number of leukocytes in the circulating blood is less than normal, the lower limit of which is generally regarded as 4000–5000 per cubic mm.

LRN–Laboratory Response Network (See Appendix L-4.)

Lumbosacral–Relating to the lumbar vertebrae and the sacrum.

Lumen, pl. lumina–The space in the interior of a tubular structure, such as an artery or the intestine.

LVS–Live vaccine strain (an IND tularemia vaccine).

Lymphadenopathy–Any disease process affecting a lymph node or lymph nodes.

Lymphopenia–A reduction, relative or absolute, in the number of lymphocytes in the circulating blood.

Macula, pl. maculae–1. A small spot, perceptibly different in color from the surrounding tissue. 2. A small, discolored patch or spot on the skin, neither elevated above nor depressed below the skin's surface.

MCBC–The week-long Medical Management of Chemical and Biological Casualties course, jointly taught by USAMRICD and USAMRIID on a quarterly basis. (See also MMBC.)

MCM–Medical countermeasure.

MD–Maryland.

Mediastinitis–Inflammation of the cellular tissue of the mediastinum.

Mediastinum–The median partition of the thoracic cavity, covered by the mediastinal pleura and containing all the thoracic viscera and structures except the lungs.

Megakaryocyte–A large cell with a polyploid nucleus that is usually multilobed; megakaryocytes are normally present in bone marrow, not in the circulating blood, and give rise to blood platelets.

Melena–Passage of dark-colored, tarry stools, due to the presence of blood altered by the intestinal juices.

Meningism–A condition in which the symptoms simulate a meningitis, but in which no actual inflammation of these membranes is present.

Meningococcemia–Presence of meningococci (*N. meningitidis*) in the circulating blood.

Meninges–Any membrane; specifically, one of the membranous coverings of the brain and spinal cord.

MERS-CoV–Middle East respiratory syndrome coronavirus.

Microcyst–A tiny cyst, frequently of such dimensions that a magnifying lens or microscope is required for observation.

Microscopy–Investigation of minute objects by means of a microscope.

Min–Minute(s).

Mm–millimeter(s).

MMBC–USAMRIID's Medical Management of Biological Casualties course, a sub-component of the MCBC (*q.v.*).

MOPP–Mission Oriented Protective Posture; US Army terminology for NBC personal protective gear (mask, hood, suit, boots).

Mo(s)–Month(s).

Mortality rate–A measure of the number of deaths (in general, or due to a specific cause) in some population, scaled to the size of that population, per unit time. (*cf.* **Case fatality rate**).

Mg–Milligram(s).

Moribund–Dying; at the point of death.

MRI–Magnetic resonance imaging.

MTF–Medical treatment facility.

Mucocutaneous–Relating to mucous membrane and skin; denoting the line of junction of the two at the nasal, oral, vaginal, and anal orifices.

MULO–Multipurpose rain/snow/CW overboots.

MVA–Modified vaccinia virus Ankara.

Myalgia–Muscular pain.

Mydriasis–Dilation of the pupil.

NA–Neuraminidase.

NAAK–Nerve Agent Antidote Kit; consists of prefilled autoinjectors for the rapid administration of atropine and pralidoxime.

NATO–North Atlantic Treaty Organization.

NBC–Nuclear, Biological and Chemical.

Narcosis–General and nonspecific reversible depression of neuronal excitability, produced by a number of physical and chemical agents, usually resulting in stupor rather than in anesthesia.

NDBR–National Drug Biological Research [Company]; used with vaccine lot numbers.

Necrosis–Pathologic death of one or more cells, or of a portion of tissue or organ, resulting from irreversible damage.

Nephropathia epidemica–A generally benign form of epidemic hemorrhagic fever reported in Scandinavia.

Neutrophilia–An increase of neutrophilic leukocytes in blood or tissues; also frequently used synonymously with leukocytosis, inasmuch as the latter is generally the result of an increased number of neutrophilic granulocytes in the circulating blood (or in the tissues, or both).

NIBC–The National Integrated Biodefense Campus at Fort Detrick, Maryland.

NICBR–The National Interagency Confederation for Biological Research.

Nosocomial–Denoting a new disorder (not the patient's original condition) associated with being treated in a hospital, such as a hospital-acquired infection.

NSAID–Non-steroidal anti-inflammatory drug.

NSB–National Strategy for Biosurveillance.

OCONUS–Outside the Continental United States.

ODP–Office of Domestic Preparedness; Overseen by both the US Department of Justice and DHS.

OHF–Omsk hemorrhagic fever [virus]; a tick-borne encephalitis.

Oliguria–Scant urine production.

Oropharynx–The portion of the pharynx that lies posterior to the mouth; it is continuous above with the nasopharynx via the pharyngeal isthmus and below with the laryngopharynx.

Orphan drug–A drug effective in a rare or exotic medical condition, but which remains commercially undeveloped owing to its limited profitability; granting "orphan status", for the creation of financial incentives, is a matter of public policy in many countries; the concept applies to many vaccines as well.

Osteomyelitis–Inflammation of the bone marrow and adjacent bone.

Outbreak–An occurrence of disease greater than expected for a particular time and place; outbreaks may be epidemics (*q.v.*), affecting a region in a country or a group of countries, or a pandemic, affecting populations globally.

PA–Physician assistant.

Pancytopenia–Pronounced reduction in the number of erythrocytes, all types of white blood cells, and the blood platelets in the circulating blood.

Pandemic–Denoting a disease affecting or attacking the population of an extensive region, country, continent; extensively epidemic.

PAPR–Powered air-purifying respirator.

Papule–A small, circumscribed, solid elevation up to 1 cm in diameter on the skin.

Parasitemia–The presence of parasites in the circulating blood; used especially with reference to malarial and other protozoan forms, and microfilariae.

Passive immunity–Providing temporary protection from disease through the administration of exogenously produced antibody (i.e., transplacental transmission of antibodies to the fetus or the injection of immune globulin for specific preventive purposes).

PBT–Pentavalent botulinum toxoid.

PCR–Polymerase chain reaction (*q.v.*).

PEP–Post-exposure prophylaxis.

Percutaneous–Denoting the passage of substances through unbroken skin, for example, by needle puncture, including introduction of wires and catheters.

Perivascular–Surrounding a blood or lymph vessel.

Petechia, pl. petechiae–Minute hemorrhagic spots, of pinpoint to pinhead size, in the skin, which are not blanched by pressure.

Pharyngeal–Relating to the pharynx.

Pharyngitis–Inflammation of the mucous membrane and underlying parts of the pharynx.

Phosgene–Carbonyl chloride; a colorless liquid below 8.2°C, but an extremely poisonous gas at ordinary temperatures; it is an insidious gas, as it is not immediately irritating, even when fatal concentrations are inhaled.

Photophobia–Light-induced pain, especially of the eyes; for example, in uveitis, the light-induced movement of the iris may be painful. SYN: photodynia, photalgia

Pleurisy–Inflammation of the pleura.

PM–afternoon or evening (Latin, *post meridiem*).

PO–By mouth; orally.

Polymerase chain reaction (PCR)–An *in vitro* molecular biology method for enzymatically synthesizing and amplifying defined sequences of DNA. Can be used for improving DNA-based diagnostic systems for identifying unknown bio-agents.

Polymorphonuclear–Having nuclei of varied forms; denoting a variety of leukocyte.

Polyuria–Excessive excretion of urine.

POW–Prisoner of war.

PPE–Personal protective equipment.

Presynaptic–Pertaining to the area on the proximal side of a synaptic cleft.

Prophylaxis, pl. prophylaxes–Prevention of disease or of a process that can lead to disease.

Prostration–A marked loss of strength, as in exhaustion.

Proteinuria–Presence of urinary protein in concentrations greater than 0.3 g in a 24-h urine collection or in concentrations greater than 1 g/l in a random urine collection on two or more occasions $\geq$ 6 h apart; specimens must be clean, voided midstream, or obtained by catheterization.

Pruritus–Syn: itching.

Ptosis, pl. ptoses–In reference to the eyes, drooping of the eyelids.

Pulmonary edema–Edema of the lungs.

Pyrogenic–Causing fever.

Q or q–Latin, *quaque*, meaning “each” or “every”.

QD or qD–Each day.

QID or qid–Four times each day.

Quarantine–The compulsory separation and confinement, with restriction of movement, of healthy individuals or groups who have potentially been exposed to a contageous disease agent to prevent further infections should infection occur. (*cf.* **biocontainment**, **isolation**).

Q.v.–Latin, *quod vide*, "which see".

Reactogenicity–The property of a vaccine of being able to produce common, "expected" adverse reactions, especially excessive immunological responses and associated signs and symptoms—fever, sore arm or redness at injection site, etc.

Retinitis–Inflammation of the retina.

Retrosternal–Posterior to the sternum.

Rhinorrhea–A discharge from the nasal mucous membrane.

RNA–Ribonucleic acid.

RT–Reverse transcriptase.

RT-PCR–Reverse transcription-polymerase chain reaction (*q.v.*)

RTA–Ricin Toxin A [chain].

RTB–Ricin Toxin B [chain].

RVF –Rift Valley fever, a VHF.

SA–Select Agent (*q.v.*).

SAP–CDC's Select Agent (*q.v.*) Program.

SAHF–South American Hemorrhagic Fevers (i.e., AHF and BHF).

Sarin–A nerve poison which is a very potent irreversible cholinesterase inhibitor and a more toxic nerve gas than tabun or soman.

SARS–Severe Acute Respiratory Syndrome [virus].

Scarification–The making of a number of superficial incisions in the skin. It is the technique used to administer tularemia and smallpox vaccines.

Scud–NATO reporting name (SS-1 Scud) for a series of tactical ballistic missiles developed by the USSR and exported widely to other countries, including Iraq.

SEB–Staphylococcal Enterotoxin B.

Select Agent–A bio-agent that, since 1997, has been declared by the DHHS, or by the USDA, to have the "potential to pose a severe threat to public health and safety". (See also BSAT and Appendix C).

Septic shock–1. Shock associated with sepsis, usually associated with abdominal and pelvic infection complicating trauma or operations; 2. Shock associated with septicemia caused by gram-negative bacteria.

Sequela, pl. sequelae–A condition after a consequence of a disease.

Shigellosis–Bacillary dysentery caused by bacteria of the genus *Shigella*, often occurring in epidemic patterns.

SNS–Strategic National Stockpile; Repository of drugs, vaccines, etc, overseen jointly by CDC and DHS.

Soman–An extremely potent cholinesterase inhibitor, similar to sarin and tabun.

SOP–Standard [or standing] operating procedure.

SQ–Subcutaneous; subcutaneously.

SRBSDS–Short Range Biological Standoff Detection System.

ST-246–The oral antiviral tecovirimat (*Arestvyr*®), an IND.

Standard precautions–A set of uniform or comprehensive measures designed to prevent the inadvertent transmission of communicable diseases between patient and HCW. They are employed during *every* patient encounter, regardless of whether or not the patient is thought to harbor an infectious disease. (See Appendix H.)

Sterile abscess–An abscess whose contents are not caused by pyogenic bacteria.

Sterilization–Process that eliminates (removes) or kills all forms of life, including transmissible agents (bacteria [including spores], viruses, fungi) present on a surface, contained in a fluid, in medication, or in a substance such as biological culture media; achieved by applying heat, chemicals, irradiation, high pressure, and/or filtration.

Stridor–A high-pitched, noisy respiration, like the blowing of the wind; a sign of respiratory obstruction, especially in the trachea or larynx.

Superantigen–An antigen that interacts with the T-cell receptor in a domain outside of the antigen recognition site. This type of interaction induces the activation of larger numbers of T cells compared to antigens that are presented in the antigen-recognition site leading to the release of numerous cytokines.

Superinfection–A new infection in addition to one already present.

Tachycardia–Rapid beating of the heart, conventionally applied to rates over 100 per minute.

TB–Tuberculosis.

TBE–Tick-borne encephalitis [viruses]; two of them cause VHF: Omsk hemorrhagic fever (OHF) virus and Kyasanur Forest disease (KFD) virus.

TEE–Transesophageal echocardiagram.

Teratogenicity–The property or capability of producing fetal malformation.

Thrombocytopenia–A condition in which there is an abnormally small number of platelets in the circulating blood.

TID or tid–Thrice each day.

TMM–The US Army's *Textbook of Military Medicine* series.

TMP-SMX–The combination antibiotic trimethoprim-sulfamethoxazole.

TMT–The DoD's Transformational Medical Technologies Initiative.

Toxin or bio-toxin–a poisonous substance produced within living cells or organisms; typically they are peptides, proteins or smaller molecules.

Toxoid–A modified bacterial toxin that has been rendered nontoxic (commonly with formaldehyde) but retains the ability to stimulate the formation of antitoxins (antibodies) and thus producing an active immunity. Examples include botulinum, tetanus, and diphtheria toxoids.

Tracheitis–Inflammation of the lining membrane of the trachea.

Transmission-based precautions–Measures implemented in addition to Standard Precautions (*q.v.*), in select circumstances, to prevent the transmission of specific disease agents known or suspected to be present in a patient; may include (1) *Contact Precautions* to preclude disease transmission via blood, body fluids, or fomites; (2) *Droplet Precautions* when transmission via macroscopic respiratory droplets is a risk, or (3) *Airborne Precautions* when microscopic (~ 3-6 micron) "droplet nuclei" provide a possible vehicle of disease transmission. (See Appendix H.)

TTE–Transthoracic echocardiagram.

TX–Texas.

UK–United Kingdom.

UN–United Nations.

UNSCOM–United Nations Special Commission; an inspection regime created by the UN to ensure Iraq's compliance with its policies concerning production and use of WMD after the Persian Gulf War.

Urticaria–An eruption of itching wheals, usually of systemic origin; it may be due to a state of hypersensitivity to foods or drugs, foci of infection, physical agents (heat, cold, light, friction), or psychic stimuli.

USAMMDA–US Army Medical Materiel Development Agency, Fort Detrick, Maryland.

USAMRICD–US Army Medical Research Institute of Chemical Defense, Aberdeen Proving Ground, Maryland.

USAMRIID–US Army Medical Research Institute of Infectious Diseases, Fort Detrick, Maryland.

USC–United States Code.

USDA–United States Department of Agriculture; oversees regulation of BSATs (*q.v.*) affecting agriculture. (See Appendix C.)

USSR–Union of Soviet Socialist Republics.

UV–Ultraviolet [light].

VA–Virginia.

Vaccine–A suspension of attenuated live or killed microorganisms (bacteria, viruses, or rickettsiae), or fractions thereof (for example, specific protein subunits or naked DNA), administered to induce immunity and thereby prevent infectious disease.

Vaccinia–An infection, primarily local and limited to a site of inoculation, induced in humans with the vaccinia virus (a relative of coxpox) to confer resistance to smallpox (variola). On about the 3rd d, papules form at the site of inoculation which become transformed into umbilicated vesicles and later pustules; they then dry up, and the scab falls off on about the 21st d, leaving a pitted scar; in some cases there are more or less marked constitutional disturbances.

Varicella–An acute contagious disease, usually occurring in children, caused by the varicella-zoster virus, a member of the family *Herpesviridae*, and marked by a sparse eruption of papules, which become vesicles and then pustules, like that of smallpox although less severe and varying in stages, usually with mild constitutional symptoms; incubation period is about 14 to 17 d. Syn: chickenpox.

Variola–Smallpox or smallpox virus.

Variolation–The historical practice of inducing immunity against smallpox by inoculating the skin with matter from skin pustules of a smallpox victim. Said to have first been done in Ancient China.

VEE/VEEV–Venezuelan Equine Encephalitis [virus].

VHC–Refers to DoD's regional Vaccine Health Centers.

VHF–Viral Hemorrhagic Fever.

VIGIV–*Vaccinia Immune Globulin, Intravenous.*

Viremia–The presence of virus in the bloodstream.

Virion–The complete virus particle that is structurally intact and infectious.

WBC–White blood cell.

WEE/WEEV–Western Equine Encephalitis [virus].

WHO–The UN's World Health Organization.

Wk(s)–Week(s).

WMD–Weapon(s) of Mass Destruction; see also NBC.

Wt–Weight.

Yr(s)–Year(s).

Zoonosis–An infection or infestation shared in nature by humans and other animals that are the normal or usual host; a disease of humans acquired from an animal source.

APPENDIX B: CDC BIO-AGENT CATEGORIES A, B & C

Categories of Bio-terrorism Agents/Diseases
(Adapted from: http://emergency.cdc.gov/agent/agentlist-category.asp)

Category	Definition	Examples
A	High-priority agents include organisms that pose a risk to national security because they … • can be easily disseminated or transmitted from person to person; • result in high fatality rates & have the potential for major public health impact; • might cause public panic & social disruption; & require special action for public health preparedness.	• Anthrax (*Bacillus anthracis*) • Botulism (*Clostridium botulinum* toxin) • Plague (*Yersinia pestis*) • Smallpox (Variola major type) • Tularemia (*Francisella tularensis*) • Viral hemorrhagic fevers (filoviruses [e.g., Ebola, Marburg] and arenaviruses [e.g., Lassa, Machupo])
B	Second highest priority agents include those that … • are moderately easy to disseminate; • result in moderate morbidity rates & low fatality rates; • require specific enhancements of CDC's diagnostic capacity & enhanced disease surveillance.	• Brucellosis (*Brucella* species) • Epsilon toxin of *Clostridium perfringens* • Food safety threats (e.g., *Salmonella* species, *Escherichia coli* O157:H7, *Shigella*) • Glanders (*Burkholderia mallei*) • Melioidosis (*Burkholderia pseudomallei*) • Psittacosis (*Chlamydia psittaci*) • Q fever (*Coxiella burnetii*) • Ricin toxin from *Ricinus communis* (castor beans) • Staphylococcal enterotoxin B • Typhus fever (*Rickettsia prowazekii*) • Viral encephalitis (alphaviruses [e.g., Venezuelan equine encephalitis, eastern equine encephalitis, western equine encephalitis]) • Water safety threats (e.g., *Vibrio cholerae*, *Cryptosporidium parvum*)
C	Third highest priority agents include emerging pathogens that could be engineered for mass dissemination in the future because of … • availability; • ease of production & dissemination; • & potential for high morbidity & fatality rates & major health impact.	Emerging infectious diseases such as … • Nipah virus • Hantavirus

APPENDIX C: BIOLOGICAL SELECT AGENTS AND TOXINS (BSATS)

Under US law, "Biological Select Agents and Toxins" (BSATs)—or simply Select Agents for short—are bio-agents which since 1997[1] have been declared by the US Department of Health and Human Services (DHHS) or by the US Department of Agriculture (USDA) to have the "potential to pose a severe threat to public health and safety". These bio-agents are divided into three broad categories: (1) DHHS select agents and toxins (affecting humans); (2) USDA select agents and toxins (affecting agriculture); and (3) Overlap select agents and toxins (affecting both).

The US Centers for Disease Control and Prevention (CDC) administers the Select Agent Program (SAP), which regulates the laboratories which may possess, use, or transfer select agents within the United States. The SAP was established to satisfy requirements of the USA PATRIOT Act of 2001 and the Public Health Security and Bioterrorism Preparedness and Response Act of 2002, which were enacted in the wake of the September 11, 2001 attacks and the subsequent 2001 anthrax attacks.

The active use of BSATs in biomedical research prompts concerns about dual use. The Federal government has created the National Science Advisory Board for Biosecurity, a critical component of a set of federal initiatives to promote biosecurity in life science research. This advisory board is composed of government, education and industry experts who provide policy recommendations on ways to minimize the possibility that knowledge and technologies emanating from vitally important biological research will be misused to threaten public health or national security.

List of Select Agents

Tier 1 BSATs are indicated by an asterisk (*).[2]

I. DHHS select agents and toxins

Pathogens

Bacteria

- Botulinum neurotoxin- species of *Clostridium**
- Coxiella burnetii
- Francisella tularensis*
- Rickettsia prowazekii
- Rickettsia rickettsii
- Yersinia pestis*

Viruses

- Coronavirus:
    - SARS-associated coronavirus (SARS-CoV)[3]
- Encephalitis viruses:
    - Eastern equine encephalitis virus (excluding South American genotypes)
    - Tick-borne encephalitis-complex viruses (3 subtypes, excluding European ones)
        - Central European tick-borne encephalitis virus
        - Far Eastern tick-borne encephalitis virus
        - Russian spring and summer encephalitis virus
- Influenza viruses:
    - Highly Pathogenic Avian Influenza H5N1 virus
    - Reconstructed 1918 influenza virus[4]
- Orthopoxviruses:
    - Monkeypox virus
    - Variola major virus* (smallpox virus)
    - Variola minor virus* (Alastrim)
- Viral hemorrhagic fever (VHF) viruses:
    - African VHF viruses:
        - Crimean-Congo haemorrhagic fever virus
        - Ebola virus*
        - Lassa fever virus
        - Lujo virus
        - Marburg virus*
    - Asian VHF viruses:
        - Kyasanur Forest disease virus
        - Omsk hemorrhagic fever virus
    - South American VHF viruses:
        - Chapare virus
        - Guanarito virus (Venezuelan hemorrhagic fever)
        - Junin virus (Argentine hemorrhagic fever)
        - Machupo (Bolivian hemorrhagic fever)
        - Sabiá virus (Brazilian hemorrhagic fever)

Toxins

- Abrin
- Botulinum neurotoxins*
- *Clostridium perfringens* epsilon toxin
- Conotoxins
- Ricin
- Saxitoxin
- Shiga-like ribosome inactivating proteins
- Shiga toxin
- Staphylococcal enterotoxins
- Tetrodotoxin
- Type A trichothecenes:
    - Diacetoxyscirpenol
    - T-2 toxin

II. Overlap select agents and toxins

Bacteria

- *Bacillus anthracis**
- *Brucella abortus*
- *Brucella melitensis*
- *Brucella suis*
- *Burkholderia mallei** (formerly *Pseudomonas mallei*)
- *Burkholderia pseudomallei** (formerly *Pseudomonas pseudomallei*)

Viruses

- Hendra virus
- Nipah virus
- Rift Valley fever virus
- Venezuelan equine encephalitis virus (excluding enzootic subtypes ID and IE)

III. USDA select agents and toxins

For animals

Bacteria

- *Mycoplasma mycoides* subspecies *mycoides* small colony (Mmm SC) (contagious bovine pleuropneumonia)

Viruses

- African horse sickness virus
- African swine fever virus
- Avian influenza virus (highly pathogenic)
- Classical swine fever virus
- Foot-and-mouth disease virus*
- Lumpy skin disease virus
- Peste des petits ruminants virus
- Rinderpest virus*
- Swine vesicular disease virus
- Virulent Newcastle disease virus 1

For plants

Bacteria

- *Ralstonia solanacearum* race 3, biovar 2
- *Rathayibacter toxicus*
- *Xanthomonas oryzae*
- *Xylella fastidiosa* (citrus variegated chlorosis strain)

Fungi or fungus-like pathogens

- *Peronosclerospora philippinensis* (*Peronosclerospora sacchari*)
- *Phoma glycinicola* (formerly *Pyrenochaeta glycines*)
- *Sclerophthora rayssiae* variety *zeae*
- *Synchytrium endobioticum*

List of former Select Agents

Select agent regulations were revised in October 2012 to remove 19 BSATs from the list (7 Human and Overlap Agents and 12 Animal Agents).[5]

Human and Overlap Agents

- *Cercopithecine herpesvirus 1* (Herpes B virus)
- *Coccidioides posadasii*
- *Coccidioides immitis*
- Eastern Equine encephalitis virus, South American genotypes
- Flexal virus
- Tick-borne encephalitis viruses, European subtypes
- Venezuelan Equine Encephalitis virus, Enzootic subtypes ID and IE

Animal Agents

- Akabane virus
- Bluetongue virus
- Bovine Spongiform Encephalitis
- Camel Pox virus
- *Erlichia ruminantium*
- Goat Pox virus
- Japanese encephalitis virus
- Malignant Catarrhal Fever virus (Alcelaphine herpesvirus type 1)
- Menangle virus
- *Mycoplasma capricolum* subspecies *capripneumoniae* (contagious caprine pleuropneumonia)
- Sheep Pox virus
- Vesicular stomatitis virus (exotic): Indiana subtypes VSV-IN2, VSV-IN3

APPENDIX D: SUMMARY OF BIO-AGENT CHARACTERISTICS

Disease	Degree of person-to-person transmission	Infective Dose (Aerosol)/ LD_{50}[1]	Incubation Period[2]	Duration of Illness	Case fatality rate (CFR)	Persistence of organism outside host	Vaccine efficacy (aerosol exposure)
Anthrax	None	8,000-50,000 spores	1-6 d	3-5 d (usually fatal if untreated)	High	Very stable - spores remain viable for > 40 yrs in soil	2 dose efficacy against up to 1,000 LD_{50} in monkeys
Brucellosis	None	10 -100 organisms	5-60 d (usually 1-2 mos)	Wks to mos	<5% untreated	Very stable	No vaccine
Glanders	Low	Unknown, Potentially low	10-14 d via aerosol	Death in 7-10 d in septicemic form	> 50%	Very stable	No vaccine
Melioidosis	Low	Unknown, Potentially low	1-21 d (up to yrs)	Death in 2-3 d with septicemic form (untreated)	19 – 50% for severe disease	Very stable; survives indefinitely in warm moist soil or stagnant water	No vaccine
Plague	Moderate (for pneumonic form)	500 - 15000 organisms	1-7 d (usually 2-3 d)	1-6 d (usually fatal)	High unless treated within 12-24 h	For up to 1 yr in soil; 270 d in live tissue	No vaccine
Tularemia	None	10-50 organisms	1-21 d (average 3-6 d)	$\geq$ 2 wks	Moderate if untreated	For mos in moist soil or other media	80% protection against 1-10 LD_{50}
Q Fever	Rare	1-10 organisms	7-41 d	2-14 d	Very low	For mos on wood & sand	94% protection against 3,500 LD_{50} in guinea pigs
Smallpox	High	Assumed low (10-100) organisms)	7-17 d (average 12 d)	4 wks	High to moderate	Very stable	Protects against large doses in primates
Venezuelan Equine Encephalitis	Rare	10-100 organisms	2-6 d	Days to wks	Low	Relatively unstable	TC 83 protects against 30-500 LD_{50} in hamsters

Disease	Degree of person-to-person transmission	Infective Dose (Aerosol)/ LD_{50}[1]	Incubation Period[2]	Duration of Illness	Case fatality rate (CFR)	Persistence of organism outside host	Vaccine efficacy (aerosol exposure)
Viral Hemorrhagic Fevers	Moderate	1-10 organisms	4-21 d	Death between 7-16 d	High to moderate (depends on agent)	Relatively unstable – (depends on agent)	No vaccine
Botulism	None	0.001 μg/kg is LD_{50} for type A (parenteral), 0.003 μg/kg (aerosol)	12 h to 5 d	Death in 24-72 h; lasts mos if not lethal	High without respiratory support	For wks in non-moving water & food if shaded from UV light	3 dose efficacy 100% against 25-250 LD_{50} in primates
Staph Enterotoxin B	None	0.03 μg / person (80kg) incapacity-ation	3-12 h after inhalation	Hours	< 1%	Unknown; Resistant to freezing	No vaccine
Ricin	None	3-5 μg/kg is LD_{50} in mice	18-24 h	Days - death within 10-12 d for ingestion	High	Stable	No vaccine
T-2 Mycotoxins	None	Moderate	2-4 h	Days to mos	Moderate	For yrs at room temp	No vaccine

[1] In this Table, "Infective Dose" refers to bacteria and viruses, while "LD50" refers to toxins.

[2] In this Table, "In Period" implies "Latent Period" where toxins are indicated.

APPENDIX E: DIFFERENTIAL DIAGNOSIS OF CHEMICAL NERVE AGENT, BOTULINUM TOXIN & SEB INTOXICATION FOLLOWING INHALATION EXPOSURE

	Chemical Nerve Agent	Botulinum Toxin	SEB
Time to Symptoms	Minutes	Hours (12-48)	Hours (1-6)
Nervous	Convulsions, Muscle twitching	Progressive, descending skeletal muscle flaccid paralysis	Headache, muscle aches
Cardiovascular	Slow heart rate	Normal rate	Normal or rapid heart rate
Respiratory	Difficult breathing, airway constriction	Normal, then progressive paralysis	Nonproductive cough; Severe cases; chest pain/difficult breathing
Gastrointestinal	Increased motility, pain, diarrhea	Decreased motility	Nausea, vomiting and/or diarrhea
Ocular	Small pupils	Droopy eyelids, large pupils, disconjugate gaze	May see "red eyes" (conjunctival injection)
Salivary	Profuse, watery saliva	Normal; difficulty swallowing	May be slightly increased quantities of saliva
Death	Minutes	2-3 d	Unlikely
Response to Atropine/2PAM-CL	Yes	No	Atropine may reduce gastrointestinal symptoms

APPENDIX F: COMPARATIVE LETHALITY OF SELECTED TOXINS & CHEMICAL AGENTS IN LABORATORY MICE*

Agent	LD50 (μg/kg)	Molecular Weight (daltons)	Source
Botulinum neurotoxin A	0.001	150,000	Bacterium
Shiga toxin	0.002	55,000	Bacterium
Tetanus toxin	0.002	150,000	Bacterium
Abrin	0.04	65,000	Plant (Rosary Pea)
Diphtheria toxin	0.10	62,000	Bacterium
Maitotoxin	0.10	3,400	Marine Dinoflagellate
Palytoxin	0.15	2,700	Marine Soft Coral
Ciguatoxin	0.40	1,000	Marine Dinoflagellate
Textilotoxin	0.60	80,000	Elapid Snake
C. perfringens toxins	0.1 – 5.0	35-40,000	Bacterium
Batrachotoxin	2.0	539	Arrow-Poison Frog
Ricin (Aerosol)	3.0	64,000	Plant (Castor Bean)
alpha-Conotoxin	5.0	1,500	Cone Snail
Taipoxin	5.0	46,000	Elapid Snake
Tetrodotoxin	8.0	319	Puffer Fish
alpha-Tityustoxin	9.0	8,000	Scorpion
Saxitoxin	10.0 (Inhal 2.0)	299	Marine Dinoflagellate
VX	15.0	267	Chemical Agent
SEB (rhesus/aerosol)	27.0 (ED_{50}~pg)	28,494	Bacterium
Anatoxin-a(S)	50.0	500	Blue-Green Algae
Microcystin	50.0	994	Blue-Green Algae
Soman (GD)	64.0	182	Chemical Agent

Agent	LD50 (µg/kg)	Molecular Weight (daltons)	Source
Sarin (GB)	100.0	140	Chemical Agent
Aconitine	100.0	647	Plant (Monkshood)
T-2 Toxin	1,210.0	466	Fungal Myotoxin

* Unless otherwise stated, LD_{50} data is determined by intravenous route, and marine toxins are determined by intraperitoneal route.

APPENDIX G: AEROSOL TOXICITY IN LD_{50} VS.QUANTITY OF TOXIN

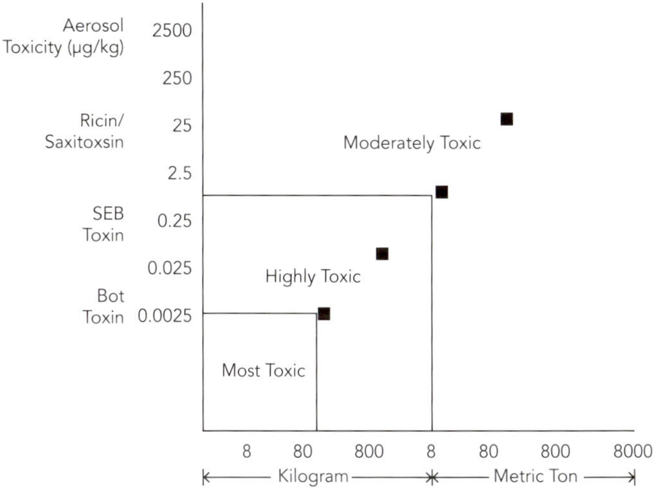

Aerosol toxicity in LD_{50} (see also Appendix F) vs. quantity of toxin required to provide a theoretically effective open-air exposure, under ideal meteorological conditions, to an area 100 km^2. Ricin, saxitoxin and botulinum toxins kill at the concentrations depicted. (Devised by William Patrick III and Richard Spertzel, 1992: Based on Cader K.L., "BWL Tech Study #3: Mathematical models for dosage and casualty resulting from single point and line source release of aerosol near ground level", DTIC #AD3 10-361, Dec 1957.)

APPENDIX H: PATIENT ISOLATION PRECAUTIONS

Standard Precautions constitute a set of "common-sense" measures designed to prevent the inadvertent transmission of communicable diseases among patients and between patient and provider. Standard Precautions should be employed during EVERY healthcare encounter, regardless of whether or not the patient is thought to harbor an infectious disease. In select circumstances, however, additional ("transmission-based") precautions are warranted; three subcategories of *Transmssion-Based Precautions* exist. (1) *Contact Precautions* are used when there is a high likelihood of disease transmission via blood, other body fluids, or fomites. (2) *Droplet Precautions* are utilized when transmission via macroscopic respiratory droplets is a risk. (3) *Airborne Precautions* are employed when microscopic (~ 3-6 micron) "droplet nuclei" provide the vehicle of disease transmission.

Standard Precautions:

- Wash hands with soap and water or use alcohol-based sanitizer before and after patient contact and between patients.
- Wear gloves when touching blood, other body fluids, secretions, excretions, and contaminated items.
- Wear a mask and eye protection, or a face shield during procedures likely to generate splashes or sprays of blood, other body fluids, secretions or excretions
- Handle used patient-care equipment and linen in a manner that prevents the transfer of microorganisms to people or equipment.
- Use safe injection practices.
- Use respiratory hygiene/cough etiquette.
- Use a mouthpiece or other ventilation device as an alternative to mouth-to-mouth resuscitation when practical.

Transmission-based Precautions:

1. Contact Precautions

Standard Precautions plus:

- Place the patient in a private room or cohort them with someone with the same infection if possible; If cohorting is employed, maintain ≥ 3 feet of spatial separation between patients.

- Wear a gown and gloves when entering the room if contact with patient is anticipated or other surfaces patient has touched especially if patient has diarrhea, a colostomy or wound drainage not covered by a dressing.
- Don personal protective equipment (PPE) upon room entry and discard before exiting the patient room to contain pathogens. Change gloves after contact with infective material.
- Limit the movement or transport of the patient from the room and if needed, lightly cover open wounds for transport.
- Ensure that patient-care items, bedside equipment, and frequently touched surfaces receive daily cleaning.
- Dedicate use of noncritical patient-care equipment (such as stethoscopes) to a single patient, or cohort patients with the same pathogen. Use single-use/ disposable equipment if possible. If not feasible, adequate disinfection between patients is necessary.

2. Droplet Precautions

Standard Precautions plus:

- Place the patient in a private room or cohort them with someone with the same infection. If not feasible, maintain $\geq$ 3 feet between patients.
- Wear a surgical mask when working within 3 feet of the patient.
- Limit movement and transport of the patient. Place a mask on the patient if they must be moved out of their room.

3. Airborne Precautions

Standard Precautions plus:

- Place the patient in a private room that has monitored negative air pressure, a minimum of 6 air changes per h, and appropriate HEPA filtration of exhausted air.
- Wear respiratory protection when entering the room. N95 masks are effective against particles as small as 1-5 micrometers.
- Limit movement and transport of the patient. Place a mask on the patient if they need to be moved (Caution- DO NOT place N95 masks on patients who have respiratory difficulty).

For more information on patient isolation guidelines, see: Siegel JD, Rhinehart E, Jackson M, Chiarello L, and the Healthcare Infection Control Practices Advisory Committee. *2007 Guideline for Isolation Precautions: Preventing Transmission of Infectious Agents in Healthcare Settings.* http://www.cdc.gov/ncidod/dhqp/pdf/isolation2007.pdf

For a general discussion of scientific and practical issues related to the air evacuation of contagious patients, see: Withers, MR and GW Christopher (2000), "Aeromedical Evacuation of Biological Warfare Casualties: A Treatise on Infectious Diseases on Aircraft", *Mil Med* 165, Suppl. 3:001.

Table. Recommended Hospital Infection Control Precautions for Selected Conventional Pathogens & Bio-agents

Standard Precautions	Contact Precautions	Droplet Precautions	Airborne Precautions
Hand washing	Gloves & Gown[A]	Private Room[B] Surgical Mask[C]	Private Room[B] Negative Pressure Room HEPA-Filter Mask
Conventional Diseases: All Patients	MRSA, VRE Enteric Infections Skin Infections Lice Scabies *C. difficile* Disease RSV, Parainfluenza	Meningococcal Disease Resistant Pneumococci Pertussis Group A Streptococci Mycoplasma Adenovirus Influenza	Pulmonary TB Measles Varicella
Bio-Agents: Anthrax Botulism Tularemia Brucellosis Q-Fever Glanders Melioidosis Ricin Intoxication SEB Intoxication T-2 Intoxication VEE, EEE, WEE	Certain VHFs -Ebola -Marburg -Lassa Fever Smallpox Melioidosis (with cutaneous lesions)	Pneumonic Plague Ebola[D]	Smallpox

A. Gloves and/or gown should also be worn as a part of standard precautions (and other forms of precaution) when contact with blood, body fluids, and other contaminated substances is likely.

B. Cohorting patients with the same disease is an acceptable alternative to a private room.

C. Surgical masks should also be employed as a part of standard and contact precautions (along with eye protection and a face shield) if procedures are likely to generate splashes or sprays of infectious material.

D. Added by the CDC in July 2014 (See *Infection Prevention and Control Recommendations for Hospitalized Patients with Known or Suspected Ebola Virus Disease in U.S. Hospitals*, <http://www.cdc.gov/vhf/ebola/hcp/infection-prevention-and-control-recommendations.html>).

APPENDIX I: BIO-AGENT PROPHYLACTICS & THERAPEUTICS

NB: (A) = Approved for this use by the FDA; (IND) = Available as an investigational new drug for this indication (i.e. NOT an FDA-approved use).

Anthrax

Vaccine/Toxoid

BioThrax® Anthrax Vaccine (AVA) (Emergent BioSolutions)

Preexposure [(A)]: licensed for adults 18-65-yr old, 0.5 mL IM @ 0, 2, 4 wk, 6, 12, 18 mo then annual boosters

Postexposure[(IND)]: DoD Contingency Use Protocol for volunteer anthrax vaccination SQ @ 0, 2, 4 wk in combination with approved & labeled antibiotics

Pediatric Annex [(IND)] for postexposure use IM @ 0, 2, 4 wk in combination with approved & labeled antibiotics.

http://www.anthrax.osd.mil/resource/policies/policies.asp

Chemoprophylaxis

NB: 60 d post-exposure prophylaxis recommended regardless of full or partial vaccination (see US Army FM 8-284)

After suspected exposure to aerosolized *B. anthracis* of unknown antibiotic susceptibility, prophylaxis with ciprofloxacin (500 mg PO q 12 h for adults, & 10-15 mg/kg PO q 12 h (up to 1 g/d) for children) OR doxycycline (100 mg PO q 12 h for adults or children > 8 yrs & >45 kg, & 2.2 mg/kg PO q 12 h (up to 200 mg/d) for children < 8 yrs) should be initiated immediately.

If antibiotic susceptibilities allow, patients who cannot tolerate tetracyclines or quinolones can be switched to amoxicillin (500 mg PO q 8 h for adults & 80 mg/kg divided q 8 h (≤ 1.5 g/d) in children).

The ACIP recommends a post-exposure regimen of 60 d of appropriate antimicrobial prophylaxis combined with 3 vaccine doses administered SQ (0, 2, & 4 wks) for previously unvaccinated persons aged > 18 yrs. The licensed vaccination schedule can be resumed at 6 mos. The first dose of vaccine should be administered within 10 d. Persons for whom vaccination was delayed should extend antimicrobial use to 14 d after the third dose (even if this practice could result in use of antimicrobials for > 60 d).

Chemotherapy

Inhalational*, Gastrointestinal, or Systemic Cutaneous Disease:

Ciprofloxacin : 400 mg IV q 12 h initially, later by mouth (adult) [(A)]
15 mg/kg/dose (up to 1 g/d) q 12 h (peds)[(A)], or

Doxycycline: 200 mg IV, then 100 mg IV q 12 h (adults) [(A)]
2.2mg/kg (100mg/dose max) q 12 h (peds < 45kg) [(A)], or (if strain susceptible),

Penicillin G Procaine: 4 million units IV q 4 h (adults) [(A)]
50,000U/kg (up to 4M U) IV q 6h (peds) [(A)]

Plus, one or two additional antibiotics with activity against *B. anthracis* (e.g. clindamycin plus rifampin could be a good empiric choice, pending susceptibilities). Potential additional antibiotics include one or more of the following: clindamycin, rifampin, gentamicin, macrolides, vancomycin, imipenem & chloramphenicol.

Convert from IV to PO therapy when the patient is stable, to complete ≥ 60 d of antibiotics.

Meningitis: Add rifampin 20 mg/kg IV q 24 h or vancomycin 1 g IV q 12 h.

*** To complete ≥ 60 d of antibiotics if aerosol exposure to *B. anthracis* has occurred.**

Comments

The ACIP recommends anthrax vaccine in a 3-dose regimen (0, 2, 4 wks) in combination with antimicrobial post-exposure prophylaxis for unvaccinated persons who have been exposed to anthrax, but only under an IND or EUA application.

Penicillins should be used for anthrax treatment or prophylaxis only if the strain is demonstrated to be PCN-susceptible. IAW CDC recommendations, amoxicillin prophylaxis is appropriate only after 14-21 d of fluoroquinolone or doxycycline & only for populations with contraindications to the other drugs (e.g. children or pregnancy). Oral dosing (versus the preferred IV) could be necessary for treatment of systemic disease in a mass casualty situation.

NB: At least 60 d of post-exposure prophylaxis required if aerosol exposure.

Cutaneous anthrax: Antibiotics for cutaneous disease (without systemic complaints) resulting from a bio-agent aerosol attack are the same as for post-exposure prophylaxis. Cutaneous anthrax acquired from natural exposure could be treated with 7-10 d of antibiotics.

Brucellosis

Vaccine/Toxoid

None

Chemoprophylaxis

A human vaccine is not available. Chemoprophylaxis is not recommended after possible exposure to endemic disease. Prophylaxis should only be considered for high-risk exposure in the following situations: (1) inadvertent wound or mucous membrane exposure to infected livestock tissues & body fluids & to livestock vaccines, (2) exposure to laboratory aerosols or to secondary aerosols generated from contaminated soil particles in calving & lambing areas, (3) confirmed bio-warfare/bio-terrorism exposure. **Despite extensive studies, optimal antibiotic therapy for brucellosis remains in dispute.**

Chemotherapy

Doxycycline & rifampin (or other antibiotics) for 6 wks is sufficient in most cases. More prolonged regimens may be required for patients with complications such as hepatitis, splenitis, meningoencephalitis, endocarditis, or osteomyelitis.

Inhalational, Gastrointestinal, or Systemic Disease

Significant infection: Doxycycline: 100 mg PO q 12 h for 4-6 wks (adults)[A], **plus** Streptomycin 1 g IM q 24 h for first 2-3 wks (adults)[A], **or** Doxycycline[A] + Gentamicin 5 mg/kg per d for 7 d (if streptomycin not available)

WHO guidelines for adults & children older than 8 yrs recommend rifampin (600-900 mg) & doxycycline q 24 h 24 h for 6 wks minimum. Treatment in children younger than 8 yrs requires rifampin & cotrimoxazole.

Less severe disease:
Doxycycline 100 mg PO q 12 h for 6 wks (adults)[A], **plus** Rifampin 600-900 mg/d PO q 24 h 24 h for 4-6 wks (adults)[A]

Long-term (up to 6 mo) therapy for meningoencephalitis, endocarditis:
Rifampin + a tetracycline + an aminoglycoside (first 3 wks)

Comments

The CDC interim PEP recommendations for high-risk exposures to *Brucella* spp. are: doxycycline 100 mg PO q 12 h, plus rifampin 600 mg PO q 24 h.

Avoid monotherapy (high relapse). Relapse common for treatments less than 4-6 wks.

Glanders & Meliodosis

Vaccine/Toxoid

None

Chemoprophylaxis

No FDA approved prophylaxis exists.

The antibiotic susceptibility pattern for *B. mallei* is similar to that of *B. pseudomallei*, with *B. mallei* exhibiting resistance to a number of antibiotics.

PO TMP/SMX (2 X 160-800 mg (960 mg tablets) if > 60 kg q 12 h plus folate 5 mg/d for 21 d should be given ASAP after exposure.

Amoxicillin/clavulanic acid (*Augmentin*) 20.5 mg/kg/dose every 8 h is an alternative, especially during pregnancy or for children < 8 yr old. Doxycycline 2.5 mg/kg (up to 100 mg) q 12 h may be considered, but carries risk of relapse. Fluoroquinolones should not be used for PEP, based upon animal studies & high relapse rates in human clinical trials for therapy.

Chemotherapy

No FDA approved therapy exists.

Ceftazidime (50 mg/kg [up to 2 g]) IV q 6 to 8 h, meropenem (25 mg/kg [up to 1 g]) IV q 8 h, or imipenem (25 mg/kg [up to 1 g]) IV q 6 h. Meropenem is advised for patients with neurologic involvement or renal insufficiency. A switch to meropenem is indicated if the patient has positive blood cultures after 7 d of therapy, or clinically deteriorates (e.g., develops organ failure or a new focus of infection) at any time during ceftaz therapy. The addition of TMP/SMX (8/40 mg/kg [up to 320/1,600 mg]) q 12 h may be considered for patients with neurologic, prostatic, bone, or joint involvement.

Continue IV therapy for ≥ 14 d & until patient clinically improved. IV therapy may be extended (4 to 8 wks) for critical illness, severe pulmonary disease, deep-seated abscesses, bone, joint, or CNS involvement. Continue with PO maintenance therapy with TMP/SMX (2 X 160-800 mg [960 mg tablets]) if > 60 kg q 12 h for 3 to 6 mos.

Comments

Both *B. mallei* & *B. pseudomallei* are sensitive to carbapenems, & most strains are also susceptible to ceftazidime & piperacillin. *B. pseudomallei* exhibits resistance to diverse antibiotics, including 1st- & 2nd-generation cephalosporins, penicillins, macrolides & aminoglycosides.

If ceftazidime or a carbapenem are not available, ampicillin/sulbactam (*Augmentin*) or other IV beta-lactam/beta-lactamase inhibitor combinations may represent viable, albeit less-proven alternatives. *Augmentin* may be an alternative to TMP/SMX, especially in pregnancy or for children < 8 yrs old. See main text for recommendations for toxicity screening & folate supplementation during prolonged courses of TMP/SMX.

Plague

Vaccine/Toxoid

None

Chemoprophylaxis

Ciprofloxacin: 500 mg PO q 12 h x 7 d (adults), 20 mg/kg (up to 500 mg) PO q 12 h (peds), **or**

Doxycycline: 100 mg PO q 12 h x 7 d (adults), 2.2 mg/kg (up to 100 mg) PO q 12 h (peds), **or**

Tetracycline: 500 mg PO q 6 hq 6 h x 7 d (adults)

Chemotherapy

Traditionally, streptomycin, tetracycline, & doxycycline are used for plague & are approved by the FDA for this purpose.

Streptomycin: 1g q 12 h IM (adults)[(A)], 15 mg/kg/d div q 12 h IM (up to 2 g/d) (peds)[(A)], **or**

Gentamicin: 5 mg/kg IM or IV q 24 h or 2 mg/kg loading dose followed by 1.7 mg/kg IM or IV (adults), 2.5 mg/kg IM or IV q 8h for 10 d (peds).

Alternatives: Doxycycline: 200 mg IV once then 100 mg IV q 12 h until clinically improved, then 100 mg PO q 12 h for total of 10-14 d (adults)[(A)], **or** ciprofloxacin: 400 mg IV q 12 h until clinically improved then 750 mg PO q 12 h for total 10-14 d, **or** chloramphenicol: 25 mg/kg IV, then 15 mg/kg q 6 h x 14 d.

A minimum of 10 d of therapy is recommended (treat for $\geq$ 3-4 d after clinical recovery). Oral dosing (versus the preferred IV) could be necessary in a mass casualty situation.

Meningitis: add chloramphenicol 25 mg/kg IV, then 15 mg/kg IV q 6 h.

Comments

Streptomycin is not widely available in the US & is of limited use. Although not licensed for use in treating plague, gentamicin is the common choice for parenteral therapy by many authorities. Reduce dosage in renal failure.

Chloramphenicol is contraindicated in children less than 2 yrs. While chloramphenicol is potentially an alternative for post-exposure prophylaxis (25 mg/kg PO q 6 h), oral formulations are available only outside the US.

Alternate therapy or prophylaxis for susceptible strains: TMP-SMX

Other fluoroquinolones or tetracyclines could represent viable alternatives to ciprofloxacin or doxycycline, respectively.

Q Fever

Vaccine/Toxoid

Inactivated Whole Cell Vaccine.

(Pre-exposure only): Licensed (Australian) *Qvax*™; IND DoD vaccine (similar to *Qvax*™) is available through USAMRIID for at-risk US laboratory personnel.

Chemoprophylaxis

Doxycycline: 100 mg PO q 12 h x 5 d (adults), 2.2 mg/kg PO q 12 h (peds), **or** tetracycline: 500 mg PO q 6 h x 5d (adults); start post-exposure prophylaxis 8-12 d postexposure.

Chemotherapy

Doxycycline is the first line treatment for all adults & for children with severe illness. Treatment should be initiated whenever Q fever is suspected & started again if the patient relapses.

Acute Q-fever: Doxycycline: 100 mg IV or PO q 12 h x $\geq$ 14 d (adults)[A], 2.2 mg/kg PO q 12 h (peds), **or**

Tetracycline: 500 mg PO q 6 h x $\geq$ 14 d

Alternatives: Quinolones (e.g., ciprofloxacin), **or** TMP-SMX, **or** Macrolides (e.g., clarithromycin or azithromycin) for 14-21 d. Patients with underlying cardiac valve defects: Doxycycline plus hydroxychloroquine 200 mg PO q 8 h for 12 mos

Chronic Q Fever: Doxycycline plus quinolones for 4 yrs, **or** doxycycline plus hydroxychloroquine for 1.5-3 yrs.

Comments

DoD Q-Fever vaccine manufactured in 1970. Significant side effects if administered inappropriately; sterile abscesses if prior exposure; skin testing required before vaccination. Time to develop immunity ~5 wks.

Initiation of post-exposure prophylaxis within 7 d of exposure merely delays incubation period of disease.

Tetracyclines are preferred antibiotic for treatment of acute Q fever except in

1. <u>Meningoencephalitis:</u> fluoroquinolones may penetrate CSF better than tetracyclines
2. <u>Children < 8 yrs (doxycycline relatively contraindicated):</u> TMP/SMX or macrolides (especially clarithromycin or azithromycin).
3. <u>Pregnancy:</u> TMP/SMX 160 mg/800 mg PO q 12 h for duration of pregnancy. If evidence of continued disease at parturition use tetracycline or quinolone for 2-3 wks. Doxycycline is contraindicated during pregnancy.

Tularemia

Vaccine/Toxoid

Live attenuated vaccine (USAMRIID-LVS, Preexposure) [IND] DoD Laboratory Use Protocol for vaccine. Single 0.1 ml dose via scarification in at-risk researchers.

Dynport Vaccine Company (DVC-LVS) undergoing Phase II trial for safety & immunogenicity in comparison with USAMRIID-LVS

Chemoprophylaxis

Ciprofloxacin: 500 mg PO q 12 h for 14 d, 15-20 mg/kg (up to 500 mg) PO q 12 h (peds), **or**

Doxycycline: 100 mg PO q 12 h x 14 d (adults), 2.2 mg/kg (up to 100 mg) PO q 12 h (peds < 45 kg), **or**

Tetracycline: 500 mg PO q 6 h x 14 d (adults)

Chemotherapy

Streptomycin: 1 g IM q 12 h for ≥ 10 d (adults)[A], 15 mg/kg (up to 2 g/d) IM q 12 h (peds)[A] , **or**

Gentamicin: 5 mg/kg IM or IV q 24 h, or 2 mg/kg loading dose followed by 1.7 mg/kg IM or IV q 8 h x ≥ 10 d (adults), 2.5 mg/kg IM or IV q 8 h (peds), **or**

Alternatives:
Ciprofloxacin 400 mg IV q 12 h for ≥ 10 d (adults); 15-20 mg/kg (up to 1 g/d) IV q 12 h (peds), **or**

Doxycycline: 200 mg IV, then 100 mg IV q 12 h x 14-21 d (adults)[A], 2.2 mg/kg (up to 100 mg) IV q 12 h (peds < 45 kg), **or**

Chloramphenicol: 15-25 mg/kg IV q 6 h x 14-21 d, **or**

Tetracycline: 500 mg PO q 6 h x 14-21 d (adults)[A]

Comments

Vaccine manufactured in 1964.

Streptomycin is not widely available in the US & is of limited use. Gentamicin, although not approved for treatment of tularemia, likely represents a suitable alternative. Adjust gentamicin dose for renal failure.

Treatment with streptomycin, gentamicin, or ciprofloxacin should be continued for 10 d; doxycycline & chloramphenicol are associated with high relapse rates with course shorter than 14-21 d. IM or IV doxycycline, ciprofloxacin, or chloramphenicol can be switched to oral antibiotic to complete course when patient clinically improved.

Chloramphenicol is contraindicated in children < 2 yrs. While chloramphenicol is potentially an alternative for post-exposure prophylaxis (25 mg/kg PO q 6 h), oral formulations are available only outside the US.

Encephalitis viruses

Vaccine/Toxoid

JE inactivated vaccine *JE-VAX*[R] (Sanofi-Pasteur) [(A)] JE inactivated vaccine *JE-VC* (Ixiaro), does not contain thimerosal [(A)]

VEE Live Attenuated Vaccine[(IND)] (DoD Laboratory Use Protocol for Pre-exposure)

TC-83 strain

VEE Inactivated Vaccine[(IND)] (DoD Laboratory Use Protocol for Pre-exposure)

C-84 strain, given only for declining titers after receiving TC-83 vaccine or as a primary vaccination series for those failing to have a titer after receiving the TC-83 vaccine.

EEE Inactivated Vaccine[(IND)] (DoD Laboratory Use Protocol for Pre-exposure)

WEE Inactivated Vaccine[(IND)] (DoD Laboratory Use Protocol for Preexposure)

Chemoprophylaxis

None

Chemotherapy

No specific therapy. Treatment consists of corticosteroids, anticonvulsants, & supportive care measures.

Comments

Adverse events for alphavirus vaccines ~ 50%

VEE TC-83 vaccine manufactured in 1965. Live attenuated vaccine, with significant side effects. About 25% of vaccine recipients experience clinical reactions requiring bed rest. No seroconversion in 20%. Only effective against subtypes 1A, 1B & 1C. VEE C-84 vaccine used for non-responders to TC-83. Preexisting immunity to a live alphavirus vaccine inhibits vaccination with a second, different alphavirus vaccine.

EEE & WEE vaccines are poorly immunogenic. Multiple boosters are required:
EEE vaccine manufactured in 1989. Antibody response is poor. Requires three-dose primary (1 mo apart) & 1-2 boosters (1 mo apart). Time to develop 'adequate' titers ~ 3 mos.

WEE vaccine manufactured in 1991. Antibody response is poor. Requires three-dose primary (1 mo apart) & 3-4 boosters (1 mo apart). Time to develop 'adequate' titers ~ 6 mos.

Hemorrhagic fever viruses

Vaccine/Toxoid

Yellow fever live attenuated 17D vaccine, given as a single shot, with a booster dose every 10 yrs. (A)

AHF vaccine[(IND)] (Cross-protection for BHF)

MP-12 attenuated RVF vaccine[(IND)] (DoD IND for high-risk laboratory workers)

TBE vaccine approved in Europe. Hantavirus vaccine approved in the Republic of Korea, reported to be 75% effective after 3 doses.

Chemoprophylaxis

Lassa fever & Crimean-Congo Hemorrhagic Fever (CCHF): Ribavirin optimal dose & duration unknown, not FDA approved for this use.

Chemotherapy

Ribavirin for confirmed or probable/suspected arenavirus (Lassa fever), nairovirus (CCHF), hantavirus (Hemorrhagic Fever with Renal Syndrome [HFRS]), or VHF of unknown etiology: IND IV Ribavirin Protocols under Force Health Protection Division/USAMMDA for 1) HFRS & 2) CCHF or Lassa fever. IV ribavirin is not licensed by FDA & must be used either under a FHP Division protocol or under FDA's expanded access.

Decision to initiate ribavirin treatment will be based on epidemiological, clinical & clinical lab results as diagnostic lab results may not be available. Always rule out malaria before starting treatment.

Treatment of HFRS with IND ribavirin:

- Loading dose: 33 mg/kg IV (max 2.64 g) once; followed by
  - Day 1-4: 16 mg/kg IV (max 1.28 gram) q 6 h (16 doses)
  - Day 5-7: 8 mg/kg IV (max 0.64 g) q 8 h (9 doses)
- If given orally: Wt > 75 kg: 600 mg PO q 12 h for 10 d; Wt < 75 kg: 400 mg PO in AM, 600 mg PO in PM for 10 d.
- Loading dose (peds): IV same as for adult. Oral 30 mg/kg PO one time.
- Maintenance dose (peds): IV same as for adult. Oral 15 mg/kg every 5 h for 4 d; 7.5 mg/kg 3x daily for 6 d*.

Treatment of CCHF or Lassa fever with IND ribavirin:

Adults:

- Loading dose: 33 mg/kg IV (max dose: 2.64g), followed by
  - Day 1-4: 16 mg/kg IV (max dose: 1.28 g) q 6 h (16 doses)
  - Day 5-10: 8mg/kg IV (max dose: 0.64 g) q 8 h (18 doses)
- Administered in 50-100 mL normal saline over 30-40 min with an infusion pump

Pediatrics:

- Loading dose peds: IV same as for adult. Oral 30 mg/kg PO one time
- Maintenance dose peds: IV same as for adult. Oral 15 mg/kg q 5 h for 4 d; 7.5 mg/kg q 8 h for 6 d*.

*Recommended dosing from WHO. See Appendix J ("Investigational New Drugs"), refs 11 & 12.

Comments

Aggressive supportive care & management of hypotension & coagulopathy very important.

Human antibody used with apparent beneficial effect in uncontrolled human trials of AHF.

For a summary of human experience with oral ribavirin use following exposures to CCHF, refer to Appendix J, refs 11 & 12.

Consensus statement (2002) in *JAMA* (see Table 2 in the VHF chapter of this book) suggests using ribavirin to treat clinically apparent VHF infection of unknown agent using doses from the CCHF/Lassa/HFRS IND stipulations.

Smallpox

Vaccine/Toxoid

Cell culture-derived vaccines (all NYCBOH strain):

- Dynport Vaccine (Pre-exposure)(IND)
- Acambis Vaccine (*ACAM2000*) (Pre-exposure)(A)

Chemoprophylaxis

- Acambis Vaccine (*ACAM2000*) (Post-exposure)(A)

Chemotherapy

IV Cidofovir for treatment of smallpox or other orthopox infection.(IND)

Probenecid 2g PO 3 h before cidofovir infusion. Infuse 1L NS 1 h before cidofovir infusion

If tolerated, infuse 2nd liter normal saline 1-3 h with/after cidofovir

Cidofovir 5 mg/kg IV over 1 h

Repeat probenecid 1g PO 2 h & 8 h after cidofovir infusion complete.

Tecovirimat. Tecovirimat (*Arestvyr®*, ST-246) is an investigational oral antiviral drug that provides an alternative to the off label use of IV cidofovir to treat orthopox infections, including smallpox & generalized vaccinia. Tecovirimat, currently under development by SIGA Technologies, Inc., with funding provided from DHHS, Biomedical Advanced Research & Development Authority (BARDA). Tecovirimat is not yet approved by FDA & is available only under an IND protocol.(IND):

Self-administered tecovirimat 600 mg/d PO with full glass of water & food for 14 d. May be extended if necessary.(IND)

For Select Vaccine Adverse reactions (Eczema vaccinatum, vaccinia necrosum, ocular vaccinia w/o keratitis, severe generalized vaccinia):1st choice: VIGIV (Vaccinia Immune Globulin, Intravenous). (Cangene Corporation) 6000U/kg IV infusion. 9000 U/kg for the patient that does not respond to the 6000 U/kg dose. See CDC guidelines at www.bt.cdc.gov/agent/smallpox/vaccination/mgmt-adv-reactions.asp

VIG is NOT recommended for mild instances of accidental implantation, implantation-associated ocular keratitis, mild or limited generalized vaccinia, erythema multiforme, or encephalitis postvaccination)

Cidofovir 5 mg/kg IV infusion (as above)(IND)

Tecovirimat (Arestvyr®, ST-246) 600 mg/d PO with full glass of water & food for 14 d. May be extended if necessary.(IND)

Comments

Pre- & post-exposure vaccination recommended if > 3 yrs since last vaccine.

Recommendations for use of smallpox vaccine in response to bio-terrorism are periodically updated by the CDC & the most recent recommendations can be found at http://www.cdc.gov.

Botulinum neurotoxin

Vaccine/Toxoid

Pentavalent (ABCDE) Botulinum Toxoid [(IND)] Vaccine (PBT) (Pre-exposure use only). IND for pre-exposure prophylaxis for high risk individuals in emergency situations only. [(IND)] Protocol for routine vaccination of laboratory workers closed by CDC in 2011.

Recombinant Botulinum Toxin Vaccine A/B (rBV A/B). IND for pre-exposure prophylaxis for high-risk individuals only. [(IND)]

Chemoprophylaxis

DoD equine antitoxins[(IND)]

In general, botulinum antitoxin is not used prophylactically. Under special circumstances, if the evidence of exposure is clear in a group of individuals, some of whom have well defined neurological findings consistent with botulism, treatment can be contemplated in those without neurological signs.

Chemotherapy

Heptavalent (A-G) equine botulinum antitoxin (H-BAT) (Cangene Corporation) available through the CDC. FDA-approved for use in the Strategic National Stockpile[(A)]

BabyBIG™, California Health Department, types A & B Human lyophilized IgG, for treatment of infant botulism[(A)]

Comments

Decline in immunogenicity of the Pentavalent Botulinum Toxoid Vaccine – current lot PBP-003 passed potency testing only to Serotypes A & B.

Could need to perform skin test for hypersensitivity before equine antitoxin administration. Antitoxin levels observed 2-4 wks after dose 3 of the primary series (wk 13).

Ricin Toxin

Vaccine/Toxoid

Genetically modified toxin subunit vaccine (RiVax) undergoing Phase 1 clinical trials at USAMRIID. No licensed FDA vaccine available.

Chemoprophylaxis

None

Chemotherapy

None

Comments

Inhalation: supportive therapy; Ingestion: gastric lavage, cathartics.

Staphylococcus Enterotoxins
Vaccine/Toxoid
Inhibitex, Inc, & Pfizer have partnered to develop a three-antigen *S. aureus* vaccine (SA3Ag), & have completed Phase 1 trials. No licensed FDA vaccine available.
Chemoprophylaxis
None
Chemotherapy
None
Comments
Inhalation: supportive therapy Ingestion: gastric lavage, cathartics.

APPENDIX J: INVESTIGATIONAL MEDICAL PRODUCTS (INDs, ETC) & EMERGENCY USE AUTHORIZATIONS (EUAs)

Overview

It is DoD policy that personnel will be provided, when operationally relevant, the best available medical countermeasures to chemical, biological, radiological, and nuclear (CBRN) agents and effects, and other health threats, per DoD Instruction (DoDI) 6200.02

The DoD Components are expected to administer or use medical products (i.e. drugs, biologics, or devices) approved, licensed, or cleared by the US Food and Drug Administration (FDA) for general commercial marketing, when available, to provide the needed medical countermeasure.

Drugs are chemical substances intended for use in the medical diagnosis, cure, treatment, or prevention of disease. ***Biologics*** are blood and blood products, vaccines, allergenics, cell and tissue-based products, and gene therapy products. A ***medical device*** is an instrument, apparatus, implement, machine, contrivance, implant, in vitro reagent, or other similar or related article, including a component part, or accessory which is:

- Recognized in the official National Formulary, or the United States Pharmacopoeia, or any supplement to them,
- Intended for use in the diagnosis of disease or other conditions, or in the cure, mitigation, treatment, or prevention of disease, in man or other animals, or
- Intended to affect the structure or any function of the body of man or other animals, and which does not achieve its primary intended purposes through chemical action within or on the body of man or other animals and which is not dependent upon being metabolized for the achievement of any of its primary intended purposes.

Unapproved medical products -- or approved medical products used “off-label” -- may be administered or used as a necessary medical countermeasure under an Emergency Use Authorizations (EUA), an Investigtional New Drug (IND) application, or investigational device exemption (IDE) issued by the FDA when such use is associated with a force health protection program and only if compliant with the regulatory requirements set forth below and with the approval of the Assistant Secretary of Defense for Health Affairs (ASD(HA)).

A medical product may be administered for a use not described in the labeling based on standard medical practice in the United States. "Standard medical practice" refers to the authority of an individual health care practitioner to prescribe or administer any legally marketed medical product to a patient for any condition or disease within a legitimate health care practitioner-patient relationship. These instances fall outside of a DoD force health protection program.

FDA regulatory requirements for INDs and EUAs apply to medical care provided to military and civilian DoD healthcare beneficiaries, DoD-affiliated personnel, and others receiving treatment at DoD medical treatment facilities located both CONUS and OCONUS.

Investigational New Drugs (IND)

INDs are drugs or biological products subject to FDA regulations at 21 CFR 312 and include:

- Drugs not approved, or biological products not licensed, by the FDA which
  - Do not yet have permission from the FDA to be legally marketed and sold in the United States ("unapproved product"), or
  - Are entirely new drugs, vaccines, or therapeutics not licensed by the FDA for any human use.
- Drugs unapproved for the applied use ("off-label"). These are FDA-approved drugs or licensed biological products administered for a use not described in the FDA-approved labeling of the drug or biological product ("unapproved use of an approved product").
- INDs can be made available under a number of mechanisms.
  - As part of a clinical research study (see 21 CFR 312 for details)
  - As part of an Expanded Access program (see 21 CFR 312 subpart I and http://www.fda.gov/downloads/Drugs/GuidanceComplianceRegulatoryInformation/Guidances/UCM351261.pdf and http://www.fda.gov/ForConsumers/ByAudience/ForPatientAdvocates/AccesstoInvestigationalDrugs/ucm176098.htm)
  - Under an Emergency Use Authorization (for details see below and refer to the following: http://www.fda.gov/regulatoryinformation/guidances/ucm125127.htm http://www.fda.gov/EmergencyPreparedness/Counterterrorism/ucm182568.htm)

Investigational Device Exemptions (IDE)

An investigational device, including *in vitro* diagnostic tests, is a device which has not been approved or cleared for marketing by the FDA. Investigational devices are regulated under 21 CFR 812. There may be circumstances under which a health care provider may wish to use an unapproved device to save the life of a patient or to help a patient suffering from a serious disease or condition for which no alternative therapy exists. Patients/physicians faced with these circumstances may have access to investigational devices under one of five main mechanisms (emergency use, emergency research compassionate use, treatment use, continued access).

These mechanisms can be utilized during a certain time-frame in the IDE process if the criteria are met. FDA approval is required except in the case of emergency use. Details of the criteria and each mechanism are defined under 21 CFR 812.36, and are described at http://www.fda.gov/medicaldevices/deviceregulationandguidance/howtomarketyourdevice/investigationaldeviceexemptionide/ucm051345.htm

Emergency Use Authorization (EUA)

An EUA is a special authority under US federal law. The FDA issues an EUA to allow use of an "unapproved medical product" or an "unapproved use of an approved medical product" during a declared emergency by the Secretary of Health and Human Services (DHHS) involving a heightened risk of attack on the public or military forces. An EUA is generally intended for situations affecting, or potentially affecting, a large number of individuals (> 10,000).

Recent examples of using medical products under an EUA come from the medical response to the 2009 H1N1 pandemic influenza. The declaration of emergency issued by the DHHS Secretary justified the authorization of the emergency use of certain approved neuraminidase inhibitors for unapproved uses (i.e. oseltamivir and zanamivir) and use of an unapproved antiviral drug, peramivir.

Another example was the authorization of the emergency use of *in vitro* diagnostics for detection of 2009 H1N1 influenza virus. This EUA impacted DoD due to using these diagnostics on our deployed Joint Biological Agent Identification Diagnostic System (JBAIDS) platforms in theater. More recently, EUAs were granted for diagnostic testing for influenza H7N9 (2013) and the Middle Eastern Respiratory Syndrome Coronavirus (MERSCoV) (2013).

Recent changes included in the Pandemic and All Hazards Preparedness Reauthorization Act (PAHPRA) of 2013 allow, under specific conditions and regulatory requirements, medical countermeasures that are not FDA-approved or cleared to be pre-positioned for use in a declared emergency. This prepositioning can be supported by the a pre-EUA submission to the FDA. This submission describes the design and manufacture of the product and provides all available safety and efficacy data for FDA review, and is periodically updated to reflect new data. Acceptance of such a submission by FDA expedites response time in case of a declared emergency.

Refer to the FDA's online materials for further guidance on "Emergency Use Authorization of Medical Products": http://www.fda.gov/regulatoryinformation/guidances/ucm125127.htm and http://www.fda.gov/EmergencyPreparedness/Counterterrorism/ucm182568.htm.

Regulatory requirements for using INDs, IDEs, and products under an EUA
Investigational medical products are subject to FDA regulations 21 CFR 312, as amended (for drugs and biologics) and 21 CFR 809 and 812 (for devices), and for all military users, DoDI 6200.02 series.

Use of products under an EUA for a force health protection program are subject to DoDI 6200.02, section 564 of the Federal Food, Drug, and Cosmetic Act [21 U.S.C.], sections 1107 and 1107a of title 10, U.S.C. and applicable FDA requirements.

DoDI 6200.02 establishes DoD policy, assigns responsibilities, and prescribes procedures concerning the application of FDA rules to DoD force health protection programs involving FDA unapproved medical products required to be used under an EUA, IND, or IDE application.

Responsibilities for the DoD Force Health Protection IND/EUA Programs
Assistant Secretary of Defense for Health Affairs (ASD(HA))
The ASD(HA), under the authority, direction, and control of the Under Secretary of Defense for Personnel and Readiness, will:

- Develop DoD FHP policy and oversee its implementation.
- Issue DoD Instructions or guidance to implement this instruction in accordance with the authority in DoDD 5136.01.
- Grant exceptions to this instruction as appropriate.
- Evaluate and, when appropriate, approve the proposed use of unapproved medical products under EUA and IND or IDE protocols as part of FHP programs, prior to submission to the FDA.
- Through the Secretary of Defense, may request that the Secretary, DHHS, declare an emergency justifying the authorization to use a medical product under an EUA as part of a force health protection program based on the determination that a military emergency, or a significant potential for a military emergency, exists involving a heightened risk to US military forces of attack with a specified biological, chemical, radiological, or nuclear agent or agents.

Heads of the DoD Components
The Heads of the DoD Components:

- Will submit all DoD EUA and IND or IDE protocols for the use of unapproved medical products as part of FHP programs, to the ASD(HA) for evaluation and approval prior to submission to the FDA.

- Will ensure all DoD EUA and IND or IDE protocols for the use of unapproved medical products as part of FHP programs:
  - Consider the available evidence of the safety and efficacy of the unapproved medical product and the nature and degree of the risk to military servicemembers and other appropriate DoD personnel.
  - Document a high risk for which the use of an unapproved medical product under an EUA or IND or IDE status is needed for the purposes of force health protection programs, take into consideration the risks and benefits of use of the unapproved medical product involved, and be in compliance with the requirements of this instruction.
  - Are coordinated with the CJCS (and if from the commander of a Combatant Command, are submitted through the CJCS), the Secretary of the Army as Lead Component, and the General Counsel of the Department of Defense.
- Will develop medical protocols, in coordination with the Secretary of the Army, and in compliance with this instruction, for use of an unapproved medical product under an EUA or IND or IDE status as part of FHP programs, and execute such protocols in strict compliance with their respective requirements.
- Will comply with Enclosure 3 of DoDI 6200.02 entitled "Procedures Applicable to EUAs for FHP Programs"; sections 564, 564A, and 564B of 21 USC Chapter 9 (Federal Food Drug, and Cosmetic Act), as amended; 10 USC 1107 and 1107a; and applicable FDA requirements when using an unapproved medical product under an EUA as part of FHP programs. As described in section 564B of the FD&C Act, it is permissible for unapproved medical products, which are intended for emergency use, to be held, positioned, and/or stockpiled, prior to an emergency; however, actual use of such unapproved medical products is still subject to all applicable legal, regulatory, and policy requirements, including the issuance of an EUA by the Commissioner of Food and Drugs authorizing the use of the medical product. For the purpose of actual use or administration of an unapproved medical product under an EUA, the use remains subject to the scope, terms, and conditions of that particular EUA.
- Will comply with Enclosure 4 of DoDI 6200.02 entitled "Procedures Applicable to IND or IDE Applications for FHP Programs" and applicable federal regulations when using unapproved medical products under IND or IDE status as part of FHP programs.
- Will comply with applicable procedures for prioritizing delivery of medical care during public health emergencies involving mass casualties in accordance with DoDI 6200.03 in order to achieve the greatest public health benefit while maintaining operational effectiveness, meeting mission requirements, and also complying with applicable laws.

- May, as part of a force health protection program, unless otherwise restricted by the ASD(HA), and subject to the scope, terms, and conditions of a particular EUA in 10 USC Chapter 9, or a specific medical protocol or device exemption, make available, to specified DoD civilian and contractor personnel unapproved medical products under an EUA or IND or IDE status should they also be at a high risk along with military servicemembers, except that the authority to waive an option to refuse under section 1107a of 10 USC or informed consent under 10 USC 1107 is inapplicable to these personnel. Specified DoD civilian and contractor personnel include:
  - Members of the DoD civilian work force, to include at least those designated as emergency-essential or non-combat essential DoD civilian employees, in accordance with DoDD 1400.31 and DoDD 1404.10.
  - Contractors performing essential services in support of mission essential functions in accordance with the Deputy Secretary of Defense Memorandum, "Continuation of Essential Contractor Services" and pursuant to 48 CFR 252.237-7023.
  - Contractors authorized to accompany the force, as appropriate, in accordance with DoDI 3020.41.
- May, unless otherwise restricted by the ASD(HA), and subject to the scope, terms, and conditions of the applicable emergency declaration, as described in 10 USC Chapter 9, and any applicable state and local laws, provide or assist in the provision of unapproved medical products to be used under an EUA as described in the applicable sections in DoDI 6200.02 Enclosure 3 entitled "Procedures Applicable to EUAs for FHP Programs", or under an IND or IDE protocol as described in the applicable sections in Enclosure 4, when offered in a voluntary manner, to organizations and categories of people who may not be explicitly part of force health protection programs, to include:
  - Individuals working in, residing on, or visiting DoD installations and commands, who are subject to the same health risks as military servicemembers, in accordance with DoDI 6200.03, and who are included within the categories of individuals specified in the scope, terms, and conditions of the applicable EUA, as described in 10 USC Chapter 9, or a specific medical protocol or device exemption. Providing these unapproved medical products to these individuals, especially in circumstances involving communicable diseases, may contribute to force health protection by mitigating the spread of the disease and the risk to operations.
  - Organizations and categories of people specified in the scope, terms, and conditions of the applicable emergency declaration, as described in 10 USC Chapter 9 or a specific medical protocol or device exemption,

who are authorized to receive unapproved medical products as part of a larger interagency public health response, such as the one described in Executive Order 13527, in which medical-related Defense Support of Civil Authorities (DSCA) is both requested and authorized in accordance with DoDD 3025.18 and DoDI 3020.52, and pursuant to applicable state and local laws. Potential limitations on DoD emergency public health powers outside the United States are described in DoDI 6200.03.

Secretary of the Army

The Secretary of the Army, in addition to the responsibilities as Head of a DoD Component, shall:

- Serve as Lead Component for synchronizing, integrating, and coordinating regulatory submissions to the FDA and developing medical protocols under this instruction for all the DoD Components.
- Develop specific medical protocols for the use of an unapproved medical product under an EUA or IND or IDE status as part of FHP programs, in coordination with the appropriate DoD Component(s) and the ASD(HA). Protocols will include appropriate record keeping, monitoring, and reporting of adverse events, and required FDA regulatory submissions for use of the unapproved medical product.
- Ensure that the Headquarters, United States Army Medical Research and Materiel Command Institutional Review Board (HQ USAMRMC IRB), under the US Army Office of The Surgeon General, carries out the procedures described in DoDI 6200.02 Enclosure entitled "Procedures Applicable to IND or IDE Applications for FHP Programs".
- Consult with the Centers for Disease Control and Prevention (CDC) on the potential for collaborative action in pursuing an EUA or IND or IDE application for an unapproved medical product intended to be used as part of force health protection programs, when the unapproved medical product has similar potential for use by the CDC to protect public health from CBRN agents and effects, or other health threats.
- Prepare and plan, in coordination with the Secretaries of the Military Departments and the CJCS, for using unapproved medical products under EUAs or IND or IDE protocols as part of FHP programs, establishing responsibilities and action timelines to make the best possible unapproved medical products available for use as part of force health protection programs.

The sponsor for all DoD IND protocols and use of medical products under an EUA is the US Army Surgeon General, whose representative is the Principal

Assistant for Acquisition, USAMRMC, acting through the US Army Medical Materiel Development Activity (USAMMDA).

The Headquarters, US Army Medical Research and Materiel Command Institutional Review Board (HQ USMRMC IRB) reviews and approves IND protocols for force health protection programs.

Force Health Protection Division, USAMMDA (FHP/USAMMDA)

- Manages DoD's Force Health Protection (FHP) program for use of investigational products under DoDI 6200.02.
- Plans, implements, and sustains DoD-directed FHP IND protocols and EUA applications.
- Synchronizes, integrates, and coordinates regulatory submissions to the FDA through USAMMDA Division of Regulated Activities and Compliance for IND/EUA applications for force health protection for all the DoD Components.
- Provides IND medical support for military personnel exposed to CBRN events and diseases endemic to the area of operation.
- Manages the Specialized MEDCOM Response Capabilities-Investigational New Drug (SMRC-IND) teams who deploy to mass casualty incidents to facilitate the administration of IND/EUAs to military and other authorized personnel.
- Assists a principal investigator (PI) and support staff in fulfillment of regulatory requirements.
- With USAMMDA Clinical Services Support Division (CSSD), monitors regulatory files and provides guidance on maintenance of regulatory files.
- Facilitates IND response and protocol management including establishing a clinical treatment site if necessary. Contact FHP for support at 301-619-1104 during duty hours or 24/7 at 301-401-2768. E-mail to usarmy.detrick.medcom-usammda.list.fhp@mail.mil.

Current IND Medical Countermeasures

Current medical countermeasures administered as INDs by FHP/USAMMDA include vaccines, drugs, and immunoglobulins to prevent and/or treat diseases caused by Category A biothreat agents, such as anthrax, botulism and smallpox, as well as for infectious diseases of military interest. Examples of drugs or biologics that could be used as INDs in the medical management of biological casualties include:

- Anthrax Vaccine Adsorbed (AVA, *BioThrax*). AVA is licensed for pre-exposure prevention of anthrax in adults. It is considered an IND when used for post-exposure prophylaxis of anthrax together with antibiotics in adults or children.

- IV cidofovir is licensed for treating cytomegalovirus retinitis in HIV patients, but not for treating generalized vaccinia. An individual physician could prescribe cidofovir "off-label" for a single case of generalized vaccinia. Because this is not an FDA-licensed indication for the drug, however, it cannot legally be official policy (e.g. of the hospital, the DoD, etc.) to treat all cases of generalized vaccinia with cidofovir. See below for details on how to obtain cidofovir in an emergency.
- Tecovirimat (*Arestvyr®*, ST-246) is an investigational oral antiviral drug that provides an alternative to IV cidofovir for the treatment of orthopox infections, including smallpox and generalized vaccinia. Tecovirimat is not yet approved by FDA and is available only under an IND protocol.
- Pentavalent Botulinum Toxoid vaccine (PBT) is an investigational vaccine that is available for emergency use only under an IND protocol.
- IV ribavirin is an investigational antiviral drug. It is not an approved drug in the US (although oral ribavirin is approved for some indications). FHP can provide it under IND protocols to treat some forms of viral hemorrhagic fever (CCHF, Lassa fever) or hemorrhagic fever with renal syndrome (hantavirus). Early treatment is critical, and the protocol can be activated so that treatment can begin prior to obtaining a positive diagnostic laboratory test result.
- Paromomycin/Gentamycin Topical Cream, in advanced development at USAMMDA, is an investigational product available under an IND protocol to treat uncomplicated cutaneous leishmaniasis.
- IV artesunate, in advanced development at USAMMDA, is an investigational anti-malarial drug available under an IND protocol to treat severe falciparum malaria.

Receipt & Administration of INDs for Military Healthcare Providers

If an IND drug or biological product protocol exists already, call USAMRIID to discuss the case with the on-call medical officer who is familiar with the protocols for administration of IND products (1-888-USA-RIID during duty hours; DSN: 343-2257 or 301-619-2257 during non-duty hours to reach the 24-hour security desk), or contact USAMMDA FHP directly at 301-619-1104 during duty hours or 24/7 at 301-401-2768. E-mail to usarmy.detrick.medcom-usammda.list.fhp@mail.mil. If the use of the IND is indicated, USAMRIID and USAMMDA will coordinate with the treatment site to ship the medical product.

There are several available options, depending on the specific product, to determine who will administer the IND product and where:

- Designate an investigator for the IND at the requesting site. The proposed investigator must meet eligibility criteria (GCP (CITI) training, signed FDA form 1572, CV, license and copy of protocol, etc…) and be approved by the sponsor. This can be arranged through USAMMDA FHP Division.

- DoD has pre-trained providers who are already established at several of the major MEDCENs who could assist with treatment or potentially travel to the patient to administer the IND product. Alternatively, the patient could be evacuated to the nearest medical center with a pre-trained, designated investigator who will administer the product. Contact USAMMDA FHP Division to determine if this is an option.
- USAMMDA FHP Division manages the Specialized MEDCOM Response Capabilities-IND (SMRC-IND) teams to administer IND products and/or implement EUAs for force health protection. For large numbers of casualties, or the need for a time-critical IND administration, USAMMDA FHP could consider sending the SMRC-IND team to oversee the protocol and administer the IND product.

If no satisfactory FDA-approved medical product is available for a medical countermeasure against a particular threat at the time of need under a force health protection program, contact USAMMDA FHP. USAMMDA FHP will coordinate with the appropriate individuals and agencies to use an unapproved product under an IND application, or to initiate the request for an EUA to treat large populations. (DoDI 6200.02 series applies).

Process for obtaining VIG-IV & cidofovir & tecovirimat

VIG-IV is a FDA-licensed medical product and is no longer administered under an IND protocol for treatment of specific smallpox vaccine adverse reactions. VIG-IV is recommended as the first line of therapy for adverse reactions caused by smallpox vaccination.

IV cidofovir is licensed to treat cytomegalovirus (CMV) retinitis (a serious eye infection) in HIV-infected people. It is not licensed to treat adverse reactions caused by smallpox vaccine (e.g. generalized vaccinia, eczema vaccinatum, progressive vaccinia), so it can only be used "off-label" (prescribed by a physician to treat a condition for which it has not been specifically approved) or through an IND protocol.

IV cidofovir is available within CONUS through the CDC under an IND protocol for treatment of smallpox and specific smallpox vaccine adverse reactions. Under the IND, cidofovir may be considered as a secondary treatment only in consultation with HHS/CDC and when VIG-IV is not efficacious. Cidofovir is released from the CDC and will be shipped by the CDC's Strategic National Stockpile (SNS). The cost of cidofovir and the cost of shipping will be covered by the US Government. Arrival of shipments should be expected within 12 h of the approval for release. The cidofovir IND protocol mandates that the treating physician must become a co-investigator primarily responsible for completing follow-up forms describing the clinical status of the patient being treated with cidofovir, including the prompt report of any significant adverse reaction in the recipient. Detailed information on the requirements of the IND will be shipped with the products.

A similar protocol is managed by USAMMDA FHP Division for OCONUS DoD health care settings. Contact FHP Division if IV cidofovir is needed to treat a smallpox vaccine adverse reaction. FHP maintains inventory of cidofovir independent of the SNS and will help to establish a site and will work with the treating physician to meet all FDA requirements to establish the physician as an investigator under the protocol, including credentials and training. OCONUS physicians requesting IV cidofovir under the IND protocol should contact USAMMDA FHP Division at 301-401-2768 (available 24/7).

CDC and USAMMDA FHP also manage similar IND protocols and inventory of tecovirimat (*Arestvyr®*, ST-246) for the same indications as IV cidofovir (orthopox infection, smallpox vaccine adverse reaction). Tecovirimat is an orally-administered antiviral drug with a reduced profile of adverse effects compared to IV cidofovir. A site can be established and tecovirmat obtained as described above for cidofovir.

Military Health Care Providers: VIG-IV stocks have been prepositioned for DOD in CONUS and OCONUS. Contact your DoD Regional Vaccine Healthcare Centers (VHC) office during normal business hours or the DoD VHC Network's Vaccine Clinical Call Center 24/7 at 1-866-210-6469 for the most current process for obtaining VIG-IV.

Military clinicians requesting use of cidofovir must consult with an infectious disease or allergy-immunology specialist. Consultations will be arranged via the DoD Vaccine Healthcare Centers (VHC) Network's Vaccine Clinical Call Center (866-210-6469, available 24/7) who will notify the Military Vaccine Agency (MILVAX) of case specifics.

The infectious disease or allergy-immunology specialist physician, in consultation with the VHC, will contact the CDC Director's Emergency Operations Center (DEOC) at 770-488-7100 and consult with on-call staff in the Division of Bioterrorism and Response (BDPR). The CDC is the release authority for cidofovir under an IND protocol in a CONUS setting and will coordinate release of this medical product from the SNS.

Civilian Health Care Providers: Civilian health care providers should first contact their State Health Department when seeking consultation for civilian patients experiencing a severe or unexpected adverse event following smallpox vaccination or when requesting cidofovir. If further consultation is required, or cidofovir is recommended, the physician and State Health Department can request consultation through the CDC Director's Emergency Operations Center as above.

Process for obtaining botulinum antitoxin

In 2013, FDA approved a new heptavalent botulinum antitoxin (HBAT, Cangene Corporation) for the treatment of botulism and for inclusion in the SNS. HBAT is the only botulinum antitoxin currently available in the US for naturally occurring non-infant botulism and is available only from the CDC.

All medical care providers who suspect a diagnosis of botulism in a patient should immediately call their state health department's emergency 24-hour telephone number. The state health department will contact the CDC DEOC (770-488-7100) to report suspected botulism cases, arrange for a clinical consultation by telephone and, if indicated, request release of HBAT. The CDC DEOC will then contact the on-call Foodborne and Diarrheal Diseases Branch medical officer.

BabyBIG® (botulism immune globulin) remains available for infant botulism through the California Infant Botulism Treatment and Prevention Program. BabyBIG® is an orphan drug that consists of human-derived botulism antitoxin antibodies and is approved by FDA for the treatment of infant botulism types A and B. To obtain BabyBIG® for suspected infant botulism, the patient's physician must contact the Infant Botulism Treatment and Prevention Program (IBTPP) on-call physician at (510) 231-7600 to review the indications for such treatment.

APPENDIX K: USE OF DRUGS/VACCINES IN SPECIAL OR VULNERABLE POPULATIONS IN THE BIO-AGENT CONTEXT

Pediatric patients

Large-scale attacks on civilian targets, as well as collateral damage inflicted during armed conflict will undoubtedly involve pediatric victims, who may be more susceptible than adults to the effects of certain biological and chemical agents for a number of anatomic, physiologic, immunologic, developmental, and programmatic reasons:

1. A thinner and less-keratinized epidermis makes dermally-active chemical (but not generally biological) agents a greater risk to children than adults.
2. A larger surface area per unit volume exacerbates problems.
3. A small relative blood volume makes children more susceptible to the volume losses associated with enteric infections such as cholera and to GI intoxications such as might be seen with exposure to the staphylococcal enterotoxins.
4. Children's high minute ventilation compared with that of adults increases the threat of agents delivered via the inhalational route.
5. The fact that children live "closer to the ground" compounds this effect when heavier-than-air substances are involved.
6. An immature blood-brain barrier may heighten the risk of CNS toxicity from nerve agents.
7. Developmental considerations make it less likely that a child would readily flee an area of danger, thereby increasing exposure to these various adverse effects.
8. Children have a unique susceptibility to certain potential bio-agents. While adults generally suffer only a brief, self-limited incapacitating illness following infection with Venezuelan equine encephalitis (VEE) virus, young children are more likely to experience seizures, permanent neurologic sequelae, and death. In the case of smallpox, waning herd immunity may disproportionately affect children. Vaccine-induced immunity to smallpox probably diminishes significantly after 3 to 10 yrs. Although most adults are considered susceptible to smallpox, given that routine civilian immunization

in the US ceased in the early 1970s, older adults may have some residual protection from death, if not from the development of disease. Today's children are among the first to grow up in a world without any individual or herd immunity to smallpox.

9. Children may experience unique disease manifestations not seen in adults; suppurative parotitis is a common characteristic occur among children with melioidosis, but is not generally seen in adults with *Burkholderia pseudomallei* infection.

10. Many of the drugs useful in treating such casualties are unfamiliar to pediatricians or have relative contraindications in childhood. The fluoroquinolones and tetracyclines are commonly cited as prophylactic and therapeutic agents of choice against anthrax, plague, tularemia, brucellosis, and Q fever. While both classes are often avoided in children, potential morbidity and mortality from these diseases far outweighs the minor risks associated with short-term use of these agents. Of note, ciprofloxacin received, as its first licensed pediatric indication, FDA approval for use in the prophylaxis of anthrax following inhalational exposure during a terrorist attack. Doxycycline and levofloxacin are now licensed specifically in children for the same indication and levofloxacin is also licensed for post-exposure prophylaxis of children against plague. Pediatric antibiotic dosing guidelines are provided in the accompanying Table.

11. Immunizations potentially useful in preventing bio-agent-induced diseases often lack approval for use in pediatric patients. The currently available anthrax vaccine is licensed only for those between 18 and 65 yrs of age. The plague vaccine, currently out of production and probably ineffective against inhalational exposures, was approved only for individuals aged 18 to 61 yrs. The smallpox vaccine, a live vaccine employing vaccinia virus, can cause fetal vaccinia and demise when given to pregnant women (see below).

12. Some useful pharmaceutical agents are not available in pediatric dosing regimens. The military distributes the Nerve Agent Antidote Kit (NAAK), consisting of prefilled autoinjectors designed for the rapid administration of atropine and pralidoxime. Many emergency departments and some ambulances stock these kits. The doses of agents contained in the NAAK are calculated for soldiers and thus are far in excess of those appropriate for young children (although separate atropine autoinjectors specifically formulated for children have been approved by the FDA).

13. Although physical protective measures and devices (e.g., "gas masks") are likely to be of little utility in a civilian bio-terrorism setting, such commercially available devices are often unavailable in pediatric sizes.

Additionally, Israeli experience during the first Gulf War suggests that frightened parents may improperly use such masks on their children, resulting in inadvertent suffocation.

14. In the event of a large-scale bioterrorist attack, there may be an insufficient number of pediatric hospital beds. In any large disaster, excess bed capacity might potentially be provided at civilian and Veterans Affairs hospitals under the auspices of the National Disaster Medical System, but that system makes no specific provision for pediatric beds.

Nursing mothers

Many pharmaceuticals are excreted in breast milk (see Table), and may thus be ingested by nursing infants. Such medications, if contraindicated in infants, should thus be avoided by breastfeeding mothers whenever possible. Specifically, it is generally recommended that fluoroquinolones, tetracyclines, and chloramphenicol be avoided by nursing mothers. As these drugs may represent the treatment of choice for many bio-agents, practitioners must weigh the risks of administering these drugs against the potential adverse consequences of using a less effective medication. In some cases, temporary cessation of nursing while taking the offending drug may be necessary. Antibiotics generally considered safe in nursing mothers include the aminoglycosides, penicillins, cephalosporins, and macrolides.

Pregnant patients

Many medications that are safe in adults may pose risks to the developing fetus. The FDA has established the following categories to qualify that risk: **A**- studies in pregnant women show no risk; **B**- animal studies show no risk, but human studies are not adequate or, alternatively, animal toxicity has been shown but human studies indicate no risk; **C**- animal studies show toxicity, human studies are inadequate but benefit of use may exceed risk; **D**- evidence of human risk exists but benefits may outweigh such risk; **X**- fetal abnormalities have been attributed to the drug and risk outweighs benefit. Pregnancy risk categories for representative therapeutics are included in the Table.

Tetracyclines and fluoroquinolones often constitute empiric therapies of choice for many bio-agent diseases yet remain relatively contraindicated during pregnancy. Animal studies indicate that tetracyclines can retard skeletal development in the fetus; embryotoxicity has also been described in animals treated early in pregnancy. There are few adequate studies of fluoroquinolones in pregnant women; existing published data, albeit sparse, do not demonstrate a substantial teratogenic risk associated with fluoroquinolone use during pregnancy. In cases for which either fluoroquinolones or tetracyclines are recommended for initial empiric prophylaxis (e.g., inhalational anthrax, plague, or tularemia), tolerated fluoroquinolone may thus represent the lower risk option. After antibiotic susceptibility data are available, antibiotics should be switched to lower risk alternatives if possible.

Live vaccines (e.g., measles-mumps-rubella) are also generally contraindicated during pregnancy, although vaccine risks must be weighed against the risk of disease (to both the vaccinated mother and her fetus). For example, the administration of smallpox vaccine (vaccinia) to pregnant women presents a very tangible risk to the fetus (in the form of fetal vaccinia infection), although that risk is likely to be less than the risk of maternal smallpox.

The immunocompromised patient

Immunocompromised individuals may be more susceptible to diseases caused by bio-agents or may develop more severe disease than immunocompetent patients. Nonetheless, consensus groups generally recommend using the same antimicrobial regimens recommended for their immunocompetent counterparts. One important difference in the management of immunocompromised patients concerns the receipt of live vaccines, such as the currently licensed smallpox vaccine, or the LVS tularemia vaccine. Generally, it is best to manage these individuals on a case-by-case basis and in concert with immunologists and/or infectious disease specialists.

Table. Antimicrobials in Special Populations

Class of Drug	Drug name	Pregnancy category	Breast milk	Pediatric oral dose	Pediatric parenteral dose
Aminoglycosides	Gentamicin	C	(+) small		3–7.5 mg/kg/d in 3 doses (IV or IM)
	Amikacin	D	(+) small		15–22.5 mg/kg/d in 3 doses (max 1.5 g/d) (IV or IM)
	Streptomycin	D	(+) small		30 mg/kg/d in 2 doses (max 2 g/d)(IM only)
	Tobramycin	D	(+) small		3–7.5 mg/kg/d in 3 doses (IV or IM)
Carbapenems	Imipenem	C	(?)		60 mg/kg/d in 4 doses (max 4 g/d) (IV or IM)
	Meropenem	B	(?)		60-120 mg/kg/d in 3 doses (max 6 g/d) (IV)

Table. Antimicrobials in Special Populations

Class of Drug	Drug name	Pregnancy category	Breast milk	Pediatric oral dose	Pediatric parenteral dose
Cephalosporins	Ceftriaxone	B	(+) trace		80–100 mg/kg in 1 or 2 doses (max 4 g/d) (IV or IM)
	Ceftazidime	B	(+) trace		125-150 mg/kg/d in 3 doses (max 6 g/d) (IV or IM)
	Cephalexin	B	(+) trace	25-50 mg/kg/d in 3-4 doses	
	Cefuroxime	B	(+) trace	20-30 mg/kg/d in 2 doses (max 2 g/d)	100-150 mg/kg/d in 3 doses (max 6 g/d) (IV or IM)
	Cefepime	B	(+) trace		150 mg in 3 doses (max 4 g/d) (IV or IM)
Chloramphenicol	Chloramphenicol	C	(+)	50-100 mg/kg/d in 4 doses (formulation not avail in US)	50-100 mg/kg/d in 4 doses (max 4 g/d) (IV)
Fluoroquinolones	Ciprofloxacin	C	(+)	30 mg/kg/d in 2 doses (max 1.5 g)	20-30 mg/kg/d in 2 doses (max 1 g/d)(IV)
	Levofloxacin	C	(+)	16 mg/kg/d in 2 doses	16 mg/kg/d in 2 doses (IV)
Glycopeptides	Vancomycin	C	(+)		40-60 mg/kg/d in 4 doses (max 4 g/d) (IV)
Lincosamides	Clindamycin	B	(+)	10-20 mg/kg/d in 3-4 doses (max 1.8 gm/d)	25-40 mg/kg/d in 3-4 doses (max 2.7 g/d) (IV or IM)
Lipopeptides	Daptomycin	B	(?)		4 mg/kg once daily (IV)

Table. Antimicrobials in Special Populations					
Class of Drug	Drug name	Pregnancy category	Breast milk	Pediatric oral dose	Pediatric parenteral dose
Macrolides	Azithromycin	B	(+)	5-12 mg/kg/d once daily (max 600 mg/d)	
	Clarithromycin	C	(?)	15 mg/kg/d in 2 doses (max 1 g/d)	
	Erythromycin	B	(+)	30-50 mg/kg/d in 2-4 doses (max 2 g/d)	15-50 mg/kg/d in 4 doses (max 4 g/d) (IV)
Monobactams	Aztreonam	B	(+) trace		90-120 mg/kg/d in 3-4 doses (max 8 g) (IV or IM)
Oxalodinones	Linezolid	C	(+)	20-30 mg/kg/d in 3 doses (max 800/mg/d)	20-30 mg/kg/d in 3 doses (max 1200/mg/d)(IV)
Penicillins	Amoxicillin	B	(+) trace	25-90 mg/kg/d in 3 doses (max 1.5 g/d)	
	Ampicillin	B	(+) trace	50-100 mg/kg/d in 4 doses (max 4 g/d)	200-400 mg/kg/d in 4 doses (max 12 g/d) (IV or IM)
	Penicillin G	B	(+) trace		25,000-400,000 U/kg/d in 4-6 doses (max 24 mil U/d) (IV or IM)
	Nafcillin	B	(+) trace		100-150 mg/kg/d in 4 doses (max 12 g) (IV or IM)
Rifampin		C	(+)	10-20 mg/kg/d in 1-2 doses (max 600 mg/d)	10-20 mg/kg/d in 1-2 doses (max 600 mg/d)

Table. Antimicrobials in Special Populations					
Class of Drug	Drug name	Pregnancy category	Breast milk	Pediatric oral dose	Pediatric parenteral dose
Streptogramins	Dalfopristin-Quinupristin	B	(+)		22.5 mg/kg/d in 3 doses (IV)
Sulfonamides	Trimethoprim/ Sulfamethoxazole	C	(+) trace	8-12 mg/ kg/d TMP in 4 doses (max 320 mg/d TMP)	8-12 mg/kg/d TMP in 4 doses (IV)
Tetracyclines	Doxycycline	D	(+)	2-4 mg/kg/d in 1-2 doses (max 200 mg/d)	2-4 mg/kg/d in 1-2 doses (max 200 mg/d)(IV)
	Tetracycline	D	(+)	20-50 mg/ kg/d in 4 doses (max 2 g)	10-25 mg/kg/d in 2-4 doses (max 2 g) (IV)
Cidofovir		C	(?)		5 mg/kg once with probenecid & hydration
Oseltamivir		C	(+)	1-12 yrs old: ≤15 kg: 30 mg twice daily; 15-23 kg: 45 mg 2X/d; 23-40 kg: 60 mg 2X/d; >40 kg: adult dose	
Ribavirin		X	(?)	30 mg/kg once, then 15 mg/kg/d in 2 doses (VHFs)	Same as for adults, dosed by weight (IV)

NB: (1) The above doses are for children outside of the neonatal period. Neonatal doses may be different. (2) Pediatric antibiotic doses included in this table represent generic doses for severe disease. They may not accurately reflect expert consensus for treatment for anthrax, plague, or tularemia. For those diseases, refer to the specific chapter for recommendations.

APPENDIX L-1: INDICATED CLINICAL SPECIMENS FOR BIO-AGENT LABORATORY DIAGNOSIS

Disease	Face or Nasal Swab[B]	Blood Culture[E]	Smear[F]	Acute & Convalescent Sera	Stool	Urine	Other Other
Anthrax	+	+	Pleural fluid & CSF; mediastinal lymph node; spleen	+	+/-	-	Cutaneous lesion aspirates or 4mm punch biopsy, toxin detection
Brucellosis	+	+	-	+	-	-	Bone marrow and blood are the most effective for culture
Glanders & Melioidosis	+	+	Sputum and abscess aspirates	+	-	+/-	Abscess culture
Plague	+	+	Sputum	+	-	-	Bubo aspirate, CSF, sputum, lesion scraping, lymph node aspirate. Never dissect bubo.
Tularemia	+	+	+	+	-	-	
Q-fever	+	D	Lesions	+	-	-	Lung, spleen, lymph nodes, bone marrow biopsies
Venezuelan Equine Encephalitis[A]	+	C	-	+	-	-	CSF
Viral Hemorrhagic Fevers[A]	+	C	-	+	-	-	Liver

Disease	Face or Nasal Swab[B]	Blood Culture[E]	Smear[F]	Acute & Convalescent Sera	Stool	Urine	Other Other
Botulism: C. botulinum toxins (A-G)	+	-	Wound tissues	+	+/-	-	Serum or other fluids for toxin detection/ mouse bioassay
Staphylococcus Enterotoxin B	+	-	-	+	+	+	Lung, kidney
Ricin Toxin	+	-	-	+	+	+	Spleen, lung, kidney
T-2 Mycotoxins	+	-	-	-	+	+	Serum, stool, or urine for metabolites

Notes:

[A] All specimens collected for viral examination should be placed into universal or viral transport media [1, 2]

[B] Swabs should all be Nylon, Rayon, or Dacron heads with plastic stems [3]

[C] Virus isolation from blood or throat swabs in appropriate containment.

[D] *C. burnetii* can persist for days in blood and resists desiccation. EDTA anti-coagulated blood preferred. Culturing should not be done except in biosafety level-3 containment.

[E] All blood for culture should be collected from ≥ 2 different sites (e.g. left arm and right arm) to control for possible skin contamination

[F] All collected sputum specimens should be graded for acceptance to rule out possible presence of normal mouth flora

APPENDIX L-2: MEDICAL & ENVIRONMENTAL BIO-AGENT SAMPLE COLLECTION, PACKAGING & SHIPMENT

This appendix provides guidance in determining which clinical samples to collect from individuals exposed to biological threat agents and when to collect them. Some of the parameters of general testing methodology and concepts of operation are also touched upon. The practical and legal parameters for packaging and shipping collected specimens are outlined. Lastly, there is a small section on which environmental samples to collect from suspect sites.

Proper collection of clinical specimens from patients in the context of possible bio-agent exposure/infection is dependent upon the time that has elapsed since the apparent exposure. Time-frames for sample collection can be succinctly categorized as "Early post-exposure," "Clinical," and "Convalescent/Terminal/Postmortem".

- ***Early post-exposure***: period immediately after exposure to a bio-agent (aerosol or otherwise); aggressively attempt to obtain samples as indicated
- ***Clinical:*** period when individuals are presenting with clinical symptoms
- ***Convalescent/Terminal/Post-mortem:*** period of convalescence, terminal stages of infection, toxicosis, or post-mortem (e.g., during autopsy)

These time-frames are not rigid and will vary according to the concentration of the agent used, the agent strain, predisposing health factors of the patient and other considerations. Tables L-2-1, 2 and 3 present recommended timing of sample collections for bacteria/rickettsia, toxins, and viruses, respectively.

Shipping Clinical Samples:

In order to maintain integrity, most specimens sent rapidly (less than 24 h) to analytical labs require only blue or wet ice or refrigeration at 2 to 8 °C. However, if the time span increases beyond 24 h or if other procedural questions do arise, contact the USAMRIID "Hot-Line" (1-888-USA-RIID) for pertinent questions.

Blood samples: Several choices are offered based on availability of the blood collection tubes. Do not send blood in all the tubes listed in the attached tables, but merely choose one. Tiger-top tubes that have been centrifuged are preferred over red-top clot tubes with serum removed from the clot, but the latter will suffice. Blood culture bottles are also preferred over citrated blood for bacterial cultures, but make sure that specimens are collected from two different sites (such as left and right arm) to mitigate blood contamination with skin flora.

Pathology specimens: Post-mortem, routinely includes liver, lung, spleen, and regional or mesenteric lymph nodes. Additional samples requested are as follows: brain tissue for encephalomyelitis cases (although fatality is rare), adrenal gland for Ebola/Marburg cases (not absolutely required) and bone marrow. Culture of bone marrow for brucellosis has higher sensitivity than blood culture.[1]

Fixatives: While 10% buffered formalin is the standard pathology fixative, it will prevent any cell culture because infections are frequently not or only intermittently bacteremic. If the transit time is short and/or refrigerated, specimens can be sent in sterile normal saline or a sterile container. Formalin is an excellent tissue penetrator, but it can interfere with PCR and RT-PCR.[2,3] Alcohols also produce excellent tissue histology, although pathologists are not used to testing samples immersed in alcohol. Alcohols have low tissue penetration, so tissue samples should be sliced thin (3-4 mm) or minced for fixation. The volume of any fixative (formalin, alcohol etc.) should be several times the volume of tissue.

The gold standard for storage of PCR samples is at -70°C or in liquid nitrogen; obviously liquid nitrogen may not always be readily available outside of fixed facilities. There are also specialized products available: Ambion's RNAlater[R] is a tissue preservative for RNA at room temperature.[4] Biomatrica[R] has a full range of products for room temperature storage of samples for molecular testing.[5] Specialized products may not be necessary, however, especially in a field-expedient situation. DNA and RNA viruses have been shown to be detectable by PCR/real time-PCR even after 6 mos of room temperature storage in alcohol. This was demonstrated in 100% ethanol, but would probably work in other alcohols.[6]

Regulatory requirements: The world has changed since the WHO Smallpox Eradication Program routinely shipped and carried thousands of live smallpox samples without creating any concern or incidents as was normal for all diagnostic and research samples. It was said in those days that samples were carried VIP ("Virus in Pocket"). Since the 2001 anthrax letter mailings, several new sets of laws and regulations from multiple authorities that control shipment of biological samples have been imposed. Although written for a study of insect vector samples, Coleman *et al.*[7] provides an excellent summary. It is exceedingly difficult to obtain reliable shipping advice for biological pathogens, particularly the Biological Select Agents and Toxins (BSATs, or SAs). The regulations are often complex, the certifications needed are difficult to obtain, and the procedures can be baffling. The effect of this complexity could impede research, put patients at medical risk, and/or place medical personnel at legal risk. Laboratory and shipper hesitation could result in a compromise of specimen integrity, such as thawing at border check points, hindrance at State boundaries, etc. Post 9/11 bio-defense legislation has resulted in more extensive regulations of SA research and/or surveillance work that affects how SAs are collected, stored, secured, and shipped.[8] All of these factors must be integrated into the sampling and specimen transportation process and awareness for planning purposes is of significant importance.

With these impediments in mind, there appear to be three basic approaches available to people left with the responsibility to do practical work: (1) Send the samples as "general diagnostic samples" without testing, or with only preliminary testing (or presumptive clinical diagnosis of a patient). However, it must be noted that these samples will most likely still fall within the category of hazardous material/dangerous goods: infectious substances/toxins. (2) Fix or otherwise kill the samples rendering them suitable only for molecular analysis, serology, or staining methods, but not any kind of assay requiring a live organism. (3) Ship samples which have been identified as SAs under the required safe guards and permits in accordance with prescribed public statutes and DoD directives. Utilization of couriers on military aircraft or the medical evacuation chain may facilitate the process, though it of course doesn't obviate regulatory requirements. Coordination with the Laboratory Response Network (LRN) and/or the Defense Laboratory Network (DLN) can also assist this process.[9]

There are several DoD regulations that govern the packaging, shipment, and receipt of SAs and/or infectious substance practices: 1) 49 CFR Parts 100-185, 2) International Air Transport Association: Dangerous Goods Regulations (IATA), 3) DoD Regulations 4500.9-R, 4) Air Force Manual 24-204, 5) International Maritime Organization Dangerous Goods Code 36-12 (IMDG), 5) 42 CFR Part 73, 6) 7 CFR Part 331, 7) 9 CFR Part 121, 8) and Army Regulation 50-1. Within all of these regulations, the materials of interest to this reading audience are broken down into the following categories of decreasing generality: (1) hazardous materials/dangerous goods, (2) infectious substances/toxins, or (3) BSATs. Thus, a BSAT is considered both an infectious substance/toxin and a hazardous material/dangerous good. 49 CFR Parts 100-185 outline the procedures and policies for packaging and receiving dangerous goods, particularly dangerous infectious substances/toxins. IATA outlines the guidelines adopted by the commercial airline industry for transport of hazardous materials/dangerous goods, particularly infectious substances/toxins, but, most importantly, lists those air carriers that will and will not transport and what their individual requirements are. DoD R4500.9-R dictates to DoD personnel the procedures for moving hazardous material/dangerous goods, including infectious substances/toxins, in accordance with US Federal law and DoD policies and also delineates the responsible parties with roles and responsibilities. AFMAN 24-204 applies both US Federal law and DoD R4500.9-R to movement of hazardous materials/dangerous goods via military aircraft and also delineates the responsible parties with roles and responsibilities. IMDG Code 36-12 describes the guidelines for movement of hazardous materials/dangerous goods via surface movement at sea. 42 CFR Part 73, 7 CFR Part 331, and 9 CFR Part 121 are the regulatory statutes that describe and control all aspects of BSATs from the perspective of US Federal law, the Centers for Disease Control and Prevention (CDC), and the US Department of Agriculture (USDA) Animal Plant Health Inspection Service (APHIS). Finally, AR 50-1 integrates US Federal law with

DoD/Army policy to build a framework of directives for US Army personnel dealing with BSATs, particularly safety and security.[10-14]

While the various regulations provide clear guidance on BSAT procedures used within or into the US, very little guidance exists regarding the packaging and shipment of BSATs in specimens during military deployments and/or other OCONUS contingency operations. Current practice during military deployments is to implement procedures that best meet the intent of relevant US BSAT laws and regulations. However, this may be mitigated by existing partner nation laws and/or regulations if they exist. An important consideration during military deployments is whether a diagnostic specimen is considered a hazardous material/infectious substance and/or a BSAT (i.e. Class 6.1 or 6.2 Dangerous Good: 49 CFR Parts 101-185), as determination triggers a variety of specific actions/responses. In general, diagnostic specimens are considered to contain BSATs if they fall under the definitions set by 42 CFR 73.3. Moreover, strong guidelines for procedures to identify specimens as highly suspicious and reportable have been set from a collaboration between the CDC, Association of Public Health Laboratories, and American Society for Microbiology, knows as Sentinel Level Clinical Laboratory Protocols for Suspected Biological Threat Agents and Emerging Infectious Diseases.[15] In a field environment during combat/contingency operations, the DoD has identified four levels of identification for bio-agents: presumptive, field confirmatory, theater validation, and definitive.[16] *Presumptive* employs one method of identification and results dictate whether further analysis and reporting needs to be performed. *Field confirmatory* employs two methods from the same technology and results dictate possible further reporting, further analysis, and certain initiated medical actions. *Theater validation* employs two methods from two complementary, but different, technologies and results dictate further reporting and analysis, wider initiation of medical actions, and commencement of force health protection measures. *Definitive* employs more than two different methods from different technologies aimed at fully characterizing the biological threat and guiding future strategic and operational medical decisions and force health protection measures.

An additional issue is that specimen preparation procedures frequently inactivate any biological pathogens that are present, so that even though a confirmatory assay identified a particular pathogen, that sample would not be considered BSAT as no viable pathogen is present. Lab personnel should exercise caution when making a determination that a positive specimen is not a BSAT as it is extremely difficult in a field setting to determine whether a viable pathogen is present. Additionally, any portion of the diagnostic sample that did not undergo nucleic acid extraction or other sterilizing procedures may, very probably, still contain viable BSATs. To further complicate matters, nucleic acid from positive-stranded RNA viruses can be used to produce infectious virus and is considered a BSAT according to 42 CFR 73.3. Clearly, military personnel conducting diagnostic testing for BSATs should understand the rules, regulations, and statutes pertaining to BSATs and how they could pertain to combat/

contingency operations. Individual unit criteria and SOPs for determining whether specimens contain a BSAT must be well articulated, as well as procedures for securing, transporting, and destroying these specimens in accordance with Army, DoD, and US laws and regulations. Personnel conducting diagnostic testing must also understand that specimens that do not meet established criteria of a BSAT may still pose a considerable safety and force health protection threat from any exposure. Personnel regularly interacting with potential infectious substances should also be fully aware of classification schemes for these substances (for purposes of packaging and transportation) and safety precautions.

Environmental Samples:
Environmental specimens should be collected ASAP after recognition of a bio-agent release to determine the nature of a bio-aerosol or other delivery system. Obviously, the sooner the environmental specimen is taken (in conjunction with early post-exposure clinical samples) the less difficult it will be to identify the agent and become aware of all important the factors surrounding the exposure.

Specimens taken well after an attack may also allow identification of the agent used. While this information would likely be too late to inform useful prophylactic measures, it may be used, when combined with other information, for intelligence purposes, the gathering of forensic evidence, the future development of countermeasures, and the prosecution of war crimes or other criminal proceedings. Although not strictly a medical responsibility, such sample collection issues are the same as for during, or shortly after, the attack, and medical personnel may be the only personnel with the requisite specimen collection expertise on site.

If time and conditions permit, medical post-exposure planning and risk assessments should be performed. As in any hazardous materials situation, a clean line and exit and entry strategy should be designed for post exposure mitigation. Depending on the situation, personnel protective equipment (PPE) should be donned. The standard M40 gas mask and Mission Oriented Protective Posture (MOPP) level 4 is effective protection against bio-agent exposure. If it is possible to have a clean line, then a three-person team is recommended, with one clean and two dirty. The former would help decontaminate the latter. Specimens may be used in a criminal prosecution, what, where, when, how, etc, of the specimen collection should be documented both in documentation and with pictures. Take into consideration that documentation materials may need to be decontaminated later, thus will have to rugged and resistant to such treatment. The types of samples taken can be extremely variable. Some of the possible samples are:

- Aerosol collections in buffer solutions
- Soil
- Swabs

- Dry powders
- Container of unknown substance
- Vegetation
- Food / water
- Body fluids or tissues

What is collected will depend on the situation. Aerosol collection during an attack would be ideal, assuming you have the appropriate collection device. Otherwise anything that appears to be contaminated can be either sampled with swabs if available, or with absorbent paper or cloth. The item itself could be collected if not too large. Well after the attack, samples from dead animals or human remains can be taken (refer to Appendix L-3, "Laboratory Assays for Bio-agent Identification", for appropriate specimens). All samples should ideally be double bagged in *Ziploc*® bags (the outside of the inner bag decontaminated with dilute bleach before placing in the second bag) labeled with time and place of collection along with any other pertinent data.

Table L-2-1 *Bacteria and Rickettsia: Timing of sample collection*		
Early postexposure	Clinical	Convalescent/Terminal/ Postmortem
Anthrax *Bacillus anthracis* 0 – 24 h Nasal & throat swabs, induced respiratory secretions for culture[1], FA & PCR	24 to 72 h Serum (TT, RT) for toxin assays; Blood (E, C, H) for PCR; Blood (BC, C) for culture[2].	3 to 10 d Serum (TT, RT) for toxin assays; Blood (BC, C) for culture; Pathology samples
Plague *Yersinia pestis* 0 – 24 h Nasal swabs, sputum, induced respiratory secretions for culture, FA & PCR	24 – 72 h Blood (BC, C) & bloody sputum for culture & FA (C); F-1 Antigen assays (TT, RT), PCR (E, C, H)	>6 d Serum (TT, RT) for IgM later for IgG; Pathology samples
Tularemia *Francisella tularensis* 0 – 24 h Nasal swabs, sputum, induced respiratory secretions for culture, FA & PCR	24 – 72 h Blood (BC, C) for culture; Blood (E, C, H) for PCR; Sputum for FA & PCR	>6 d Serum (TT, RT) for IgM & later IgG, agglutination titers; Pathology samples
Glanders *Burkholderia mallei* 0 – 24 h Nasal swabs, sputum, induced respiratory secretions for culture & PCR.	24 – 72 h Blood (BC, C) for culture; Blood (E, C, H) for PCR; Sputum & drainage from skin lesions for PCR & culture.	>6 d Blood (BC, C) & tissues for culture; Serum (TT, RT) for immunoassays; Pathology samples.
Brucellosis *Brucella abortus, suis, & melitensis* 0 – 24 h Nasal swabs, sputum, induced respiratory secretions for culture & PCR.	24 – 72 h Blood (BC, C) for culture; Blood (E, C, H) for PCR.	>6 d Blood (BC, C) & tissues for culture; Serum (TT, RT) for immunoassays; Pathology samples
Q-Fever *Coxiella burnetii* 0 – 24 h Nasal swabs, sputum, induced respiratory secretions for culture & PCR.	2 to 5 d Blood (BC, C) for culture in eggs or mouse inoculation; Blood (E, C, H) for PCR.	>6 d Blood (BC, C) for culture in eggs or mouse inoculation; Pathology samples.
BC: Blood culture bottle C: Citrated blood (3-ml)	E: EDTA (3-ml) H: Heparin (3-ml)	TT: Tiger-top (5–10 ml) RT: Red top if no TT

1: Sputum specimens for culture should always be evaluated/scored for contamination with saliva. Negative results from sputum specimens not graded to be clinically relevant could still be positive, but may not be perceived as such due to salivary contamination.[17]

2: Blood for culture should be collected in the appropriate blood culture media and should be collected from > 2 different sites to control for contamination. No more than 3 sets of blood culture specimens should be taken in a 24 h period.

Table L-2-2 *Toxins: Timing of sample collection*		
Early postexposure	Clinical	Convalescent/Terminal/ Postmortem
Botulism Botulinum toxin from *Clostridium botulinum* 0 – 24 h Nasal swabs, induced respiratory secretions for PCR (contaminating bacterial DNA) & toxin assays; Serum (TT, RT) for toxin assays	24 to 72 h Nasal swabs, respiratory secretions for PCR (contaminating bacterial DNA) & toxin assays.	>6 d Usually no IgM or IgG; Pathology samples (liver & spleen for toxin detection)
Ricin Intoxication Ricin toxin from castor beans 0 – 24 h Nasal swabs, induced respiratory secretions for PCR (contaminating castor bean DNA) & toxin assays; Serum (TT) for toxin assays	36 to 48 h Serum (TT, RT) for toxin assay; Tissues for immunohisto-logical stain in pathology samples.	>6 d Serum (TT, RT) for IgM & IgG in survivors
Staph enterotoxicosis *Staphylococcus* Enterotoxin B 0 – 3 h Nasal swabs, induced respiratory secretions for PCR (contaminating bacterial DNA) & toxin assays; Serum (TT, RT) for toxin assays	2–6 h Urine for immunoassays; Nasal swabs, induced respiratory secretions for PCR (contaminating bacterial DNA) & toxin assays; Serum (TT, RT) for toxin assays	>6 d Serum for IgM & IgG; Note: Only paired antibody samples will be of value for IgG assays...most adults have antibodies to staph enterotoxins.
T-2 toxicosis 0 – 24 h postexposure Nasal & throat swabs, induced respiratory secretions for immunoassays, HPLC/ mass spectrometry (HPLC/MS).	1 to 5 d Serum (TT, RT), tissue for toxin detection	>6 d post-exposure Urine for detection of toxin metabolites
BC: Blood culture bottle C: Citrated blood (3-ml)	E: EDTA (3-ml) H: Heparin (3-ml)	TT: Tiger-top (5–10 ml) RT: Red top if no TT

Table L-2-3 *Viruses: Timing of sample collection*

Early postexposure	Clinical	Convalescent/Terminal/ Postmortem
Equine Encephalomyelitis VEE, EEE and WEE viruses 0 – 24 h Nasal swabs & induced respiratory secretions for RT-PCR & viral culture (in viral transport media)	24 to 72 h Serum & throat swabs for culture (TT, RT), RT-PCR (E, C, H, TT, RT) & Antigen ELISA (TT, RT), CSF, Throat swabs up to 5 d	>6 d Serum (TT, RT) for IgM; Pathology samples plus brain
Ebola/Marburg 0 – 24 h Nasal swabs & induced respiratory secretions for RT-PCR & viral culture (in viral transport media)	2 to 5 d Serum (TT, RT) for viral culture	>6 d Serum (TT, RT) for viral culture; Pathology samples plus adrenal gland.
Pox (Smallpox, monkeypox) *Orthopoxvirus* 0 – 24 h Nasal swabs & induced respiratory secretions for PCR & viral culture (in viral transport media)	2 to 5 d Serum (TT, RT) for viral culture	>6 d Serum (TT, RT) for viral culture; Drainage from skin lesions/ scrapings for microscopy, EM, viral culture, PCR; Pathology samples

BC: Blood culture bottle C: Citrated blood (3-ml)	E: EDTA (3-ml) H: Heparin (3-ml)	TT: Tiger-top (5–10 ml) RT: Red top if no TT

APPENDIX L-3: LABORATORY ASSAYS FOR BIO-AGENT IDENTIFICATION

Disease	Agent	Gold Standard	Antigen Detection	IgG	IgM	PCR
Anthrax	*Bacillus anthracis*	Culture[1]	X	X	X	X
Brucellosis	*Brucella* spp.	Culture[1]	X	X	X	X
Glanders	*Burkholderia mallei*	Culture[1]		X	X	X
Melioidosis	*Burkholderia pseudomallei*	Culture[1]		X	X	X
Plague	*Yersinia pestis*	Culture or 4-fold increase in Ab titer to F1 antigen[1]	X	X	X	X
Tularemia	*Francisella tularensis*	Culture (Chocolate Agar or BYCE) or 4 fold increase in Ab titer to *F. tularensis* antigen[1]	X	X	X	X
Q Fever	*Coxiella burnetii*	Acute: 4-fold increase in Ab titer to *C. burnetii*. Chronic: IFA to phase I antigen >1:800[1]	X	X	X	X
Smallpox	Orthopoxviruses	Reference laboratory testing only; generally PCR assays[1]	X	X		X
Venezuelan Equine Encephalitis	VEE virus	Paired Sera Serology or Virus Specific IgM in sera or CSF[2]	X	X	X	X
Viral Hemorrhagic Fevers	Filoviruses	Serology/PCR[3]	X	X	X	X
	Hantaviruses	Serology/PCR[3]	X	X	X	X
Botulism	Bot Toxins (A-G)/ *Clostridium botulinum*	Toxin Present in Sera (Serology Test) or Isolation of *C. botulinum* from sample[1]	X			*
Saxitoxin	Saxitoxin	HPLC-MS[4]				X

Disease	Agent	Gold Standard	Antigen Detection	IgG	IgM	PCR
Staph Enterotoxin B	SEB Toxin	ELISA[4]	X	X		*
Ricin	Ricin Toxin	ELISA[4]	X	X	X	X
T-2 Mycotoxins	T-2 Mycotoxins	LC-MS or HPLC-MS[4]	X			
Tetrodototoxin	Tetrodotoxins	HPLC-MS[4]	X			

* Toxin gene detected – only works if cellular debris including genes present as contaminant. Purified toxin does not contain detectable genes.

See Glossary (App. A) for acronyms/initialisms.

Not all of the indicated assays are available in field laboratories.

APPENDIX L-4: THE LABORATORY RESPONSE NETWORK (LRN)

http://www.bt.cdc.gov/lrn/

History

The Laboratory Response Network (LRN) was established by the Department of Health and Human Services, Centers for Disease Control and Prevention (CDC) in accordance with Presidential Decision Directive 39, which outlined national anti-terrorism policies and assigned specific missions to federal departments and agencies.

Through a collaborative effort involving LRN founding partners, the FBI and the Association of Public Health Laboratories, the LRN became operational in August 1999. Its objective was to ensure an effective laboratory response to bio-terrorism by helping to improve the nation's public health laboratory infrastructure, which had limited ability to respond to bio-terrorism.

Today, the LRN is charged with the task of maintaining an integrated network of state and local public health, federal, military, and international laboratories that can respond to bio-terrorism, chemical terrorism and other public health emergencies. The LRN is a unique asset in the nation's growing preparedness for biological and chemical terrorism. The linking of state and local public health laboratories, veterinary, agriculture, military, and water- and food-testing laboratories is unprecedented.

In the years since its creation, the LRN has played an instrumental role in improving the public health infrastructure by helping to boost laboratory capacity. Laboratories are better equipped, their staff levels are increasing, and laboratories are employing advanced technologies.

Public health infrastructure refers to essential public health services, including the people who work in the field of public health, information and communication systems used to collect and disseminate accurate data, and public health organizations at the state and local levels.

LRN Mission

The LRN is a national security asset that, with its partners, will develop, maintain and strengthen an integrated domestic and international network of laboratories to respond quickly to biological, chemical, and radiological threats and other high priority public health emergencies needs through training, rapid testing, timely notification and secure messaging of laboratory results.

National Laboratories

National laboratories, including those operated by CDC, USAMRIID, and the Naval Medical Research Center (NMRC), are responsible for specialized strain characterizations, bioforensics, select agent activity, and handling highly infectious biological agents.

Reference Laboratories

Reference laboratories are responsible for investigation and/or referral of specimens. They are made up of more than 150 state and local public health, military, international, veterinary, agriculture, food, and water testing laboratories. In addition to laboratories located in the United States, facilities located in Australia, Canada, the United Kingdom, Mexico and South Korea serve as reference laboratories abroad.

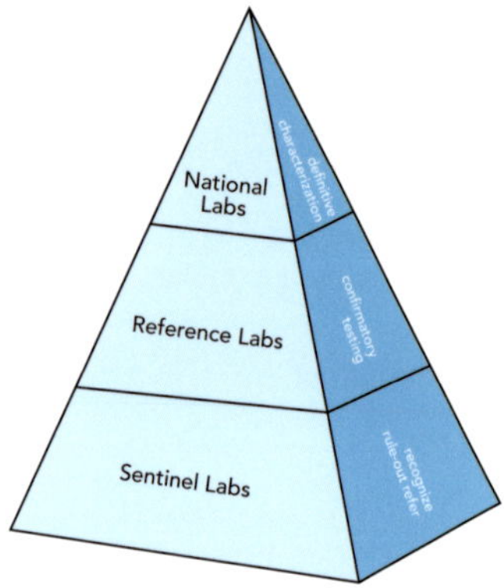

Sentinel Laboratories

The LRN is currently working with the American Society for Microbiology and state public health laboratory directors to ensure that private and commercial laboratories are part of the LRN. There is an estimated 25,000 private and commercial laboratories in the United States. The majority of these laboratories are hospital-based, clinical institutions, and commercial diagnostic laboratories.

Sentinel laboratories play a key role in the early detection of biological agents. Sentinel laboratories provide routine diagnostic services, rule-out, and referral steps in the identification process. While these laboratories may not be equipped to perform the same tests as LRN reference laboratories, they can test samples.

> **Note:** If you believe that you have been exposed to a biological or chemical agent, or if you believe an intentional biological threat will occur or is occurring, please contact your local health department and/or your local police or other law enforcement agency.

For specific contact information for local FBI offices and State Public Health Departments, see Appendix M.

Local public health laboratories (LRN), private laboratories, and commercial laboratories with questions about the LRN should contact their state public health laboratory director or the Association of Public Health Laboratories.

Centers for Disease Control and Prevention
Laboratory Preparedness and Response Branch
Division of Preparedness and Emerging Infection
National Center for Emerging, Zoonotic and Infectious Disease
1600 Clifton Road NE, Mailstop C-18
Atlanta, GA 30333
Email: *LRN@cdc.gov*

Association of Public Health Laboratories
8515 Georgia Ave, Suite 700
Silver Spring, MD 20910
Website: *www.aphl.org*
Email: *info@aphl.org*

APPENDIX M: EMERGENCY RESPONSE CONTACTS – FBI & PUBLIC HEALTH

Federal Bureau of Investigation (FBI) Field Offices (by state)

Alabama

FBI Birmingham
1000 18th Street North
Birmingham, AL 35203
birmingham.fbi.gov
(205) 326-6166

FBI Mobile
200 N. Royal Street
Mobile, AL 36602
mobile.fbi.gov
(251) 438-3674

Alaska

FBI Anchorage
101 East Sixth Avenue
Anchorage, AK 99501-2524
anchorage.fbi.gov
907-276-4441

Arizona

FBI Phoenix
Suite 400
201 East Indianola Avenue
Phoenix, AZ 85012-2080
phoenix.fbi.gov
(602) 279-5511

Arkansas

FBI Little Rock
#24 Shackleford West Boulevard
Little Rock, AR 72211-3755
littlerock.fbi.gov
(501) 221-9100

California

FBI Los Angeles
Suite 1700, FOB
11000 Wilshire Boulevard
Los Angeles, CA 90024-3672
losangeles.fbi.gov
(310) 477-6565

FBI Sacramento
4500 Orange Grove Avenue
Sacramento, CA 95841-4205
sacramento.fbi.gov
(916) 481-9110

FBI San Diego
Federal Office Building
9797 Aero Drive
San Diego, CA 92123-1800
sandiego.fbi.gov
(858) 565-1255

FBI San Francisco
450 Golden Gate Avenue, 13th. Floor
San Francisco, CA 94102-9523
sanfrancisco.fbi.gov
(415) 553-7400

Colorado

FBI Denver
8000 East 36th Avenue
Denver, CO 80238
denver.fbi.gov
(303) 629-7171

Connecticut

FBI New Haven
600 State Street
New Haven, CT 06511-6505
newhaven.fbi.gov
(203) 777-6311

District of Columbia

FBI Washington
Washington Metropolitan Field Office
601 4th Street, N.W.
Washington, D.C. 20535-0002
washingtondc.fbi.gov
(202) 278-2000

Florida

FBI Jacksonville
6061 Gate Parkway
Jacksonville, FL 32256
jacksonville.fbi.gov
(904) 248-7000

FBI North Miami Beach
16320 Northwest Second Avenue
North Miami Beach, FL 33169-6508
miami.fbi.gov
(305) 944-9101

FBI Tampa
5525 West Gray Street
Tampa, FL 33609
tampa.fbi.gov
(813) 253-1000

Georgia

FBI Atlanta
Suite 400
2635 Century Parkway, Northeast
Atlanta, GA 30345-3112
atlanta.fbi.gov
(404) 679-9000

Hawaii

FBI Honolulu
Room 4-230,
Prince Kuhio FOB
300 Ala Moana Boulevard
Honolulu, HI 96813
honolulu.fbi.gov
(808) 566-4300

Illinois

FBI Chicago
2111 West Roosevelt Road
Chicago, IL 60608-1128
chicago.fbi.gov
(312) 421-6700

FBI Springfield
900 East Linton Avenue
Springfield, IL 62703
springfield.fbi.gov
(217) 522-9675

Indiana

FBI Indianapolis
Room 679, FOB
575 North Pennsylvania Street
Indianapolis, IN 46204-1585
indianapolis.fbi.gov
(317) 639-3301

Kentucky

FBI Louisville
12401 Sycamore Station Place
Louisville , KY
40299-6198
louisville.fbi.gov
(502) 263-6000

Louisiana

FBI New Orleans
2901 Leon C. Simon Dr.
New Orleans, LA 70126
neworleans.fbi.gov
(504) 816-3000

Maryland

FBI Baltimore
2600 Lord Baltimore Drive
Baltimore, MD 21244
baltimore.fbi.gov
(410) 265-8080

Massachusetts

FBI Boston
Suite 600
One Center Plaza
Boston, MA 02108
boston.fbi.gov
(617) 742-5533

Michigan

FBI Detroit
26th. Floor, P. V. McNamara FOB
477 Michigan Avenue
Detroit, MI 48226
detroit.fbi.gov
(313) 965-2323

Minnesota

FBI Minneapolis
Suite 1100
111 Washington Avenue, South
Minneapolis, MN 55401-2176
minneapolis.fbi.gov
(612) 376-3200

Mississippi

FBI Jackson
1220 Echelon Parkway
Jackson, MS 39213
jackson.fbi.gov
(601) 948-5000

Missouri

FBI Kansas City
1300 Summit St.
Kansas City, MO 64105-1362
kansascity.fbi.gov
(816) 512-8200

FBI St. Louis
2222 Market Street
St. Louis, MO 63103-2516
stlouis.fbi.gov
(314) 231-4324

Nebraska

FBI Omaha
4411 South 121st Court
Omaha, NE 68137-2112
omaha.fbi.gov
(402) 493-8688

Nevada

FBI Las Vegas
John Lawrence Bailey Building
1787 West Lake Mead Boulevard
Las Vegas, NV 89106-2135
lasvegas.fbi.gov
(702) 385-1281

New Jersey

FBI Newark
11 Centre Place
Newark, NJ 07102-9889
newark.fbi.gov
(973) 792-3000

New Mexico

FBI Albuquerque
4200 Luecking Park Ave. NE
Albuquerque, NM 87107
albuquerque.fbi.gov
(505) 889-1300

New York

FBI Albany
200 McCarty Avenue
Albany, NY 12209
albany.fbi.gov
(518) 465-7551

FBI Buffalo
One FBI Plaza
Buffalo, NY 14202-2698
buffalo.fbi.gov
(716) 856-7800

FBI New York
26 Federal Plaza, 23rd Floor
New York, NY 10278-0004
newyork.fbi.gov
(212) 384-1000

North Carolina

FBI Charlotte
7915 Microsoft Way
Charlotte, NC 28273
charlotte.fbi.gov
(704) 672-6100

Ohio

FBI Cincinnati
Room 9000
550 Main Street
Cincinnati, OH 45202-8501
cincinnati.fbi.gov
(513) 421-4310

FBI Cleveland
Federal Office Building
1501 Lakeside Avenue
Cleveland, OH 44114
cleveland.fbi.gov
(216) 522-1400

Oklahoma

FBI Oklahoma City
3301 West Memorial Drive
Oklahoma City, OK 73134
oklahomacity.fbi.gov
(405) 290-7770

Oregon

FBI Portland
Suite 400, Crown Plaza Building
1500 Southwest 1st Avenue
Portland, OR 97201-5828
portland.fbi.gov
(503) 224-4181

Pennsylvania

FBI Philadelphia
8th. Floor
William J. Green Jr. FOB
600 Arch Street
Philadelphia, PA 19106
philadelphia.fbi.gov
(215) 418-4000

FBI Pittsburgh
3311 East Carson St.
Pittsburgh, PA 15203
pittsburgh.fbi.gov
(412) 432-4000

Puerto Rico

FBI San Juan
Room 526, US Federal Bldg.
150 Carlos Chardon Avenue
Hato Rey
San Juan, PR 00918-1716
sanjuan.fbi.gov
(787) 754-6000

South Carolina

FBI Columbia
151 Westpark Blvd
Columbia, SC 29210-3857
columbia.fbi.gov
(803) 551-4200

Tennessee

FBI Knoxville
1501 Dowell Springs Boulevard
Knoxville, TN 37909
knoxville.fbi.gov
(865) 544-0751

FBI Memphis
Suite 3000, Eagle Crest Bldg.
225 North Humphreys Blvd.
Memphis, TN 38120-2107
memphis.fbi.gov
(901) 747-4300

Texas

FBI Dallas
One Justice Way
Dallas, Texas 75220
dallas.fbi.gov
(972) 559-5000

FBI El Paso
660 S. Mesa Hills Drive
El Paso, Texas 79912-5533
elpaso.fbi.gov
(915) 832-5000

FBI Houston
1 Justice Park Drive
Houston, TX 77092
houston.fbi.gov
(713) 693-5000

FBI San Antonio
5740 University Heights Boulevard
San Antonio, TX 78249
sanantonio.fbi.gov
(210) 225-6741

Utah

FBI Salt Lake City
Suite 1200, 257 Towers Bldg.
257 East, 200 South
Salt Lake City, UT 84111-2048
saltlakecity.fbi.gov
(801) 579-1400

Virginia

FBI Norfolk
150 Corporate Boulevard
Norfolk, VA 23502-4999
norfolk.fbi.gov
(757) 455-0100

FBI Richmond
1970 E. Parham Road
Richmond, VA 23228
richmond.fbi.gov
(804) 261-1044
For Northern Virginia, contact the Washington Field Office.

Washington

FBI Seattle
1110 Third Avenue
Seattle, WA 98101-2904
seattle.fbi.gov
(206) 622-0460

Wisconsin

FBI Milwaukee
Suite 600
330 East Kilbourn Avenue
Milwaukee, WI 53202-6627
milwaukee.fbi.gov
(414) 276-4684

State Health Departments

Alabama

Department of Public Health
The RSA Tower
201 Monroe Street
Montgomery, Alabama 36104
334-206-5300
(800) ALA-1818
www.adph.org

Alaska

Division of Public Health
350 Main Street, Room 508
Juneau, Alaska 99801
(907) 465-3090
Fax: (907) 465-4632
http://health.hss.state.ak.us

Arizona

Department of Health Services
150 North 18th Avenue
Phoenix, Arizona 85007
(602) 542-1025
Fax: (602) 542-0883
http://www.azdhs.gov

Arkansas

Department of Health
4815 West Markham Street
Little Rock, Arkansas 72205
1-501-661-2000 or
1-800-462-0599
www.healthy.arkansas.gov

California

Department of Public Health
PO Box 997377 MS 0500
Sacramento, CA 95899-7377
(916) 558-1784
http://www.cdph.ca.gov

Colorado

Department of Public Health and Environment
4300 Cherry Creek Drive South
Denver, Colorado 80246-1530
303- 692-2000
(800) 886-7689 (In-state)
http://www.cdphe.state.co.us/

Connecticut

Department of Public Health
410 Capitol Avenue
Hartford, CT 06134
Phone: (860) 509-8000
http://www.ct.gov/dph/

Delaware

Division of Public Health
417 Federal Street
Jesse Cooper Building
Dover, DE 19901
(302) 744-4700
FAX: (302) 739-6659
http://www.dhss.delaware.gov/dhss/dph/

Florida

Department of Health
2585 Merchants Row Boulevard Tallahassee, Florida 32399
(850) 245-4444
http://www.doh.state.fl.us/

Georgia

Department of Public Health
Two Peachtree Street, NW
Atlanta, Georgia 30303-3186
Phone: (404) 657-2700
http://health.state.ga.us/
Hawaii

Department of Public Health
Kinau Hale
1250 Punchbowl Street
Honolulu, HI 96813
(808) 586-4400
http://hawaii.gov/health

Idaho

Department of Health and Welfare
PO Box 83720
Boise, ID 83720-0036
(208) 334-5500
http://www.healthandwelfare.idaho.gov/

Illinois

Department of Public Health
535 West Jefferson Street
Springfield, Illinois 62761
(217) 782-4977
Fax (217) 782-3987
http://www.idph.state.il.us/

Indiana

State Department of Health
2 North Meridian Street
Indianapolis, IN 46204
(317) 233-1325
http://www.state.in.us/isdh/

Iowa

Department of Public Health
321 E. 12th Street
Des Moines, Iowa, 50319-0075
(515) 281-7689
toll-free at (866) 227-9878
http://www.idph.state.ia.us/

Kansas

Department of Health and Environment
Curtis State Office Building
1000 SW Jackson
Topeka, Kansas 66612
(785) 296-1500
http://www.kdheks.gov/

Kentucky

Department for Public Health
275 East Main Street
Frankfort, KY 40621
(502) 564-3970
http://chfs.ky.gov/dph/

Louisiana

Department of Health and Hospitals
P.O. Box 629
Baton Rouge, LA 70821-0629
(225) 342-9500
http://new.dhh.louisiana.gov/

Maine

Department of Health and
Human Services
221 State Street
Augusta, ME 04333
(207) 287-3707
Fax: (207) 287-3005
http://www.maine.gov/dhhs/

Maryland

Department of Health and Mental Hygiene
201 West Preston Street
Baltimore, MD 21201
(410) 767-6500 or (877) 463-3464
http://www.dhmh.state.md.us/

Massachusetts

Department of Public Health
250 Washington Street
Boston, Massachusetts 02108
http://www.mass.gov/

Michigan

Department of Community Health
Capitol View Building
201 Townsend Street
Lansing, Michigan 48913
(517) 373-3740
http://www.michigan.gov/mdch/

Minnesota

Department of Health
P.O. Box 64975
St. Paul, MN 55164-0975
(651) 201-5000
(888) 345-0823
http://www.health.state.mn.us/

Mississippi

State Department of Health
570 East Woodrow Wilson Drive
Jackson, MS 39216
(601)576-7400
(866) 458-4948
http://msdh.ms.gov/index.htm

Missouri

Department of Health and Senior Services
912 Wildwood
P.O. Box 570
Jefferson City, Missouri 65102
Phone: (573) 751-6400
Fax: (573) 751-6010
Email: info@health.mo.gov
http://health.mo.gov/

Montana

Department of Public Health and Human Services
111 North Sanders, Room 301
Helena, MT 59620
(406) 444-5622
Fax: (406) 444-1970
http://www.dphhs.mt.gov/

Nebraska

Department of Health & Human Services
301 Centennial Mall South
Lincoln, Nebraska 68509
(402) 471-3121
http://www.hhs.state.ne.us/

Nevada

Department of Health & Human Services
4126 Technology Way, Suite 100
Carson City, Nevada 89706-2009
(775) 684-4000
(775) 684-4010 Fax
http://dhhs.nv.gov/

New Hampshire

Division of Public Health Services
NH Department of Health & Human Services
29 Hazen Drive
Concord, NH 03301
(603) 271-4501
(800) 852-3345 Ext. 4501
http://www.dhhs.nh.gov/dphs/

New Jersey

Department of Health and Senior Services
P. O. Box 360,
Trenton, NJ 08625-0360
Phone: (609) 292-7837
Toll-free in NJ: (800) 367-6543
http://www.state.nj.us/health/

New Mexico

Department of Health
1190 South St. Francis Drive
Santa Fe, NM 87502
Phone: (505) 827-2613
FAX: (505) 827-2530
http://nmhealth.org/

New York State

Department of Health
Corning Tower
Empire State Plaza,
Albany, NY 12237
Public Health Duty Officer Helpline
(866) 881-2809
http://www.health.state.ny.us/

North Carolina

Division of Public Health
1931 Mail Service Center
Raleigh, NC 27699-1931
(919) 707-5000
Fax: (919) 870-4829
http://publichealth.nc.gov/

North Dakota

Department of Health
600 East Boulevard Avenue
Bismarck, ND 58505-0200
(701) 328-2372
Fax: (701) 328-4727
http://www.ndhealth.gov/

Ohio

Department of Health
246 N. High St.
Columbus, Ohio 43215
(614) 466-3543
mailto: Director@odh.ohio.gov
http://www.odh.ohio.gov/

Oklahoma

State Department of Health
1000 NE 10th
Oklahoma City, OK 73117
(405) 271-5600
(800) 522-0203
http://www.ok.gov/health/

Oregon

Public Health Division
800 NE Oregon Street
Portland, OR 97232
(971) 673-1222
Fax: (971) 673-1299
http://public.health.oregon.gov/

Pennsylvania

Department of Health
Health and Welfare Building
8th Floor West
625 Forster Street
Harrisburg, PA 17120
(877) 724-3258
http://www.portal.state.pa.us/portal/server.pt/community/department_of_health_home/

Rhode Island

Department of Health
3 Capitol Hill
Providence, RI 02908
(401) 222-5960
http://www.health.ri.gov/

South Carolina

Department of Health and Environmental Control
2600 Bull Street
Columbia, SC 29201
(803) 898-DHEC (3432)
http://www.scdhec.gov/

South Dakota

Department of Health
600 East Capitol Ave.
Pierre, SD 57501-2536
(605) 773-3361
(800) 738-2301 (in state)
http://doh.sd.gov/

Tennessee

Department of Health
425 5th Avenue North
Cordell Hull Building, 3rd Floor
Nashville, TN 37243
(615) 741-3111
http://health.state.tn.us/

Texas

Department of State Health Services
1100 West 49th Street
Austin, Texas 78756-3199
(512) 458-7111
(888) 963-7111
http://www.dshs.state.tx.us/

Utah

Department of Health
P.O. Box 141010
Salt Lake City, UT 84114-1010
(801) 538-6003
http://health.utah.gov/

Vermont

Department of Health
108 Cherry Street
Burlington, VT 05402
Voice: (802) 863-7200
In Vermont (800) 464-4343
Fax: (802) 865-7754
http://healthvermont.gov/

Virginia

Department of Health
P.O. Box 2448
Richmond, Virginia 23218-2448
109 Governor Street
Richmond, Virginia 23219
(804) 864-7002
http://www.vdh.state.va.us/

District of Columbia

Department of Health
899 North Capitol Street, NE
Washington, DC 20002
(202) 442-5955
http://dchealth.dc.gov/doh/

Washington State

Department of Health
101 Israel Road SE
Tumwater, Washington 98501
PO Box 47890
Olympia, Washington 98504-7890
(360) 236-4030
http://www.doh.wa.gov/

West Virginia

Department of Health and Human Resources
Bureau for Public Health
Room 702
350 Capitol Street
Charleston, WV 25301-3712
Telephone: (304) 558-2971
Fax: (304) 558-1035
http://www.wvdhhr.org/bph/

Wisconsin

Department of Health Services
1 West Wilson Street
Madison, WI 53703
(608) 266-1865
http://www.dhs.wisconsin.gov/

Wyoming

Department of Health
401 Hathaway Building
Cheyenne, WY 82002
(307) 777-7656
(866) 571-0944
Fax: (307) 777-7439
http://www.health.wyo.gov/

APPENDIX N: REFERENCES

Introduction

1. Gilman JK, Wright M, Land HC, Schoomaker EB. A model of federal interagency cooperation: The National Interagency Confederation for Biological Research. Biosecur Bioterror 2014;12(3):144–50. (Accessed April 10, 2015, at http://www.pubfacts.com/detail/24819736/A-model-of-federal-interagency-co-operation:-the-National-Interagency-Confederation-for-Biological-Re.)

History of Biological Warfare and the Current Threat

1. Mayor A. *Greek fire, poison arrows and scorpion bombs: Biological and chemical warfare in the ancient world.* New York: The Overlook Press, 2003.

2. Trevisanato SI. The "Hittite Plague," an epidemic of tularemia and the first record of biological warfare. *Med Hypotheses* 2007;69(6):1371–4.

3. Mayor, *Op. cit.,* pp 100-101.

4. Wheelis M. Biological warfare at the 1346 Siege of Caffa. *Emerg Infect Dis* 2002;8(9):971–5.

5. Price DA. *Love and hate in Jamestown: John Smith, Pocahontas, and the heart of a new nation.* New York: Knopf, 2003:204.

6. Ranlet P. The British, the Indians, and smallpox: What actually happened at Fort Pitt in 1763? *Pennsylvania History* 2000:427–41.

7. Fenn EA. *Pox Americana: The great smallpox epidemic of 1775–82.* Hill & Wang, 2002: 88–92, 132–3.

8. Koenig R. *The fourth horseman: One man's secret campaign to fight the Great War in America.* New York: Public Affairs, 2006.

9. Guillemin J. *Biological weapons: From the invention of state-sponsored programs to contemporary bioterrorism.* New York: Columbia University Press, 2005:24–5.

10. Harris SH (1994), *Factories of Death.* New York, New York: Routledge.

11. Barenblatt D. *A plague upon humanity: The hidden history of Japan's biological warfare program.* New York: Harper Perennial, 2005:xii–xiii.

12. Covert NM. *Cutting edge: A history of Fort Detrick, Maryland.* 4th ed. 2000.

13. Meselson M, Guillemin J, Hugh-Jones M, et al. The Sverdlovsk anthrax outbreak of 1979. *Science* 1994;266:1202–8.

14. Cook MS, Woolf AF. *Preventing proliferation of biological weapons: U.S. assistance to the former Soviet states.* Washington, DC: Congressional Research Service, 2002:3.

15. Leitenberg M, Zilinskas RA. *The Soviet biological weapons program: A history.* Cambridge, MA: Harvard University Press, 2012.

16. Alibek K. *Biohazard: The chilling true story of the largest covert biological weapons program in the world—told from inside by the man who ran it.* New York: Random House, 1999.

17. Zilinskas RA. Puzzling policy trends in Russia related to the biosciences and biosecurity. Paper presented at *The 11th CBW Protection Symposium, Swedish Defense Research Agency (Totalförsvarets forskningsinstitut, FOI),* Stockholm, 3–5 June 2013. (Accessed April 10, 2015, at http://www.foi.se/Global/V%C3%A5ra%20 tj%C3%A4nster/Konferenser%20och%20seminarier/CBW%20symposium/Proceedings/Zilinskas.pdf.)

18. Colvin M, Mahnaimi U. Saddam tested anthrax on human guinea pigs. *London Sunday Times,* 18 January 1998.

19. Takahashi H, Keim P, Kaufmann AF, et al. Bacillus anthracis incident, Kameido, Tokyo, 1993. *Emerg Infect Dis* 2004;10:117–20.

20. CDC. Investigation of a ricin-containing envelope at a postal facility—South Carolina, 2003. *MMWR Morb Mortal Wkly Rep* 2003;52:1129–31.

22. Associated Press. James Everett Dutschke sentenced in ricin case. *Politico.com*, 19 May 2014.

23. Kerr PK. *Nuclear, biological, and chemical weapons and missiles: Status and trends.* Washington, DC: U.S. Congressional Research Service, 20 February 2008. (Accessed April 10, 2015, at http://usiraq.procon.org/sourcefiles/CRS_2-20-08.pdf.)

Further Reading

Carus WS. *Bioterrorism and biocrimes: The illicit use of biological agents since 1900.* Amsterdam: Fredonia Books, 2002.

Christopher GW, Cieslak TJ, Pavlin JA, Eitzen EM. Biological warfare. A historical perspective. *JAMA* 1997;278:412–7.

Geissler E, van Courtland Moon JE, eds. *Biological and toxin weapons: Research, development and use from the Middle Ages to 1945.* Oxford, U.K.: Oxford University Press, 1999.

Noah DL, Huebner KD, Darling RG, Waeckerle J. The history and threat of biological warfare and terrorism. *Emerg Med Clin North Am* 2002;20:255–71.

Speirs EM. *A history of chemical and biological weapons.* London: Reaktion Books, 2010.

Torok TJ, Tauxe RV, Wise RP, et al. A large community outbreak of salmonellosis caused by intentional contamination of restaurant salad bars. *JAMA* 1997;278:389–95.

Distinguishing Between Natural and Intentional Disease Outbreaks

1. Hugh-Jones M. Distinguishing between natural and unnatural outbreaks of animal diseases. *Rev Sci Tech* 2006;25:173–86.

2. Dembek ZF, Pavlin JA, Kortepeter MG. Epidemiology of biowarfare and bioterrorism. In: Dembek ZF, ed. *Medical aspects of biological warfare.* Textbooks of Military Medicine Series. Washington, DC: Borden Institute; Office of the Surgeon General, U.S. Army, 2007:39–68.

3. Mauer WA, Kaneene JB. Integrated human-animal disease surveillance. *Emerg Infect Dis* 2005;11(9):1490–1. (Accessed March 15, 2014, at http://dx.doi.org/10.3201/eid1109.050180.)

4. CDC. National Notifiable Diseases Surveillance System (NNDSS). (Accessed April 10, 2015, at http://wwwn.cdc.gov/nndss/script/nedss.aspx.)

5. http://www.cdc.gov/excite/classroom/outbreak/steps.htm.

6. Dembek ZF, Kortepeter MG, Pavlin, JA. Discernment between deliberate and natural infectious disease outbreaks. *Epidemiol Infect* 2007;137:353–71.

7. WHO. Disease outbreaks. (Accessed April 10, 2015, at http://www.who.int/topics/disease_outbreaks/en/.)

Biosurveillance

1. CDC. Emergency preparedness and response. (Accessed April 10, 2015, at www.bt.cdc.gov.)

2. WHO. Global Alert and Response (GAR): Integrated disease surveillance. (Accessed April 10, 2015, at http://www.who.int/csr/labepidemiology/projects/diseasesurv/en/.)

3. WHO. *Global infectious disease surveillance.* Fact Sheet, No. 200. (Accessed April 10, 2015, at http://www.who.int/mediacentre/factsheets/fs200/en/.)

4. http://www.publichealth.hscni.net/directorate-public-health/health-protection/surveillance-data.

5. Food and Agriculture Organization of the United Nations. Challenges of animal health information systems and surveillance for animal diseases and zoonoses. *Proceedings of the international workshop organized by FAO, Rome, November 23–26, 2010.* FAO Animal Production and Health Proceedings, No. 14. Rome: FAO, 2011. (Accessed April 10, 2015, at http://www.fao.org/docrep/014/i2415e/i2415e00.htm.)

6. White House. *National Strategy for Biosurveillance.* Washington, DC: The White House, July 2012. (Accessed April 10, 2015, at http://www.whitehouse.gov/sites/default/files/National_Strategy_for_Biosurveillance_July_2012.pdf.)

7. National Security Council. *National Strategy for Countering Biological Threats.* Washington, DC: The White House, November 2009. (Accessed April 10, 2015, at http://www.whitehouse.gov/sites/default/files/National_Strategy_for_Countering_BioThreats.pdf.)

8. Deputy Secretary of Defense. *Interim guidance for implementing the National Strategy for Biosurveillance.* Washington, DC: U.S. Department of Defense, June 2013.

Ten Steps in the Management of Potential Biological Casualties

1. For example:

- U.S. Army. *Field manual: Treatment of biological warfare agent casualties.* Washington, DC: Headquarters, Departments of the Army, the Navy, and the Air Force, and Commandant, Marine Corps, July 2000. (FM 8-284, NAVMED P-5042, AFMAN (I) 44-156, MCRP 4-11.1C.)
- U.S. Army. *Field manual: NATO handbook on the medical aspects of NBC defensive operations.* Washington, DC: Departments of the Army, the Navy, and the Air Force, February 1996. (FM 8-9, NAVMED P-5059, AFJMAN 44-151, AMedP-6.)

2. Committee on Trauma, American College of Surgeons. *Advanced trauma life support for doctors: Student course manual.* 8th ed. Chicago: American College of Surgeons, 2008.

3. Binder P, Attre O, Boutin JP, et al. Medical management of biological warfare and bioterrorism: Place of the immunoprevention and the immunotherapy. *Comp Immunol Microbiol Infect Dis* 2003; 26:401–21.

4. Cieslak TJ, Rowe JR, Kortepeter MG, et al. A field-expedient algorithmic approach to the clinical management of chemical and biological casualties. *Mil Med* 2000; 165:659–62.

5. Cieslak TJ, Henretig FM. Medical consequences of biological warfare: The ten commandments of management. *Mil Med* 2001; 166(suppl 2):11–12.

6. Henretig FM, Cieslak TJ, Kortepeter MG, Fleisher GR. Medical management of the suspected victim of bioterrorism: An algorithmic approach to the undifferentiated patient. *Emerg Med Clin North Am* 2002; 20:351–64.

7. Cieslak TJ, Christopher GW. Medical management of potential biological casualties: A stepwise approach. In: Dembek ZF, ed. *Medical aspects of biological warfare.* Textbooks of Military Medicine Series. Washington, DC: Borden Institute; Office of the Surgeon General, U.S. Army, 2007:443–63.

8. Scarfone RJ, Madsen JM, Cieslak TJ, et al. Emergency department recognition and management of victims of biological and chemical terrorism. In: Fleisher GR, Ludwig S, Henretig FM, eds. *Textbook of pediatric emergency medicine.* 7th ed. Philadelphia, PA: Lippincott Williams & Wilkins, in press.

9. Cone DC, Koenig KL. Mass casualty triage in the chemical, biological, radiological, or nuclear environment. *Eur J Emerg Med* 2005; 6:287–302.

10. Siegel JD, Rhinehart E, Jackson M, Chiarello L, and the Healthcare Infection Control Practices Advisory Committee. *2007 guideline for isolation precautions: Preventing transmission of infectious agents in healthcare settings.* (Accessed April 10, 2015, at http://www.cdc.gov/hicpac/pdf/isolation/Isolation2007.pdf).

11. CDC. Investigating an outbreak. In: *Principles of epidemiology: Self study course SS3030.* 2nd ed. Atlanta, GA: Centers for Disease Control and Prevention, 1998:347–424.

12. Pavlin JA. Epidemiology of bioterrorism. *Emerg Infect Dis* 1999; 5:528–30.

13. Holloway HL, Norwood AE, Fullerton CS, et al. The threat of biological weapons: Prophylaxis and mitigation of psychological and social consequences. *JAMA* 1997; 278:425–7.

14. Franz DR, Jahrling PB, Friedlander AM, et al. Clinical recognition and management of patients exposed to biological warfare agents. *JAMA* 1997; 278:399–411.

15. Cieslak TJ, Henretig FM. Biological and chemical terrorism. In: Kliegman RM, Stanton BMD, St. Geme J, and Schor NF, eds. *Nelson textbook of pediatrics.* 20th ed. Philadelphia, PA: W.B. Saunders, in press: Chapter 724.

16. Dembek ZF, Cieslak TJ. Biological events. In: Koenig K, Schultz C, eds. *Disaster medicine.* : Cambridge University Press, in press: Chapter 32.

17. U.S. Army Medical Research Institute of Infectious Diseases. USAMRIID: *Biodefense solutions to protect our nation.* (Accessed April 10, 2015, at www.usamriid.army.mil.)

18. Cieslak TJ. Medical management of potential biological casualties: A stepwise approach. In: xxxx, ed. *Medical aspects of biological warfare.* Textbooks of Military Medicine Series. Washington, DC: Borden Institute; Office of the Surgeon General, U.S. Army, in press: Chapter xx.

Anthrax

1. Inglesby TV, Henderson DA, Bartlett JG, et al., for the Working Group on Civilian Biodefense. Anthrax as a biological weapon. *JAMA* 1999; 281:1735–45.

2. Inglesby TV, O'Toole T, Henderson, DA, for the Working Group on Civilian Biodefense. Anthrax as a biological weapon, 2002: Updated recommendations for management. *JAMA* 2002; 287:2236–52.

3. Dewan PK, Fry AM, Laserson K, et al., and members of the Washington, DC, Anthrax Response Team. Inhalational anthrax outbreak among postal workers, Washington, DC, 2001. *Emerg Infect Dis* 2002; 8:1066–72.

4. Fennelly KP, Davidow AL, Miller SL, Connell N, Ellner J. Airborne infection with *Bacillus anthracis*—from mills to mail. *Emerg Infect Dis* 2004; 10:996–1001.

5. Fasanella A, Galante D, Garafolo D, Jones MH. Anthrax undervalued zoonosis. *Vet Microbiol* 2010; 140:318–31.

6. Gold H. Anthrax: A report of one hundred seventeen cases. AMA *Arch Intern Med* 1955; 96:387–96.

7. Chitlaru T, Altboum Z, Reuveny S, Shafferman A. Progress and novel strategies in vaccine development and treatment of anthrax. *Immunol Rev* 2011; 239:221–36.

8. Cybulski RJ Jr., Sanz P, O'Brien AD. Anthrax vaccination strategies. *Mol Aspects Med* 2009; 30:490–502.

9. Migone TS, Subramanian GM, Zhong J, et al. Raxibacumab for the treatment of inhalational anthrax. *N Engl J Med* 2009; 361(2):135–44.

10. Friedlander AM, Little SF. Advances in the development of next-generation anthrax vaccines. *Vaccine* 2009; 27(suppl 4):D28–32.

11. Dupuy LC, Schmaljohn CS. DNA vaccines for biodefense. *Expert Rev Vaccines* 2009; 8:1739–54.

12. Klinman DM, Yamamoto M, Tross D, Tomaru K. Anthrax prevention and treatment: Utility of therapy combining antibiotic plus vaccine. *Expert Opin Biol Ther* 2009; 9:1477–86.

13. Vietri NJ, Purcell BK, Tobery SA, et al. A very short course in antibiotic treatment is effective in preventing death from experimental inhalational anthrax after discontinuing antibiotics. *J Infect Dis* 2009; 199:336–41.

14. Vietri NJ, Purcell BK, Lawler LJ, et al. Short-course postexposure antibiotic prophylaxis combined with vaccination protects against experimental inhalational anthrax. *Proc Natl Acad Sci USA* 2006;103:7813–16.

15. Anthrax Vaccine Immunization Program. *FDA issues final order—AVA safe and effective, protects individuals at high risk for anthrax disease; DoD resumes mandatory anthrax vaccinations for select groups.* (Accessed April 10, 2015, at http://www.anthrax.osd.mil/resource/policies/policies.asp.)

16. CDC. Use of anthrax vaccine in the United States: Recommendations of the Advisory Committee on Immunization Practices (ACIP), 2009. *MMWR Recomm Rep* 2010; 59 (RR-6):1–30.

Brucellosis

1. Moreno E. Retrospective and prospective perspectives on zoonotic brucellosis. *Front Microbiol* 2014; 5:1–18.

2. Teske SS, Huang Y, Tamraker SB, Bartrand TA, Weir MH, Haas CN. Animal and human dose–response models for Brucella species. *Risk Anal* 2011; 31(10):1576–96.

3. Rubach MP, Halliday JEB, Cleaveland S, Crump JA. Brucellosis in low-income and middle-income countries. *Curr Opin Infect Dis* 2013; 26:404–12.

4. Burns DS, Bailey MS. Undifferentiated febrile illnesses in military personnel. *J R Army Med Corps* 2013; 159:200–5.

5. Young EJ, Corbel MJ, eds. *Brucellosis: Clinical and laboratory aspects.* Boca Raton, FL: CRC Press, LLC, 1989.

6. Colmenero JD, Reguera JM, Martos F, et al. Complications associated with Brucella melitensis infection: A study of 530 cases. *Medicine* 1996; 75:195–211.

7. McLean DR, Russell N, Khan MY. Neurobrucellosis: Clinical and therapeutic features. *Clin Infect Dis* 1992; 15:582–90.

8. CDC. Suspected brucellosis case prompts investigation of possible bioterrorism-related activity—New Hampshire and Massachusetts, 1999. *MMWR Morb Mortal Wkly Rep* 2000; 49:509–12.

9. Solera J, Martinez-Alfaro E, Espinosa A. Recognition and optimum treatment of brucellosis. *Drugs* 1997; 53:245–56.

10. Traxler RM, Guerra MA, Morrow HG, et al. Review of brucellosis cases from laboratory exposures in the United States in 2008 to 2011 and improved strategies for disease prevention. *J Clin Microbiol* 2013; 51:3132–6.

11. Wang Z, Wu Q. Research progress in live attenuated Brucella vaccine development. *Curr Pharm Biotechnol* 2013; 14:887–96.

Glanders/Melioidosis

1. Van Zandt KE, Greer MT, Gelhaus HC. Glanders: An overview of infection in humans. *Orphanet J Rare Dis* 2013; 8:131.

2. Currie BJ. Burkholderia pseudomallei and Burkholderia mallei: Melioidosis and glanders. In: Mandell GL, Bennett JE, Dolin R, eds. *Principles and practice of infectious diseases.* 7th ed. Philadelphia, PA: Churchill Livingstone, 2010: 2869–79.

3. Wiersinga WJ, Currie BJ, Peacock SJ. Melioidosis. *N Engl J Med* 2012; 367:1035–1044.

4. CDC. Laboratory-acquired human glanders—Maryland, May 2000. *MMWR Morb Mortal Wkly Rep* 2000; 49(24):532–5.

5. Srinivasan A, Kraus CN, DeShazer D, et al. Glanders in a military research microbiologist. *N Engl J Med* 2001; 345:256–8.

6. Leitenberg M, Zilinskas RA. *The Soviet biological weapons program: A history.* Cambridge, MA: Harvard University Press, 2012:287–8.

7. Limmathurotsukol D, Chaowagul W, Chiefakul W, et al. Risk factors for recurrent melioidosis in northeast Thailand. *Clin Infect Dis* 2006; 43:979–86.

8. Peacock SJ, Schweizer HP, Dance DAB, et al. Management of accidental laboratory exposure to Burkholderia pseudomallei and B. mallei. *Emerg Infect Dis* 2008; 14(7):e2.

9. Peacock SJ, Cheng AC, Currie BJ, Dance DAB. The use of serological tests as evidence of exposure to Burkholderia pseudomallei. *Am J Trop Med Hyg* 2011; 84:1021–2.

10. Cheng AC, Currie BJ, Dance DAB, et al. Clinical definitions of melioidosis. *Am J Trop Med Hyg* 2013;88:411–13.

11. Meumann EM, Cheng AC, Ward L, Currie BJ. Clinical features and epidemiology of melioidosis pneumonia: Results from a 21-year study and review of the literature. *Clin Infect Dis* 2012;54:362–9.

12. Larsen JC, Johnson NH. Pathogenesis of Burkholderia pseudomallei and Burkholderia mallei. *Mil Med* 2009;174:647–51.

13. Lipsitz R, Garges S, Aurigemma R, et al. Workshop on treatment of and postexposure prophylaxis for Burkholderia pseudomallei and B. mallei infection, 2010. *Emerg Infect Dis* 2012;18(2):e2.

14. Sim SH, Jasper LC, Wang D, Liu Y, Ooi EE. Pre- and post-exposure prophylaxis of experimental Burkholderia pseudomallei infection with doxycycline, amoxicillin/clavulanic acid and co-trimoxazole. *J Antimicrob Chemother* 2008;61:674–8.

15. Russell P, Eley SM, Ellis J, et al. Comparison of efficacy of ciprofloxacin and doxycycline against experimental melioidosis and glanders. *J Antimicrob Chemother* 2000;45:813–18.

16. Siegel JD, Rhinehart E, Jackson M, Chiarello L, and the Healthcare Infection Control Practices Advisory Committee. *2007 guideline for isolation precautions: Preventing transmission of infectious agents in healthcare settings.* (Accessed March 14, 2014, at http://www.cdc.gov/ncidod/dhqp/pdf/isolation2007.pdf.)

Plague

1. Gage KL, Kosoy MY. Natural history of plague: Perspectives from more than a century of research. *Annu Rev Entomol* 2005;50:505–28.

2. Dennis, DT, Gage KL, Gratz N, Poland JD, Tikhomirov E. *Plague manual: Epidemiology, distribution, surveillance and control.* Geneva: World Health Organization, 1999. (WHO/CDS/CSR/EDC/99.2.)

3. Bei L, Chunhong D, Lei Z, et al. Humoral and cellular immune responses to Yersinia pestis infection in long-term recovered plague patients. *Clin Vaccine Immun* 2012;19:228–34.

4. Stenseth NC, Atshabar BB, Begon M, et al. Plague: Past, present, and future. *PLoS Med* 2008;5(1):1e.

5. Smiley ST. Immune defense against pneumonic plague. *Immunol Rev* 2008;225:256–71.

6. Guillemin J. *Biological weapons: From the invention of state-sponsored programs to contemporary bioterrorism.* New York: Columbia University Press, 2005:84.

7. Inglesby TV, Dennis DT, Henderson DA, et al. (2000), Plague as a biological weapon: Medical and public health management. *JAMA* 2000;283:2281–90.

8. Campbell GL, Dennis DT. (1998) Plague and other Yersinia infections. In: Kasper DL, et al.; eds. *Harrison's principles of internal medicine.* 14th ed. New York: McGraw Hill, 1998:975–83.

9. Mandell GL, Bennett JE, Dolin R, eds. *Mandell, Douglas, and Bennett's principles and practice of infectious diseases.* 7th ed. Philadelphia, PA: Churchill Livingstone Elsevier, 2010:2945.

10. Perry RD, Fetherston JD. Yersinia pestis—etiologic agent of plague. *Clin Microbiol Rev* 1997;10:35–66.

11. Crook LD, Tempest B. Plague: A clinical review of 27 cases. *Arch Intern Med* 1992;152:1253–6.

12. Borio L, Hynes NA. Plague as a bioterrorism weapon. In: Mandell GL, Bennett JE, Dolin R, eds. *Mandell, Douglas, and Bennett's principles and practice of infectious diseases.* 7th ed. Philadelphia, PA: Churchill Livingstone Elsevier, 2010:3965–70.

13. Dennis DT, Mead PS (2010), Yersinia species, including plague. In: Mandell GL, Bennett JE, Dolin R, eds. *Mandell, Douglas, and Bennett's principles and practice of infectious diseases.* 7th ed. Philadelphia, PA: Churchill Livingstone Elsevier, 2010:2943–53.

14. Wanger A. Yersinia. In: Murray PR, Baron EL, Landry ML, Jorgensen, JH and Pfaller MA, eds. *Manual of Clinical Microbiology.* 9th ed. Washington, DC: ASM Press, 2007:688–97.

15. Heath, David G. Personal observation, 2014.

16. Butler T. Plague into the 21st century. *Clin Infect Dis* 2009;49:736–42.

17. Boulanger LL, Ettestad P, Fogarty JD, Dennis DT, Romig D, Mertz G. (2004), Gentamicin and tetracyclines for the treatment of human plague: Review of 75 cases in New Mexico, 1985–1999. *Clin Infect Dis* 2004;38:663–9.

18. CDC. (1996) Prevention of plague. Recommendations of the Advisory Committee on Immunization Practices (ACIP). *MMWR Recomm Rep* 1996;45(RR-14):1–15.

19. Heath DG, Anderson GW, Mauro JM, et al. (1998) Protection against experimental bubonic and pneumonic plague by a recombinant capsular F1-V antigen fusion protein vaccine. *Vaccine* 1998;16(11/12):1131–7.

20. Fellows P, Price J, Lin W, et al. Animal models supporting bridge ELISA titers as a correlate of protection for a recombinant plague vaccine (rF1V). Poster presented at the *11th ASM Biodefense and Emerging Diseases Meeting*, Washington, DC, 25–27 February 2013.

Q Fever

1. Anderson A, Bijlmer H, Fournier PE, et al. Diagnosis and management of Q fever—United States 2013: Recommendations from CDC and the Q Fever Working Group. *MMWR Recomm Rep* 2013;62(RR03):1–23.

2. Hartzell JD, Gleeson T, Scoville S, et al. Practice guidelines for the diagnosis and management of patients with Q fever by the Armed Forces Infectious Diseases Society. *Mil Med* 2012;5:484–94.

3. Maurin M, Raoult D. Q fever. *Clin Microbiol Rev* 1999;12:518–53.

4. Parker N, Barralet JH, Bell AM. Q fever. *Lancet.* 2006;367:679–88.

5. Kampschreur LM, Dekker S, Hagenaars JC, et al. Identification of risk factors for chronic Q fever, the Netherlands. *Emerg Infect Dis* 2012;18:563–70.

6. Schimmer B, Dijkstra F, Vellema P, et al. Sustained intensive transmission of Q fever in the south of the Netherlands. *Euro Surveill* 2009;14:3.

7. Anderson AD, Baker TR, Littrell AC, et al. Seroepidemiologic survey for *Coxiella burnetii* among hospitalized U.S. troops deployed to Iraq. *Zoonoses Publ Health* 2011;58:276–83.

8. Bailey MS, Trinick TR, Dunbar JA, et al. Undifferentiated febrile illnesses amongst British troops in Helmand, Afghanistan. *J R Army Med Corps* 2011;157:150–5.

9. Faix DJ, Harrison DJ, Riddle MS, et al. Outbreak of Q fever among U.S. military in western Iraq, June–July 2005. *Clin Infect Dis* 2008;46(7):e46–48.

10. Hamilton LR, George DL, Scoville SL, et al. PCR for rapid diagnosis of acute Q fever at a combat support hospital in Iraq. *Mil Med* 2011;176:103–5.

11. Hartzell JD, Peng SW, Wood-Morris RN, et al. Atypical Q fever in U.S. soldiers. *Emerg Infect Dis* 2007;13:1247–9.

12. Raoult D, Fenollar F, Stein A. Q fever during pregnancy: Diagnosis, treatment, and follow-up. *Arch Intern Med* 2002;162:701–4.

13. Fenollar F, Fournier P, Carrieri M, et al. Risks factors and prevention of Q fever endocarditis. *Clin Infect Dis* 2001;33:312–6.

14. Gikas A, Kokkini S, Tsioutis C. Q fever: Clinical manifestations and treatment. *Expert Rev Anti Infect Ther* 2010;8:529–39.

15. Maltezou HC, Raoult D. Q fever in children. *Lancet Infect Dis* 2002;2:686–91.

16. Fournier P-E, Marrie TJ, Raoult D. Diagnosis of Q fever. *J Clin Microbiol* 1998;36:1823–34.

17. Marmor MF, Kellner U, Lai TY. Revised recommendations on screening for chloroquine and hydroxychloroquine retinopathy. *Ophthalmology* 2011;118:415–22.

18. Million M, Thuny F, Richet H, Raoult D. Long-term outcome of Q fever endocarditis: A 26-year personal survey. *Lancet Infect Dis* 2010;10:527–35.

19. Marrie TJ. Q fever endocarditis. *Lancet Infect Dis* 2010;10:507–9.

20. Gefenaite G, Munster JM, van Houdt R. Effectiveness of the Q fever vaccine: A meta-analysis. *Vaccine.* 2011;29:295–8.

21. Benenson AS, Tigertt WD. Studies on Q fever in man. *Trans Assoc Am Physics* 1956;69:98–104.

22. Moodie CE, Thompson HA, Meltzer MI, Swerdlow DL. Prophylaxis after exposure to Coxiella burnetii. *Emerg Infect Dis* 2008;14:1558–66.

Tularemia

1. Evans ME, Gregory DW, Schaffner W, McGee ZA. Tularemia: A 30-year experience with 88 cases. *Medicine (Baltimore)* 1985;64:251–69.

2. Feldman KA, Enscore RE, Lathrop SL, et al. An outbreak of primary pneumonic tularemia on Martha's Vineyard. *N Engl J Med* 2001;345:1601–16.

3. Dennis DT, Inglesby TV, Henderson DA, et al. Tularemia as a biological weapon: Medical and public health management. *JAMA* 2001;285:2763–73.

4. Leitenberg M, Zilinskas RA, Kuhn JH. *The Soviet biological weapons program: A history.* Cambridge, MA: Harvard University Press, 2012.

5. Penn RL. Francisella tularensis (tularemia). In: Mandell GL, Bennett JE, Dolin R, eds. *Mandell, Douglas, and Bennett's principles and practice of infectious diseases.* 7th ed. Philadelphia, PA: Churchill Livingstone Elsevier, 2010:2927–37.

6. CDC. Tularemia—United States, 2001–2010. *MMWR Morb Mortal Wkly Rep* 2013;62:963–6.

7. Public Health Agency of Canada. *Francisella tularensis—Material Safety Data Sheets (MSDS).* (Accessed March 28, 2014, at http://www.phac-aspc.gc.ca/lab-bio/res/psds-ftss/msds68e-eng.php.)

8. Francis E. Tularemia. *JAMA* 1925;84:1243–50.

9. Croddy E, Krcalova S. Tularemia, biological warfare, and the Battle for Stalingrad (1942–1943). *Mil Med* 2001;166:837–8.

10. Thomas LD, Schaffner W. Tularemia pneumonia. *Infect Dis Clin North Am* 2010;24:43–55.

11. Shapiro DS, Schwartz DR. Exposure of laboratory workers to Francisella tularensis despite a bioterrorism procedure. *J Clin Microbiol* 2002;40:2278–81.

12. Siegel JD, Rhinehart E, Jackson M, Chiarello L, and the Healthcare Infection Control Practices Advisory Committee. *2007 guideline for isolation precautions: Preventing transmission of infectious agents in healthcare settings.* (Accessed March 18, 2014, at http://www.cdc.gov/hicpac/2007IP/2007isolationPrecautions.html.)

13. Rusnak J, Kortepeter M, Hawley R, Andersen A, Boudeau E, Eitzen E. Risk of occupationally acquired illnesses from biological threat agents in unvaccinated laboratory workers. *Biosecur Bioterror* 2004;2:1–13.

Smallpox

1. Fenner F, Henderson DA, Arita I, Jezek A, Ladnyi ID. *Smallpox and its eradication.* Geneva: World Health Organization, 1988.

2. Bray M, Buller M. Looking back at smallpox. *Clin Infect Dis* 2004;38:882–9.

3. Breman JG, Henderson DA. Diagnosis and management of smallpox. *N Engl J Med* 2002;346:1300–8.

4. Prichard MN, Kern ER. Orthopoxvirus targets for the development of antiviral therapies. *Curr Drug Targets Infect Disord* 2005;5:17–28.

5. Fenn EA. *Pox Americana: The great smallpox epidemic of 1775–82.* New York: Hill and Wang, 2001:88–89.

6. Henderson DA, Inglesby TV, Bartlett JG, et al. Smallpox as a biological weapon: Medical and public health management. *JAMA* 1999;281:2127–37.

7. Khalil AS, Collins JJ. Synthetic biology: Applications come of age. *Nature reviews. Genetics* 2010;11:367–79.

8. Esposito JJ, Sammons SA, Frace AM, et al. Genome sequence diversity and clues to the evolution of variola (smallpox) virus. *Science* 2006;313:807–12.

9. McFadden G. Poxvirus tropism. *Nat Rev Microbiol* 2005;3:201–13.

10. Damon IK, Esposito JJ. *Poxvirus infections in humans.* Washington, DC: American Society for Microbiology Press, 2003.

11. Downie AW, Fedson DS, Saint Vincent L, Rao AR, Kempe CH. Haemorrhagic smallpox. *J Hyg (Lond)* 1969;67:619–29.

12. Downie AW, Saint Vincent L, Goldstein L, Rao AR, Kempe CH. Antibody response in non-haemorrhagic smallpox patients. *J Hyg (Lond)* 1969;67:609–18.

13. Zaucha GM, Jahrling PB, Geisbert TW, Swearengen JR, Hensley L. The pathology of experimental aerosolized monkeypox virus infection in cynomolgus monkeys (*Macaca fascicularis*). *Lab Invest* 2001;81:1581–1600.

14. Reed KD, Melski JW, Graham MB, et al. The detection of monkeypox in humans in the Western Hemisphere. *N Engl J Med* 2004;350:342–50.

15. Di Giulio DB, Eckburg PB. Human monkeypox: An emerging zoonosis. *Lancet Infect* Dis 2004;4:15–25.

16. Chen N, Li G, Liszewski MK, et al. Virulence differences between monkeypox virus isolates from West Africa and the Congo basin. *Virology* 2005;340:46–63.

17. CDC. Evaluating patients for smallpox [poster]. (Accessed April 10, 2015, at http://www.bt.cdc.gov/agent/smallpox/diagnosis/pdf/spox-poster-full.pdf.)

18. Ibrahim SM, Kulesh DA, Saleh SS, et al. Real-time PCR assay to detect smallpox virus. *J Clin Microbiol* 2003;41:3835–9.

19. Kulesh DA, Baker RO, Loveless BM, et al. Smallpox and pan-orthopox virus detection by real-time 3'-minor groove binder TaqMan assays on the Roche LightCycler and the Cepheid Smart Cycler platforms. *J Clin Microbiol* 2004;42:601–9.

20. McClain DJ, Harrison S, Yeager CL, et al. Immunologic responses to vaccinia vaccines administered by different parenteral routes. *J Infect Dis* 1997;175:756–63.

21. Painter W, Robertson A, Trost LC, Godkin S, Lampert B, Painter G. First pharmacokinetic and safety study in humans of the novel lipid antiviral conjugate CMX001, a broad-spectrum oral drug active against double-stranded DNA viruses. *Antimicrob Agents Chemother* 2012;56:2726–34.

22. Lederman ER, Davidson W, Groff HL, et al. Progressive vaccinia: Case description and laboratory-guided therapy with vaccinia immune globulin, ST-246, and CMX001. *J Infect Dis* 2012;206:1372–85.

23. Greenberg RN, Kennedy JS. ACAM2000: A newly licensed cell culture–based live vaccinia smallpox vaccine. *Expert Opin Investig Drugs* 2008;17:555–64.

24. CDC. Supplemental recommendations on adverse events following smallpox vaccine in the pre-event vaccination program: Recommendations of the Advisory Committee on Immunization Practices. *MMWR Morb Mortal Wkly Rep* 2003;52:282–4.

25. CDC. Smallpox vaccine adverse events monitoring and response system for the first stage of the smallpox vaccination program. *MMWR Morb Mortal Wkly Rep* 2003;52:88–9, 99.

26. Chen RT, Lane JM. Myocarditis: The unexpected return of smallpox vaccine adverse events. *Lancet* 2003;362:1345–6.

27. Redfield RR, Wright DC, James WD, Jones TS, Brown C, Burke DS. Disseminated vaccinia in a military recruit with human immunodeficiency virus (HIV) disease. *N Engl J Med* 1987;316:673–6.

28. Frey SE, Winokur PL, Salata RA, et al. Safety and immunogenicity of IMVAMUNE(R) smallpox vaccine using different strategies for a post event scenario. *Vaccine* 2013;31:3025–33.

29. Reidmann EM. FDA Fast Track status for IMVAMUNE. *Hum Vaccin* 2010;6(5):368–72.

30. Kennedy JS, Greenberg RN. IMVAMUNE: Modified vaccinia Ankara strain as an attenuated smallpox vaccine. *Expert Rev Vaccines* 2009;8:13–24.

Equine Encephalitides (VEE, EEE, and WEE)

1. Griffin D. Alphaviruses. In: Knipe DM, Howley PM, eds. *Fields virology.* Philadelphia, PA: Lippincott Williams & Wilkins, 2007:1023–68.

2. Weaver SC, Winegar R, Manger ID, Foreester NL. Alphaviruses: Population genetics and determinants of emergence. *Antiviral Res* 2012;94(3):242–57.

3. Steele KE, Reed DS, Glass PJ, et al. Alphavirus encephalitides. In: Dembek ZF, ed. *Medical aspects of biological warfare.* Textbooks of Military Medicine Series. Washington, DC: Borden Institute; Office of the Surgeon General, U.S. Army, 2007:241–70.

4. Weaver SC, Barrett AD. Transmission cycles, host range, evolution and emergence of arboviral disease. *Nat Rev Microbiol* 2004;2(10):789–801.

5. Arrigo NC, Adams AP, Weaver SC. Evolutionary patterns of eastern equine encephalitis virus in North versus South America suggest ecological differences and taxonomic revision. *J Virol* 2010;84(2):1014–25.

6. Brault AC, Powers AM, Chavez CLV, et al. Genetic and antigenic diversity among eastern equine encephalitis viruses from North, Central, and South America. *Am J Trop Med Hyg* 1999;61(4):579–86.

7. Steele KE, Twenhafel N. Review paper: Pathology of animal models of alphavirus encephalitis. *Vet Pathol* 2010;45(7):790–805.

8. Calisher CH. Medically important arboviruses of the United States and Canada. *Clin Microbiol Rev* 1994;7(1):89–116.

9. National Security Agency. *National security decision memorandum, November 25.* Washington, DC: NSA, 1969.

10. Meyer KF, Haring CM, Howitt B. The etiology of epizootic encephalomyelitis of horses in the San Joaquin Valley, 1930. *Science* 1931;74(1913):227–8.

11. Tenbroeck C, Hurst EW, Traub E. Epidemiology of equine encephalomyelitis in the eastern United States. *J Exp Med* 1935;62(5):677–85.

12. Giltner LT, Shahan MS. The immunological relationship of eastern and western strains of equine encephalomyelitis virus. *Science* 1933;78(2034):587–8.

13. Giltner LT, Shahan MS. Transmission of infectious equine encephalomyelitis in mammals and birds. *Science* 1933;78(2012):63–4.

14. Giltner LT, Shahan MS. The 1933 outbreak of infectious equine encephalomyelitis in the eastern states. *North American Veterinarian* 1933;14:25–7.

15. Kubes V, Rios FA. The causative agent of infectious equine encephalomyelitis in Venezuela. *Science* 1939;90:20–1.

16. Rivas F, Diaz LA, Cardenas VM, et al. Epidemic Venezuelan equine encephalitis in La Guajira, Colombia, 1995. *J Infect Dis* 1997;175(4):828–32.

17. Quiroz E, Aguilar PV, Cisneros J, Tesh RB, Weaver SC. Venezuelan equine encephalitis in Panama: Fatal endemic disease and genetic diversity of etiologic viral strains. *PLoS Negl Trop Dis* 2009;3(6):e472.

18. Navarro JC, Medina G, Vasquez C, et al. Postepizootic persistence of Venezuelan equine encephalitis virus, Venezuela. *Emerg Infect Dis* 2005;11(12):1907–15.

19. Richmond JY, McKinney RW, eds. *Biosafety in microbiological and biomedical laboratories.* 4th ed. Washington, DC: U.S. Government Printing Office, 1999.

20. Reisen WK, Monath TP. Western equine encephalomyelitis. In: Monath TP, ed. *The arboviruses: Epidemiology and ecology.* Boca Raton, FL: CRC Press, Inc., 1988:89–137.

21. Reisen WK, Kramer LD, Chiles RE, Green EGN, Martinez VM. Encephalitis virus persistence in California birds: Preliminary studies with house finches. *J Med Entomol* 2001;38(3):393–9.

22. CDC. Confirmed and probable western equine encephalitis virus neuroinvasive disease cases, H, United States, 1964–2010, by state. [April 15, 2014]; (Accessed month day, year, at http://www.cdc.gov/ncidod/dvbid/arbor/arbocase/wee_cases.)

23. Mossel EC, Ledermann JP, Phillips AT, Borland EM, Powers AM, Olson KE. Molecular determinants of mouse neurovirulence and mosquito infection for western equine encephalitis virus. *PLoS One* 2013;8(3):e60427.

24. Franck PT, Johnson KM. An outbreak of Venezuelan encephalitis in man in the Panama Canal Zone. *Am J Trop Med Hyg* 1970;19(5):860–5.

25. Martin DH, Sudia WD, Eddy GA, Reeves WC, Johnson KM, Newhouse VF. An epidemiologic study of Venezuelan equine encephalomyelitis in Costa Rica, 1970. *Am J Epidemiol* 1972;95(6):565–78.

26. Bowen GS, Fashinell TR, Dean PB, Gregg MB. Clinical aspects of human Venezuelan equine encephalitis in Texas. *Bull Pan Am Health Organ* 1976;10(1):46–57.

27. Sanmartin C, MacKenzie RB, Trapido H, et al. [Venezuelan equine encephalitis in Colombia, 1967]. *Bol Oficina Sanit Panam* 1973;74(2):108–37.

28. Charles PC, Walters E, Margolis F, Johnston RE. Mechanism of neuroinvasion of Venezuelan equine encephalitis virus in the mouse. *Virology* 1995;208(2):662–71.

29. Ryzhikov AB, Ryabchikova EI, Sergeev AN, Tkacheva NV. Spread of Venezuelan equine encephalitis virus in mice olfactory tract. *Arch Virol* 1995;140(12):2243–54.

30. Ryzhikov AB, Tkacheva NV, Sergeev AN, Ryabchikova EI. Venezuelan equine encephalitis virus propagation in the olfactory tract of normal and immunized mice. *Biomed Sci* 1991;2(6):607–14.

31. Steele KE, Davis KJ, Stephan K, Kell W, Vogel P, Hart MK. Comparative neurovirulence and tissue tropism of wild-type and attenuated strains of Venezuelan equine encephalitis virus administered by aerosol in C3H/HeN and BALB/c mice. *Vet Pathol* 1998;35(5):386–97.

32. Vogel P, Abplanalp D, Kell W, et al. Venezuelan equine encephalitis in BALB/c mice: Kinetic analysis of central nervous system infection following aerosol or subcutaneous inoculation. *Arch Pathol Lab Med* 1996;120(2):164–72.

33. Danes L, Kufner J, Hruskova J, Rychtero V. The role of the olfactory route on infection of the respiratory tract with Venezuelan equine encephalomyelitis virus in normal and operated Macaca rhesus monkeys. I. Results of virological examination. *Acta Virol* 1973;17(1):50–6.

34. Johnson KM, Shelokov A, Peralta PH, Dammin GJ, Young NA. Recovery of Venezuelan equine encephalomyelitis virus in Panama. A fatal case in man. *Am J Trop Med Hyg* 1968;17(3):432–40.

35. Leon CA. Sequelae of Venezuelan equine encephalitis in humans: A four year follow-up. *Int J Epidemiol* 1975;4(2):131–40.

36. Weaver SC, Salas R, RicoHesse R, et al. Re-emergence of epidemic Venezuelan equine encephalomyelitis in South America. VEE Study Group. *Lancet* 1996;348:436–40.

37. Goldfield M, Welsh JN, Taylor BF. The 1959 outbreak of Eastern encephalitis in New Jersey. 5. The inapparent infection:disease ratio. *Am J Epidemiol* 1968;87(1):32–3.

38. Goldfield M, Taylor BF, Welsh JN. The 1959 outbreak of Eastern encephalitis in New Jersey. 6. The frequency of prior infection. *Am J Epidemiol* 1968;87(1):39–49.

39. CDC. Eastern equine encephalitis—New Hampshire and Massachusetts, August–September 2005. *MMWR Morb Mortal Wkly Rep* 2006;55(25):697–700.

40. Hart KL, Keen D, Belle EA. An outbreak of eastern equine encephalomyelitis in Jamaica, West Indies. I. Description of human cases. *Am J Trop Med Hyg* 1964;13:331–4.

41. Deresiewicz RL, Thaler SJ, Hsu LG, Zamani AA. Clinical and neuroradiographic manifestations of eastern equine encephalitis. *N Engl J Med* 1997;336(26):1867–74.

42. Przelomski MM, Orourke E, Grady GF, Berardi VP, Markley HG. Eastern equine encephalitis in Massachusetts: A report of 16 cases, 1970–1984. *Neurology* 1988;38(5):736–9.

43. Silverman MA, Misasi J, Smole S, et al. Eastern equine encephalitis in children, Massachusetts and New Hampshire, USA, 1970–2010. *Emerg Infect Dis* 2013;19(2):194–201; quiz 352.

44. Hanson RP, Sulkin SE, Buescher EL, Hammon WM, McKinney RW, Work TH. Arbovirus infections of laboratory workers. Extent of problem emphasizes the need for more effective measures to reduce hazards. *Science* 1967;158(806):1283–6.

45. Reed DS, Larsen T, Sullivan LJ, et al. Aerosol exposure to western equine encephalitis virus causes fever and encephalitis in cynomolgus macaques. *J Infect Dis* 2005;192(7):1173–82.

46. Reeves WC, Hammon WM, Longshore WA Jr., McClure HE, Geib AF. *Epidemiology of the arthropod-borne viral encephalitides in Kern County, California, 1943–1952*. Publications in Public Health University of California 1962;4:1–257.

47. Shinefield HR, Townsend TE. Transplacental transmission of western equine encephalomyelitis. *J Pediatr* 1953;43(1):21–5.

48. Calisher CH, Emerson JK, Muth DJ, Lazuick JS, Monath TP. Serodiagnosis of western equine encephalitis virus infections: Relationships of antibody titer and test to observed onset of clinical illness. *J Am Vet Med Assoc* 1983;183(4):438–40.

49. Bartelloni PJ, McKinney RW, Duffy TP, Cole FE. An inactivated eastern equine encephalomyelitis vaccine propagated in chick-embryo cell culture. II. Clinical and serologic responses in man. *Am J Trop Med Hyg* 1970;19(1):123–6.

50. Bartelloni PJ, McKinney RW, Calia FM, Ramsburg HH, Cole FE. Inactivated western equine encephalomyelitis vaccine propagated in chick embryo cell culture. Clinical and serological evaluation in man. *Am J Trop Med Hyg* 1971;20(1):146–9.

51. Lukaszewski RA, Brooks TJ. Pegylated alpha interferon is an effective treatment for virulent Venezuelan equine encephalitis virus and has profound effects on the host immune response to infection. *J Virol* 2000;74(11):5006–15.

Viral Hemorrhagic Fevers (VHFs)

1. Leitenberg M, Zilinskas RA, Kuhn JH. *The Soviet biological weapons program: A history.* Cambridge, MA: Harvard University Press, 2012:253.

2. Jahrling PB, Marty AM, Geisbert TW. Viral hemorrhagic fevers. In: Dembek ZF, ed. *Medical aspects of biological warfare.* Textbooks of Military Medicine Series. Washington, DC: Bordon Institute; Office of the Surgeon General, U.S. Army, 2007:271–310.

3. Charrel RN, de Lamballerie X. Arenaviruses other than Lassa virus. *Antiviral Res* 2003;57:89–100.

4. CDC. Update: Management of patients with suspected viral hemorrhagic fever—United States. *MMWR Morb Mortal Wkly Rep* 1995;44:475–9.

5. Garner JS. Guideline for isolation precautions in hospitals. Part I. Evolution of isolation practices, Hospital Infection Control Practices Advisory Committee. *Am J Infect Control* 1996;24:24–31.

6. Yun NE, Walker DH. Pathogenesis of Lassa fever. *Viruses* 2012;4:2031–48.

7. CDC. Lassa fever. (Accessed April 13, 2015, at http://www.cdc.gov/vhf/lassa/.)

8. Whitehouse CA. Crimean–Congo hemorrhagic fever. *Antiviral Res* 2004;64:145–60.

9. CDC. Rift Valley fever (RVF). (Accessed March 12, 2014, at http://www.cdc.gov/vhf/rvf/.)

10. CDC. CDC Select Agent Program. Atlanta, GA: CDC. (Accessed March, 14, 2014, at http://www.cdc.gov/phpr/documents/DSAT_brochure_July2011.pdf.)

11. Schmaljohn C, Hjelle B. Hantaviruses: A global disease problem. *Emerg Infect Dis* 1997;3:95–104.

12. Miettinen MH, Makela SM, Ala-Houhala IO, et al. Ten-year prognosis of Puumala hantavirus-induced acute interstitial nephritis. *Kidney Int* 2006;69:2043–8.

13. Bukreyev AA, Chandran K, Dolnik O, et al. Discussions and decisions of the 2012–2014 International Committee on Taxonomy of Viruses (ICTV) Filoviridae Study Group, January 2012–June 2013. *Arch Virol* 2014;159:821–30.

14. Khan AS, Tshioko FK, Heymann DL, et al. The reemergence of Ebola hemorrhagic fever, Democratic Republic of the Congo, 1995. Commission de Lutte contre les Epidemies a Kikwit. *J Infect Dis* 1999;179(suppl 1):S76–86.

15. CDC. Outbreaks chronology: Ebola virus disease. 2014. (Accessed April 13, 2015, at http://www.cdc.gov/vhf/ebola/outbreaks/history/chronology.html.)

16. Marsh GA, Haining J, Robinson R, et al. Ebola Reston virus infection of pigs: Clinical significance and transmission potential. *J Infect Dis* 2011;204(Suppl 3):S804–9.

17. Formenty P, Hatz C, Le Guenno B, Stoll A, Rogenmoser P, Widmer A. Human infection due to Ebola virus, subtype Côte d'Ivoire: Clinical and biologic presentation. *J Infect Dis* 1999;179 Suppl 1:S48–53.

18. Roddy P, Howard N, Van Kerkhove MD, et al. Clinical manifestations and case management of Ebola haemorrhagic fever caused by a newly identified virus strain, Bundibugyo, Uganda, 2007–2008. *PloS One* 2012;7:e52986.

19. Ligon BL. Outbreak of Marburg hemorrhagic fever in Angola: A review of the history of the disease and its biological aspects. *Semin Pediatr Infect Dis* 2005;16:219–24.

20. CDC. Imported case of Marburg hemorrhagic fever—Colorado, 2008. *MMWR Morb Mortal Wkly Rep* 2009;58:1377–81.

21. Mahanty S, Bray M. Pathogenesis of filoviral haemorrhagic fevers. *Lancet Infect Dis* 2004;4:487–98.

22. Borio L, Inglesby T, Peters CJ, et al. Hemorrhagic fever viruses as biological weapons: Medical and public health management. *JAMA* 2002;287:2391–405.

23. Buchmeier MJ, de la Torre JC, Peters CJ. Arenaviridae: The viruses and their replication. In: Knipe DM, Howley PM, eds. *Fields Virology*. Philadelphia, PA: Lippincott, Williams & Wilkins, 2007:1791–827.

24. CDC. Crimean–Congo hemorrhagic fever (CCHF): Signs and symptoms. (Accessed March 18, 2014, at http://www.cdc.gov/vhf/crimean-congo/symptoms/index.html.)

25. Schmaljohn CS, Nichol ST. Bunyaviridae. In: Knipe DM, Howley PM, eds. *Fields Virology*. Philadelphia, PA: Lippincott, Williams & Wilkins, 2007:1741–89.

26. CDC. Yellow fever: Symptoms and treatment. (Accessed March 19, 2014, at http://www.cdc.gov/yellowfever/symptoms/index.html#symptoms.)

27. Tuboi SH, Costa ZG, da Costa Vasconcelos PF, Hatch D. Clinical and epidemiological characteristics of yellow fever in Brazil: Analysis of reported cases 1998–2002. *Trans R Soc Trop Med Hyg* 2007;101:169–75.

28. CDC. Omsk hemorrhagic fever (OHF): Signs and symptoms. (Accessed March 19, 2014, at http://www.cdc.gov/vhf/omsk/symptoms/index.html.)

29 CDC. Kyasanur Forest disease (KFD). (Accessed March 19, 2014, at http://www.cdc.gov/vhf/kyasanur/.)

30. Kortepeter MG, Bausch DG, Bray M. Basic clinical and laboratory features of filoviral hemorrhagic fever. *J Infect Dis* 2011;204(Suppl 3):S810–6.

31. Borio L, Inglesby T, Peters CJ, et al. Hemorrhagic fever viruses as biological weapons—Medical and public health management. *JAMA* 2002; 287:2391–405.

32. CDC. Infection prevention and control recommendations for hospitalized patients under investigation (PUIs) for Ebola virus disease (EVD) in U.S. hospitals. (Accessed October 18, 2014, at http://www.cdc.gov/vhf/ebola/hcp/infection-prevention-and-control-recommendations.html.)

Botulism

- Angulo FJ, Getz J, Taylor JP, et al. A large outbreak of botulism: The hazardous baked potato. *J Infect Dis* 1998;178:172–7.
- Arnon SS, Schecter R, Inglesby TV, et al. Botulism toxin as a biological weapon: Medical and public health management. *JAMA* 2001;285:1059–70.
- Arnon SS, Schechter R, Maslanka SE, et al. Human botulism immune globulin for the treatment of infant botulism. *N Engl J Med* 2006;354:462–71.
- Bleck TP. Botulism as a potential agent of bioterrorism. In: Fong IW, Alibek K, eds. *Bioterrorism and infectious agents: A new dilemma for the 21st century*. New York: Springer, 2005:194–5.
- CDC. Investigational heptavalent botulinum antitoxin (HBAT) to replace licensed botulinum antitoxin AB and investigational botulinum antitoxin E. *MMWR Morb Mortal Wkly Rep* 2010;59(10):299.
- Dembek ZF, Smith LA, Rusnak JM. Botulism: Its cause, effects, diagnosis, clinical and laboratory identification and treatment modalities. *Disaster Med Public Health Prep* 2007;1:122–134.
- CDC. Botulism in the United States 1899–1996. In: *Handbook for epidemiologists, clinicians, and laboratory workers*. Atlanta, GA: CDC, 1998.

- Hakami RM, Ruthel G, Stahl AM, Bavari S. Gaining ground: Assays for therapeutics against botulinum neurotoxin. *Trends Microbiol* 2010;18:164–72.
- Rusnak JM, Smith LA. Botulinum neurotoxin vaccines: Past history and recent developments. *Hum Vacc* 2009;5:794–805.
- Shapiro RL, Hatheway C, Becher J, Swerdlow DL. Botulism surveillance and emergency response: A public health strategy for a global challenge. *JAMA* 1997;278:433–5.
- Shapiro RL, Hatheway C, Swerdlow DL. Botulism in the United States: A clinical and epidemiologic review. *Ann Intern Med* 1998;129:221–8.
- Smith LA. Botulism and vaccines for its prevention. *Vaccine* 2009;27(Suppl 4):D33–D39.
- CDC. Wound botulism—California, 1995. *MMWR Morb Mortal Wkly Rep* 1995;44:200–202.

Ricin

1. Griffiths GD. Understanding ricin from a defensive viewpoint. *Toxins* 2011;3:1373–92.

2. Griffiths GD, Phillips GJ, Holley J. Inhalation toxicology of ricin preparations: Animal models, prophylactic and therapeutic approaches to protection. *Inhal Toxicol* 2007;19:873–87.

3. Spivak L, Hendrickson RG. Ricin. *Crit Care Clin* 2005;21:815–24.

4. Musshoff F, Madea B. Ricin poisoning and forensic toxicology. *Drug Test Anal* 2009;1:184–91.

5. Smart JK. History of chemical and biological warfare: An American perspective. In: Sidell FR, Takafuji ET, Franz DR, eds. *Medical aspects of chemical and biological warfare.* Textbook of Military Medicine. Part I: Warfare, weaponry, and the casualty. Washington, DC: Borden Institute; Office of the Surgeon General, U.S. Army, 1997:9–86.

6. CDC. Investigation of a ricin-containing envelope at a postal facility—South Carolina, 2003. *MMWR Morb Mortal Wkly Rep* 2003;52:1129–31.

7. Olsnes S, Kozlov JV. Ricin. *Toxicon* 2001;39:1723–8.

8. Kortepeter M, Parker G. Potential biological weapons threats. *Emerg Infect Dis* 1999;5:523–7.

9. Audi J, Belson M, Patel M, Schier J, Osterloh J. Ricin poisoning: A comprehensive review. *JAMA* 2005;294:2342–51.

10. Roy CJ, Hale M, Hartings JM, Pitt L, Duniho S. Impact of inhalation exposure modality and particle size on the respiratory deposition of ricin in BALB/c mice. *Inhal Toxicol* 2003;15:619–38.

11. Bradberry SM, Dickers KJ, Rice P, Griffiths GD, Vale JA. Ricin poisoning. *Toxicol Rev* 2003;22(1):65–70.

12. Bigalke H, Rummel A. Medical aspects of toxin weapons. *Toxicology* 2005;214:210–20.

13. Worbes S, Kohler K, Pauly D, et al. Ricinus communis intoxications in human and veterinary medicine—a summary of real cases. *Toxins* 2011;3:1332–72.

14. Ramsden C, Drayson M, Bell E. The toxicity, distribution, and excretion of ricin holotoxin in rats. *Toxicology* 1989;55:161–71.

15. He X, McMahon S, Henderson TD II, Griffey SM, Cheng LW. Ricin toxicokinetics and its sensitive detection in mouse sera or feces using immuno-PCR. *PLoS ONE* 2010;5(9):e12858.

16. Holley JL, Poole SJC, Cooper IAM, Griffiths GD, Simpson AJ. (2007). The production and evaluation of ricin antitoxins. In: *Defence against the effects of chemical hazards: Toxicology, diagnosis and medical countermeasures. Proceedings of the Human Factors and Medicine Panel (HFM) Symposium, Edinburgh, Scotland, October 8–10, 2007.* Neuilly-sur-Seine, France: Research and Technology Organisation, 2007:12-1–12-8. (RTO-MP-HFM-149, paper 12).

17. Kortepeter M, Cieslak T, Eitzen E. Bioterrorism. *J Environ Health* 2001;63: 21–4.

18. Marsden CJ, Smith DC, Roberts LM, Lord JM. Ricin: Current understanding and prospects for an antiricin vaccine. *Expert Rev Vaccines* 2005;4:229–37.

19. Smith, LA. *Efforts to develop a recombinant ricin toxin A-chain 1–33/44–198 (rRTA 1–33/44–198) Vaccine (RVEc™)*. FY2013 Annual Report, December 2013. Unpublished report.

Staphylococcal Enterotoxin B

1. Lina G, Bohach GA, Nair SP, Hiramatsu K, Jourvin-Marche E, Mariuzza R. Standard nomenclature for the superantigens expressed by Staphylococcus. *J Infect Dis* 2004;189:2334–6.

2. Ono HK, Omoe K, Imanishi K, et al. Identification and characterization of two novel staphylococcal enterotoxins, types S and T. *Infect Immun* 2008;76:4999–5005.

3. Chiang YC, Liao WW, Fan CM, Pai WY, Chiou CS, Tsen HY. PCR detection of staphylococcal enterotoxins (SEs) N, O, P, P, R, U, and survey of SE types in Staphylococcus aureus isolates from food-poisoning cases in Taiwan. *Int J Food Microbiol* 2008;121:66–73.

4. Letertre C, Perelle S, Kilasser F, Fach P. Identification of a new putative enterotoxin SEU encoded by the egc cluster of Staphylococcus aureus. *J Appl Microbiol* 2003;95:38–43.

5. Balaban N, Rasooly A. Staphylococcal enterotoxins. *Int J Food Microbiol* 2000;61:1–10.

6. Krakauer T, Stiles BG. The staphylococcal enterotoxin (SE) family. SEB and siblings. *Virulence* 2013;4:759–73.

7. Raj HD, Berfdoll MS. Effect of enterotoxin B on human volunteers. *J Bacteriol* 1969;90:833–4.

8. Rusnak JM, Kortepeter M, Ulrich R, Poli M, Boudreau E. Laboratory exposures to staphylococcal enterotoxin B. *Emerg Infect Dis* 2004;10:1544–9.

9. U.S. Department of Health and Human Services. *Biosafety in microbiological and biomedical laboratories.* 5th ed. Washington DC: U.S. Government Printing Office, 2007. (HHS Publication no. (CDC) 21-1112.) (Accessed March 24, 2014, at http://www.cdc.gov/biosafety/publications/bmbl5/BMBL.pdf.)

10. LeClaire RD, Pitt MLM. Biological weapons defense: Effect levels. In: Lindler LE, Lebeda FJ, Korch GW, eds. *Biological weapons defense: Infectious diseases and counter bioterrorism.* Totowa, NJ: Humana Press, Inc., 2005:41–61.

11. Argudin MA, Mendoza MC, Rodicio MR. Food poisoning and *Staphylococcus aureus* enterotoxins. *Toxins* 2010;2:1751–73.

12. Krakauer T. Immune response to staphylococcal superantigens. *Immunol Res* 1999;29:163–73.

13. Schwabe, Notermans S, Boot R, et al. Inactivation of staphylococcal enterotoxins by heat and reactivation by high pH treatment. *Int J Food Microbiol* 1990;10:33–42.

14. Genigeorgis CA. Present state of knowledge on staphylococcal intoxication. *Int J Food Microbiol* 1989;9:327–60.

15. Strange P, Skov L, Lisby S, Nielsen PL, Baadsgaard O. Staphylococcal enterotoxin B applied to normal and intact atopic skin induces dermatitis. *Arch Dermatol* 1996;132:27–33.

16. Wedum AG. The Detrick experience as a guide to the probable efficacy of P4 microbiological containment facilities for studies in microbial recombinant DNA molecules. *J Am Biol Saf Assoc* 1996;1:7–25.

17. Hursh SR, McNally RP, Fanzone JF Jr., Mershon MM. *Staphylococcal enterotoxin B battlefield challenge modeling with medical and nonmedical countermeasures: Computerized simulations of staphylococcal enterotoxin B aerosol dosage impacts on casualty levels and preservation of unit effectiveness by countermeasures.* Joppa, MD: Science Applications International Corporation, 1995. (Technical Report MBDRP-95-2).

18. Dinges MM, Orwin PM, Schlievert PM. Exotoxins of *Staphylococcus aureus. Clin Microbiol Rev* 2000;13:16–34.

19. Seprenyi G, Shibata T, Onody R, Kohsaka T. In staphylococcus enterotoxin B (SEB)–stimulated human PBMC, the LAK activity of non–T cells might have a major role in the mechanism of glomerular endothelial cells' injury. *Immunobiology* 1997;197:44–54.

20. Ulrich RG, Wilhelmsen CL, Krakauer TD. Staphylococcal enterotoxin B and related toxins. In: Dembek ZF, ed. *Medical aspects of biological warfare*. Textbooks of Military Medicine Series. Washington, DC: Borden Institute; Office of the Surgeon General, U.S. Army, 2007:311–22.

21. Ahanotu E, Alvelo-Ceron D, Ravita T, Gaunt E. Staphylococcal enterotoxin B as a biological weapon: Recognition, management, and surveillance of staphylococcal enterotoxin. *Appl Biosaf* 2006;11:120–6.

22. Krakauer T, Stiles BG. Staphylococcal enterotoxins, toxic shock syndrome toxin-1, and streptococcal pyrogenic exotoxins: Some basic biology of bacterial superantigens. *Recent Res Dev Infect Immun* 2003;1:1–27.

23. Mattix ME, Hunt R, Wilhelmsen C, Johnson A, Baze W. Aerosolized staphylococcal enterotoxin B–induced pulmonary lesions in rhesus monkeys (*Macaca mulatta*). *Toxicol Pathol* 1995;23:262–8.

24. Madesen JM. Toxins as weapons of mass destruction. A comparison and contrast with biological-warfare and chemical warfare agents. *Clin Lab Med* 2001;21:593–605.

25. Peruski AH, Peruski LF. Immunological methods for detection and identification of infectious disease and biological warfare agents. *Clin Diagn Lab Immunol* 2003;10:506–13.

26. Peruski LF, Peruski AH. Rapid diagnostic assays in the genomic biology era: Detection and identification of infectious disease and biological weapon agents. *BioTechniques* 2003;35:840–6.

27. Boyle T, Njoroge JM, Jone RL, Principato M. Detection of staphylococcal enterotoxin B in milk and milk products using immunodiagnostic lateral flow devices. *J AOAC Int* 2010;93:569–75.

28. Tsui P-Y, Chiao D-J, Wey J-J, Liu C-C, Yu C-P, Shyu R-H. Development of staphylococcal enterotoxin B detection strips and application of SEB detection strips in food. *J Med Sci* 2013;33:285–91.

29. Schotte U, Langfeldt N, Peruski AH, Meyer H. Detection of staphylococcal enterotoxin B (SEB) by enzyme-linked immunosorbent assay and by a rapid hand-held assay. *Clin Lab* 2002;48:395–400.

30. Lapeyre C. Immunoenzymatic detection of Staphylococcal enterotoxins: International interlaboratory study. *J AOAC Int* 1996;79:1095–1101.

31. Bennett RW. Staphylococcal enterotoxin and its rapid identification in foods by enzyme-linked immunosorbent assay–based methodology. *J Food Prot* 2005;68:1264–75.

32. Cook E, Wang X, Robiou N, Fries BC. Measurement of staphylococcal enterotoxin B in serum and other supernatant with a capture enzyme-linked immunosorbent assay. *Clin Vaccine Immunol* 2007;14:1094–1101.

33. Thompson NE, Razdan M, Kuntsmann G, Aschenbach JM, Evenson ML, Gergdoll MS. Detection of staphylococcal enterotoxins by enzyme-linked immunosorbent assays and radioimmunoassay: Comparison of monoclonal and polyclonal antibody systems. *Appl Environ Microbiol* 1986;51:885–90.

34. Sasaki T, Terano Y, Shibata T, et al. Establishment of highly specific and quantitative immunoassay systems for staphylococcal enterotoxin A, B, and C using newly-developed monoclonal antibodies. *Microbiol Immunol* 2005;49:589–97.

35. Peruski AH, Johnson LH, Peruski LF. Rapid and sensitive detection of biological warfare agents using time-resolved fluorescence assays. *J Immunol Meth* 2002;263:35–41.

36. Bruno JG, Kiel JL. Use of magnetic beads in selection and detection of biotoxin aptamers by electrochemiluminescence and enzymatic methods. *BioTechniques* 2002;32:178-83.

37. Liu F, Li Y, Song C, et al. Highly sensitive microplate chemiluminescence enzyme immunoassay for the determination of staphylococcal entertoxin B based on a pair of specific monoclonal antibodies and its application to various matrices. *Anal Chem* 2010;82:7758–65.

38. Fischer A, von Eiff C, Kuezius T, Omoe K, Peters G, Becker K. A quantitative real-time immune-PCR approach for detection of staphylococcal enterotoxins. *J Mol Med* 2007;85:461–9.

39. Panneerseelan L, Muriana PM. An immunomagnetic PCR signal amplification assay for sensitive detection of Staphylococcal aureus enterotoxins in foods. *J Food Protect* 2009;72:2538–46.

40. Nedelkov D. Rasooly A, and Nelson RW. Multitoxin biosensor-mass spectrometry analysis: A new approach for rapid, real-time, sensitive analysis of staphylococcal toxins in food. *Int J Food Microbiol* 2000;60:1–13.

41. Nedelkov D, Nelson RW. Detection of staphylococcal enterotoxin B via biomolecular interaction analysis mass spectrometry. *Appl Environ Microbiol* 2003;69:5212–15.

42. Lin C-M, Chiang Y-C, Tsen H-Y. Development and use of a chromogenic macroarray system for the detection of Staphylococcus aureus with enterotoxin A, B, D, D, E, and G genes in food and milk samples. *Foodborne Pathog Dis* 2009;6:445–52.

43. Velusamy V, Arshak K, Korostynska O, Oliwa K, Adley C. An overview of foodborne pathogen detection: In the perspective of biosensors. *Biotechnol* 2010;28:232–54.

44. Tempelman LA, King KD, Anderson GP, Ligler FS. Quantitating staphylococcal enterotoxin B in diverse media using a portable fiber-optic biosensor. *Anal Biochem* 1996;233:50–7.

45. Ruan C, Zeng K, Varghese OK, Grimes CA. A staphylococcal enterotoxin B magnetoelastic immunosensor. *Biosens Bioelectron* 2004;20:485–91.

46. Gupta G, Singh PK, Boopathi SM, Kamboj DV, Singh B, Vijayaraghavan R. Surface Plasmon resonance detection of biological warfare agent Staphylococcal enterotoxin B using high antibody monoclonal antibody. *Thin Solid Films* 2010;519:1171–7.

47. Azuma K, Koike K, Kobayashi T, Mochizuki T, Mashiko K, Yamamoto Y. Detection of circulating superantigens in an intensive care unit population. *Int J Infect Dis* 2004;8:202–90.

48. Holtfreter SK, Roschack K, Eichler K, et al. Staphylococcus aureus carriers neutralize superantigens by antibodies specific for their colonizing strain: A potential explanation for their improved prognosis in severe sepsis. *J Infect Dis* 2006;193:1275–8.

49. Mantis NJ. Vaccines against the category B toxins: Staphylococcal enterotoxin B, epsilon toxin and ricin. *Adv Drug Deliv Rev* 2005;57:1424–39.

50. Boles JW, Pitt ML, LeClaire RD, et al. Generation of protective immunity by inactivated recombinant staphylococcal enterotoxin B vaccine in nonhuman primates and identification of correlates of immunity. *Clin Immunol* 2003;108:51–9.

51. Coffman JD, Zhu J, Roach JM, Bavari S, Ulrich RG, Giardina SL. Production and purification of a recombinant Staphylococcal enterotoxin B vaccine candidate expressed in *Escherichia coli. Protein Expr Purif* 2002;24:302–12.

52. Ulrich RC, Olson MA, Bavari S. Development of engineered vaccines effective against structurally related bacterial superantigens. *Vaccine* 1998;16:1857–64.

53. LeClaire RD, Hunt RE, Bavari S. Protection against bacterial superantigen staphylococcal enterotoxin B by passive vaccination. *Infect Immun* 2002; 70:2278–81.

54. LeClaire RD, Bavari S. Human antibodies to bacterial superantigens and their ability to inhibit T-cell activation and lethality. *Antimicrob Agents Chemother* 2001;45:460–3.

55. Karauzum H, Chen G, Abaandou L, et al. Synthetic human monoclonal antibodies toward staphylococcal enterotoxin B (SEB) protective against toxic shock syndrome. *J Biol Chem* 2012; 287:25203–15.

56. Drozdowski B, Zhou Y, Kline B, et al. Generation and characterization of high affinity human monoclonal antibodies that neutralize staphylococcal enterotoxin B. *J Immune Based Ther Vaccines* 2010;8:1–9.

57. Chow S, Casadevall A. Monoclonal antibodies and toxins—a perspective on function and isotype. *Toxins* 2012;4:430–54.

58. Verkaik NJ, de Vogel CP, Boelens, et al. Anti-staphylococcal humoral immune response in persistent nasal carriers and noncarriers of *Staphylococcus aureus. J Infect Dis* 2009;199:625–32.

T-2 Mycotoxins

1. Boonen J, Malysheva SV, Taevernier L, et al. Human skin penetration of selected model mycotoxins. *Toxicology* 2012;301(1-3):21–32.

2. Ciegler A. (1975) Mycotoxins: Occurrence, chemistry, biological activity. *Lloydia* 1975;38:21–35.

3. Ciegler A, Bennett JW. Mycotoxins and mycotoxicoses. *BioScience* 1980;30:512–15.

4. Huebner KD, Wannemacher RW Jr., Stiles BG, et al. Additional toxins of clinical concern. In: Dembek ZF, ed. *Medical aspects of biological warfare.* Textbooks of Military Medicine Series. Washington, DC: Bordon Institute; Office of the Surgeon General, U.S. Army, 2007:355–89.

5. Joffe AZ. Alimentary toxic aleukia. In: Kadis S, Ciegler A, Ajl SJ, eds. *Microbiol toxins. Vol VII. Algal and fungal toxins.* New York: Academic Press, 1971:139–89.

6. Katz R, Singer B. Can an attribution assessment be made for yellow rain? Systematic reanalysis in a chemical-and-biological-weapons use investigation. *Politics Life Sci* 2007;26(1):24–42.

7. Haig AM Jr. Chemical warfare in Southeast Asia and Afghanistan. *Report to the Congress from Secretary of State Haig, 22 March 1982.* Washington, DC: U.S. Government Printing Office, 1982. (Special Report 98.)

8. Meselson MS, Perry J. The yellow rain affair: Lessons learned from a discredited allegation. In: Clunan AL, et al., eds. *Terrorism, war, or disease? Unraveling the use of biological weapons.* Redwood City, CA: Stanford University Press, 2008:72–96.

9. Watson SA, Mirocha CJ, Hayes AW. Analysis for trichothecenes in samples from Southeast Asia associated with "yellow rain." *Fundam Appl Toxicol* 1984;4:700–17.

10. Ember LR. Yellow rain. *Chem Eng News* 1984;62:8–34.

11. Seagrave S. *Yellow rain. A journey through the terror of chemical warfare.* New York: M Evans and Co., Inc., 1981.

12. Wannemacher RW Jr., Wiener SL. Threat from trichothecenes mycotoxins and their countermeasures. In: Sidell FR, Takafuji ET, Franz DR, eds. *Medical aspects of chemical and biological warfare. Textbook of Military Medicine. Part I: Warfare, weaponry, and the casualty.* Washington, DC: Borden Institute; Office of the Surgeon General, U.S. Army, 1997:655–76.

13. Leitenberg M, Zilinskas RA, Kuhn JH. *The Soviet biological weapons program: A history.* Cambridge, MA: Harvard University Press, 2012, pg 456.

14. Martin JW, Christopher GW, Eitzen EM. History of biological weapons: From poisoned darts to intentional epidemics. In: Dembek ZF, ed. *Medical aspects of biological warfare.* Textbooks of Military Medicine Series. Washington, DC: Bordon Institute; Office of the Surgeon General, U.S. Army, 2007:1–20.

15. Zilinskas RA. Iraq's biological warfare program: The past as future? In: Lederberg J ed. *Biological weapons: Limiting the threat.* Cambridge, MA: MIT Press, 1999: Chapter 8.

16. Dearborn DG, Smith PG, Brooks LJ, et al. Update: Pulmonary hemorrhage/ hemosiderosis among infants—Cleveland, Ohio 1993–1996. *MMWR Morb Mortal Wkly Rep* 1997;46:33–5.

17. Richards CA. Stachybotrys atra suspected in three infant deaths: 18 others sickened. *Pediatr Infect Dis J* 1997;10:1–8.

18. Joffee A. *Fusarium species: Their biology and toxicology.* New York: John Wiley & Sons, 1986.

19. Blazes DL, Lawler JV, Lazarus AA. When biotoxins are tools of terror. Early recognition of intentional poisoning can attenuate effects. *Postgrad Med* 2002;112(2):89–92, 95–6, 98.

20. Wu J, Jing L, Yuan H, Peng SQ. T-2 toxin induces apoptosis in ovarian granulosa cells of rats through reactive oxygen species-mediated mitochondrial pathway. *Toxicol Lett* 2011;202(3):168–77.

21. Bunner DL, Upshall DG, Bhatti AR. Toxicology data on T-2 toxin. In: *Report of Focus Officers Meeting on Mycotoxin Toxicity, September 23–24, 1985.* Suffield, AB, Canada: Defense Research Establishment at Suffield, 1985.

22. Wannemacher RW. Dermal toxicity of T-2 toxin in guinea pigs, rats and cynomolgus monkeys. In: Lacey J, ed. *Trichothecenes and Other Mycotoxins: Proceedings of the International Mycotoxin Symposium, Sydney, Australia, August 1984.* Chichester, U.K.: Wiley, 1985:423–32.

23. Poppenga RH, Lundeen GR, Beasley VR, Buck WB. Assessment of a general therapeutic protocol for the treatment of acute T-2 toxicosis in swine. *Vet Hum Toxicol* 1987;29(3):237–9.

24. U.S. Army. *Field Manual: Multiservice tactics, techniques, and procedures for treatment of chemical agent casualties and conventional military chemical injuries.* Washington, DC: Department of the Army; Quantico,

VA: Marine Corps Combat Development Command; Newport, Rhode Island: Navy Warfare Development Command; Maxwell Air Force Base, AL: Air Force Doctrine Center, 18 September 2007. (FM 4-02.285 (FM 8-285), MCRP 4-11.1A, NTRP 4-02.22, AFTTP (I) 3-2.69.), Appendix D.

25. Schwartz MD, Hurst CG, Kirk MA, Reedy SD, Braue EH Jr. Reactive skin decontamination lotion (RSDL) for the decontamination of chemical warfare agent (CWA) dermal exposure. *Curr Pharm Biotechnol* 2012;13(10):1971–9.

Emerging Threats: Novel Infectious Diseases and New Potential Bioweapons

1. Lederberg J, Shope RE, Oaks S. *Emerging infections: Microbial threats to health in the United States.* Washington, DC: Institute of Medicine, National Academy of Sciences, 1992.

2. Jones KE, Patel NG, Levy MA, et al. Global trends in emerging infectious diseases. *Nature* 2008;451:990–3.

3. Garten RJ, Davis CT, Russell CA, et al. Antigenic and genetic characteristics of swine-origin 2009 A(H1N1) influenza viruses circulating in humans. *Science* 2009;325:197–201.

4. WHO. Cumulative number of confirmed human cases for avian influenza A(H5N1) reported to WHO, 2003–2013 [data tables]. Geneva: WHO. (Accessed April 14, 2015, at http://www.who.int/influenza/human_animal_interface/EN_GIP_20130604CumulativeNumberH5N1cases.pdf.)

5. WHO. Influenza: Avian influenza A(H7N9) virus. (Accessed April 14, 2015, at http://www.who.int/influenza/human_animal_interface/influenza_h7n9/en/.)

6. WHO. Global Alert and Response (GAR): Summary of probable SARS cases with onset of illness from 1 November 2002 to 31 July 2003. (Accessed April 14, 2015, at http://www.who.int/csr/sars/country/table2004_04_21/en/.)

7. Zaki AM, van Boheemen S, Bestebroer TM, Osterhaus AD, Fouchier RA. Isolation of a novel coronavirus from a man with pneumonia in Saudi Arabia. *N Engl J Med* 2012;367:1814–20.

8. CDC. Updated information on the epidemiology of Middle East respiratory syndrome coronavirus (MERS-CoV) infection and guidance for the public, clinicians, and public health authorities, 2012–2013. *MMWR Morb Mortal Wkly Rep* 2013;62:793–6.

9. Perera R, Wang P, Gomaa M, et al. Seroepidemiology for MERS coronavirus using microneutralisation and pseudoparticle virus neutralisation assays reveal a high prevalence of antibody in dromedary camels in Egypt, June 2013. *Euro Surveill* 2013;18(36):8–14.

10. Reusken CB, Haagmans BL, Muller MA, et al. Middle East respiratory syndrome coronavirus neutralising serum antibodies in dromedary camels: A comparative serological study. *Lancet Infect Dis* 2013;13:859–66.

11. Buchholz U, Bernard H, Werber D, et al. German outbreak of Escherichia coli O104:H4 associated with sprouts. *N Engl J Med.* 2011;365:1763–70.

12. Gault G, Weill FX, Mariani-Kurkdjian P, et al. Outbreak of haemolytic uraemic syndrome and bloody diarrhoea due to Escherichia coli O104:H4, south-west France, June 2011. *Euro Surveill* 2011;16(26):5–7.

13. Pastorino B, Muyembe-Tamfum JJ, Bessaud M, et al. Epidemic resurgence of chikungunya virus in Democratic Republic of the Congo: Identification of a new central African strain. *J Med Virol* 2004;74:277–82.

14. Sergon K, Yahaya AA, Brown J, et al. Seroprevalence of chikungunya virus infection on Grande Comore Island, Union of the Comoros, 2005. *Am J Trop Med Hyg* 2007;76:1189–93.

15. Josseran L, Paquet C, Zehgnoun A, et al. Chikungunya disease outbreak, Reunion Island. *Emerg Infect Dis* 2006;12:1994–5.

16. Schuffenecker I, Iteman I, Michault A, et al. Genome microevolution of chikungunya viruses causing the Indian Ocean outbreak. *PLoS Med* 2006;3:e263.

17. Tsetsarkin KA, Vanlandingham DL, McGee CE, Higgs S. A single mutation in chikungunya virus affects vector specificity and epidemic potential. *PLoS Pathog* 2007;3:e201.

18. European Centre for Disease Prevention and Control. Chikungunya. (Accessed April 14, 2015, at http://www.ecdc.europa.eu/en/healthtopics/chikungunya_fever/pages/index.aspx.)

19. Cello J, Paul AV, Wimmer E. Chemical synthesis of poliovirus cDNA: Generation of infectious virus in the absence of natural template. *Science* 2002;297:1016–8.

20. Kobasa D, Takada A, Shinya K, et al. Enhanced virulence of influenza A viruses with the haemagglutinin of the 1918 pandemic virus. *Nature* 2004;431:703–7.

21. Vogel G. Infectious diseases. WHO gives a cautious green light to smallpox experiments. *Science* 2004;306:1270–1.

22. Imai M, Watanabe T, Hatta M, et al. Experimental adaptation of an influenza H5 HA confers respiratory droplet transmission to a reassortant H5 HA/H1N1 virus in ferrets. *Nature* 2012;486:420–8.

23. Herfst S, Schrauwen EJ, Linster M, et al. Airborne transmission of influenza A/H5N1 virus between ferrets. *Science* 2012;336:1534–41.

24. Gibson DG, Benders GA, Andrews-Pfannkoch C, et al. Complete chemical synthesis, assembly, and cloning of a Mycoplasma genitalium genome. *Science* 2008;319:1215–20.

25. Gibson DG, Glass JI, Lartigue C, et al. Creation of a bacterial cell controlled by a chemically synthesized genome. *Science* 2010;329:52–6.

Field Detection

1. Gibbs PJ. The evolution of one health: A decade of progress and challenges for the future. *Vet Rec* 2014;174(4):85–91.

2. Asokan GV, Kasimanickam RK, and Asokan V. Surveillance, response systems, and evidence updates on emerging zoonoses: The role of one health. *Infect Ecol Epidemiol* 2013;3:21386.

3. U.S. Army. *Multi-service tactics, techniques, and procedures for chemical, biological, radiological, and nuclear reconnaissance and surveillance.* Fort Monroe, VA: U.S. Army Training and Doctrine Command; Quantico, VA: Marine Corps Combat Development Command; Norfolk, VA: Navy Warfare Development Command; Tyndall Air Force Base, FL: Air Force Civil Engineer Support Agency, 2011. (ATP 3-11.37, MCWP 3-37.4, NTTP 3-11.29, AFTTP 3-2.44.), pg 5-3.

4. Ackelsberg J, Leykam FM, Hazi Y, et al. The NYC native air sampling pilot project: Using HVAC filter data for urban biological incident characterization. *Biosecur Bioterror* 2011;9(3):213–24.

5. Begier EM, Barrett NL, Mshar PA, et al. Connecticut bioterrorism field epidemiology response team. *Emerg Infect Dis* 2005;11:1483–6.

6. Bravata DM, Sundaram V, McDonald KM, et al. Evaluating detection and diagnostic decision support systems for bioterrorism response. *Emerg Infect Dis* 2004;10:100–8.

7. Espy MJ, Cockerill III FR, Meyer RF, et al. Detection of smallpox virus DNA by LightCycler PCR. *J Clin Microbiol* 2002;40:1985–8. Erratum in: *J Clin Microbiol* 2002;40:4405.

8. Field PR, Mitchell JL, Santiago A, et al. Comparison of a commercial enzyme-linked immunosorbent assay with immunofluorescence and complement fixation tests for detection of *Coxiella burnetii* (Q fever) immunoglobulin M. *J Clin Microbiol* 2000;38:1645–7.

9. Johnasson A, Berglund L, Erikkson U, et al. Comparative analysis of PCR versus culture for diagnosis of ulceroglandular tularemia. *J Clin Microbiol* 2000;38:22–6.

10. Kulesh DA, Baker RO, Loveless BM, et al. Smallpox and pan-orthopox virus detection by real-time 3'-minor groove binder TaqMan assays on the Roche LightCycler and the Cepheid Smart Cycler platforms. *J Clin Microbiol* 2004;42:601–9.

11. Kraft AE, Kulesh DA. Applying molecular biological techniques to detecting biological agents. *Clin Lab Med* 2001;21:631–60.

12. Seiner DR, Colburn HA, Baird C, et al. Evaluation of the FilmArray system for detection of *Bacillus anthracis, Francisella tularensis,* and *Yersinia pestis. J Appl Microbiol* 2012;114:992.